Reflux Oesophagitis

Reflux Oesophagitis

T. P. J. Hennessy, MA MCh, FRCS, FRCSI
Regius Professor of Surgery, St James's Hospital and Trinity College, Dublin

A. Cuschieri, MD, ChM, FRCS(Ed), FRCS(Eng)
Professor of Surgery, Ninewells Hospital and Medical School, University of Dundee

J. R. Bennett, MD, FRCP
Consultant Physician, Hull Royal Infirmary

Butterworths
London Boston Singapore Sydney Toronto Wellington

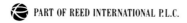 PART OF REED INTERNATIONAL P.L.C.

First published 1989

© **Butterworth & Co. (Publishers) Ltd, 1989**

British Library Cataloguing-in Publication Data
Hennessy, T. P. J. (Thomas P J)
  Reflux oesophagitis.
  1. Man. Gastrointestinal tract. Reflux
  gastroesophagitis
  I. Title II. Cuschieri, A. (Alfred) III. Bennett,
  J. R.
  616.3'3'

  ISBN 0–407–01445–4

Library of Congress Cataloguing-in-Publication Data
Hennessy, T. P. J. (Thomas Patrick Joseph)
  Reflux oesophagitis / T. P. J. Hennessy, A. Cuschieri, J. R. Bennett.
    p.   cm.
  Includes bibliographical references.
  ISBN 0-407-01445-4:
  1. Gastroesophageal reflux. I. Cuschieri, A. (Alfred)
  II. Bennett, John R. (John Roderick) III. Title.
    [DNLM: 1. Esophagitis, Peptic. WI 250 H515r]
  RC815.7.H47   1989
  616.3'2—dc19
  DNLM/DLC for Library of Congress   89-17481 CIP

Filmset by Bath Typesetting Ltd, Bath, Avon
Printed and bound in Great Britain by Courier International Ltd, Tiptree, Essex

Preface

The technological advances in investigating techniques—endoscopy, solid state portable loggers for ambulatory monitoring, radiosondes, miniature catheter-mounted transducers, radio-isotope methods of transit etc.—have generated a marked resurgence of interest in the pathophysiology and management of common oesophageal disorders, particularly gastro-oesophageal reflux disease and its complications. This has been accompanied by a standardization of assessment of disease severity, with the acceptance and usage of internationally agreed definitions which have undoubtedly facilitated cooperative ventures and multicentre prospective studies. The outcome of this research effort is a better appreciation of the nature of this complex condition, more effective drugs for the control of acid reflux including newer prokinetic agents to improve oesophageal clearance. The complex relation between reflux disease, motility disorders, abnormal visceral microcirculation and chest pain is being unravelled, although the picture is by no means clear and several issues still require clarification.

Changes have also been witnessed in the surgical management of reflux disease and its complications. The efficacy of established operations can now be better evaluated and more recently introduced procedures assessed with greater objectivity. There has also been a growing realization that specialist treatment of the complications of oesophageal reflux disease is necessary if the morbidity associated with treatment is to decline, and the benefit to the patient increase. There is no doubt that from the surgical standpoint, the oesophagus remains an unforgiving organ.

The aim of this book is to provide a balanced and concise account of current thinking on the nature and problems of gastro-oesophageal reflux disease, which has replaced peptic ulceration as one of the most frequently encountered disorders of the upper gastro-intestinal tract in the Western hemisphere.

Contributors

John R. Bennett MD, FRCP
Consultant Physician, Hull Royal Infirmary, Hull

Alfred Cuschieri MD, ChM, FRCS(Ed.), FRCS(Eng.)
Professor of Surgery, Ninewells Hospital and Medical School, University of Dundee, Dundee

John S. de Caestecker MA, MRCP
Senior Registrar in Medicine, Department of Medicine II, St George's Hospital Medical School, London

Craig A. Eriksen MD, FRCS(Ed.)
Clinical Fellow in Surgery, Ninewells Hospital and Medical School, University of Dundee, Dundee

Peter Gillen MCh, FRCSI
Senior Surgical Registrar, Regional Hospital, Cork, Eire

Robert C. Heading BSc, MD, FRCP
Senior Lecturer, University Department of Medicine, Royal Infirmary, Edinburgh

Thomas P. J. Hennessy MA, MCh, FRCS, FRCSI
Regius Professor of Surgery, St James's Hospital and Trinity College, Dublin, Eire

Contents

Chapter 1

The pathophysiology of reflux

J. S. de Caestecker and R. C. Heading

Introduction

The relationship of refluxed gastric contents to distal oesophagitis is a relatively recent concept. Perhaps the first milestone was the recognition in 1935 of peptic oesophagitis as a distinct entity, and the suggestion that it might be the result of the action of gastric acid and pepsin on the oesophageal muscosa [1]. Since this time, the mechanisms responsible for preventing gastro-oesophageal reflux (GOR) have been a focus for research and controversy, mirrored by changing attitudes towards surgical and medical treatment of the condition [2–7].

It is clear that the pathophysiology of GOR and its consequences is multifactorial, including factors permitting reflux of gastric contents, those normally promoting oesophageal clearance and properties of the refluxate itself [8,9]. An understanding of current concepts of pathophysiology requires first a clear definition of the termin-ology. 'Hiatus hernia' is not, as was once supposed, a synonym for GOR or oesophagitis [2,3,10], nor is oesophagitis an all embracing term descriptive of all cases of GOR [9]. 'Oesophagitis' describes the mucosal inflammation and ulceration which can, but does not always, accompany GOR [11]. 'Gastro-oesophageal reflux' is a quantitative rather than an 'all-or-none' phenomenon, and refers to the process of reflux of stomach contents into the oesophagus. This may be physiological, occurring in small amounts in healthy individuals, or pathological, observed in abnormally large quantities in symptomatic patients [11]. The whole disease spectrum, including symptomatic refluxers without oesophagitis, and those with oesophagitis or its complications (such as benign stricture or Barrett's oesophagus), is embraced by the term 'gastro-oesophageal reflux disease' [9].

In this chapter, the role of several factors in GOR disease will be examined in turn: the lower oesophageal sphincter as a barrier to reflux, oesophageal acid clearance mechanisms, the importance of mechanical factors and hiatus hernia, oesophageal mucosal resistance, gastric factors, including the nature of the refluxate, and the part played by oesophageal sensory pathways.

The patterns of gastro-oesophageal reflux and factors implicated in the develop-ment of complications of oesophagitis will be reviewed. Finally, a summary will attempt to draw together several of the more important factors and to formulate a unifying hypothesis linking the principal oesophageal and gastric abnormalities underlying the development of GOR disease.

The lower oesophageal sphincter

Although no anatomical lower oesophageal sphincter (LOS) has been demonstrated in humans, a physiological sphincter undoubtedly exists, extending over the terminal 1–4 cm of the oesophagus [12–16]. The circular smooth muscle of this area is functionally distinct from that of the adjacent stomach and oesophagus, having a lower transmembrane potential [12], different length–tension relationships in vitro [18,19] and in vivo [20] and increased sensitivity to gastrin [21] and cholinergic agents [22]. Recently a quantitative difference was found in the structure of a subunit of myosin isolated from LOS circular muscle compared to that of the oesophageal body [23]. A high density of VIP (vasoactive intestinal polypeptide) containing nerve fibres has been demonstrated in the LOS [24], a feature in common with gastrointestinal sphincters [25].

Basal lower oesophageal sphincter pressure

The LOS exhibits tonic basal tone in vivo. Although insertion of a manometry catheter probably alters sphincter tension by exerting stretch, infused catheter systems have been shown to estimate accurately the 'yield pressure' within the LOS by comparison with a model in vitro system [26]. Additional evidence for the close correlation between measurements of LOS pressure and sphincter strength comes from a study comparing the force required to pull a Teflon ball through the sphincter with LOS pressure [27].

The marked axial and radial asymmetry of the LOS [28] underlines the problem of obtaining a representative sample of LOS pressure. The inference is that multiple recordings should be taken with perfused catheters having different radial orientations in order to obtain more representative readings. Dent has designed a perfused sleeve device which measures the average sphincter pressure [29]. In fact, it probably records the highest pressure within the sphincter and, being of larger diameter than most other perfused catheters, probably itself alters sphincter tension. Using multiple perfused catheters with different radial orientations, two methods of pressure measurements have been described: the 'rapid pull-through' and 'station pull-through' techniques [30,31]. Because diaphragmatic contraction contributes to LOS pressure [32,33], intrinsic sphincter pressure is best estimated by measurements obtained in end expiration (when the diaphragm is relaxed), whichever technique is used. Nevertheless, measurements obtained during station pull-through are consistently lower than those obtained during rapid pull-through [30,34]. The rapid pull-through technique is quicker and easy to perform and interpret, and has been said to provide more reproducible measurements than station pull-through [30], although this has been disputed [31]. The poor reproducibility of repeated measurements over a period of weeks in the same individuals found with the rapid pull-through technique [35] is not surprising, as prolonged studies using Dent's sleeve have shown marked diurnal variations in basal LOS pressure in relation to posture [36] and meals [37]. During fasting, increases in basal LOS pressure have been observed in relation to the gastric migrating motor complex recorded in phase III of the interdigestive cycle [38]. Even in patients with oesophagitis who have long periods of very low basal LOS pressure, the sphincter pressure can often be observed to rise into the normal range [39].

The significance of low basal LOS pressure needs to be seen in the light of the

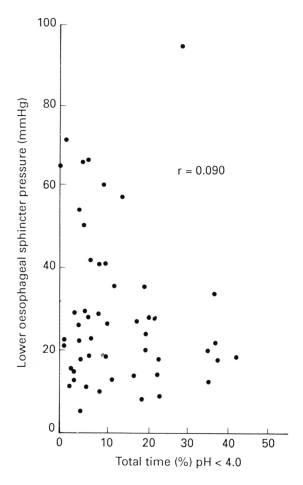

Figure 1.1 Relationship between basal lower oesophageal sphincter pressure (rapid pull-through technique) and percentage total time pH is less than 4 during 23-hour pH monitoring in 52 subjects investigated for chest pain or reflux symptoms (unpublished data)

variability of sphincter pressure within individuals and the drawbacks of the various techniques of measurement.

A low basal LOS pressure measured by perfused catheters has been said to discriminate between patients with GOR disease and controls, regardless of the presence of a hiatus hernia [40,41]. This confirmed the earlier findings of Atkinson and colleagues, using water-filled but unperfused catheters [14]. Subsequent larger studies have found substantial overlap in basal LOS pressures between controls and GOR patients [42,43] and, although low basal sphincter pressures are often found in patients with severe oesophagitis [44], it is clear that abnormal GOR can occur over a wide range of basal LOS pressure (Figure 1.1).

Other mechanisms have been shown to be responsible for reflux events, but before these are discussed, it is appropriate here to review briefly the factors influencing LOS pressure. Cholinergic and α-adrenergic agents increase LOS pressure, whilst β-adrenergic agonists decrease it [45]. Atropine in humans reduces but does not abolish LOS basal pressure [46]. Of the gastrointestinal hormones, gastrin increases LOS pressure, while secretin, cholecystokinin, and glucagon decrease it, the first two by competitive antagonism of the effect of gastrin [47]. Pancreatic polypeptide, bombesin and motilin also contract the LOS, while GIP and VIP are inhibitory [48]. None of these factors has been shown to be of major importance in the maintenance of basal LOS pressure in humans.

In humans and the North American opossum (whose oesophageal muscular coat closely resembles its human counterpart), basal sphincter tone is unlikely to be primarily neurogenic in origin [48]. It may be determined by an active myogenic mechanism, perhaps dependent on slow depolarization of the transmembrane potential, which is lower in resting LOS muscle than in the adjacent oesophagus [17]. A passive mechanism dependent on the property of LOS muscle to exert tension in response to stretch may also come into play [18–20]. In this respect, it has been suggested that the 'mucosal plug' created by mucosal folds in the collapsed oesophagus may stretch the LOS muscle sufficient to bring this mechanism into play.

With regard to GOR, a number of foodstuffs and pharmacological substances affects resting LOS pressure. Thus, fatty foods decrease sphincter pressure, possibly via release of cholecystokinin [49], while protein and alkalis are reported to increase it [49,50]. The pressure falls, however, with a mixed meal [51]. Substances increasing intracellular cyclic AMP decrease LOS pressure [52] including β-adrenergic agonists and methyl xanthines [45]. This is the probable mechanism for the effect of coffee [53] and chocolate [52]. Smoking reduces LOS pressure [54] and promotes GOR [55]. Anticholinergic drugs exert an inhibitory effect on the LOS [45,46,56] as do calcium channel antagonists [56].

The lower oesophageal sphincter and mechanisms of gastro-oesophageal reflux

Dent's sleeve device has extended understanding of the mechanisms operating at the level of the LOS during the occurrence of GOR [29], overcoming the difficulties encountered during prolonged studies with perfused catheter systems of axial LOS movements related to swallowing and breathing [57]. Several studies have now confirmed the original findings of the Milwaukee group [37] that the majority of episodes of GOR occur during periods of transient LOS relaxation (TLOSR) regardless of basal LOS pressure in both normal controls [36,37,58,59] and GOR patients [36,39,51,60]. An increased frequency of TLOSRs occurs in controls and GOR patients after meals [37,38,51] compared to the fasting state in recumbent patients and about two-thirds of TLOSRs are accompanied by GOR in reflux patients, compared with approximately one-third in normal controls [51,60]. More TLOSRs after meals are accompanied by GOR than TLOSRs occurring during fasting [51]. An increased frequency of TLOSRs in reflux patients [59] has not been confirmed by all groups [36,60]. There is evidence that, at least in healthy controls, GOR occurs during fasting in association with the gastric component of the migrating motor complex [61], although these findings are at variance with those of an earlier study [38], which found (using a Dent sleeve to monitor LOS pressure) that sphincter pressure rose in association with increased gastric motor activity. Although GOR patients have not been studied with respect to fasting gastroduodenal motor activity in relation to episodes of GOR, the latter group proposes that this adaptive response may fail in reflux patients [38].

In healthy controls, TLOSRs are almost the only mechanism for GOR [37,59], whilst they account for only 65–73% of reflux episodes in GOR patients [57,60]. Other mechanisms include:

1. Free reflux across an LOS with absent basal pressure, which is found more commonly in patients with the most severe degree of oesophagitis [39].
2. Reflux at the moment of deep inspiration.
3. Reflux accompanying a transient increase in intra-abdominal pressure.

These mechanisms are summarized in Figure 1.2. With regard to the last mechanism, an adaptive and protective increase in LOS pressure in response to increase in intra-abdominal pressure has been demonstrated in several studies [16,40,41,62,63]. This response is deficient in GOR patients [16,41,64] and is probably mediated by a cholinergic vagal reflex [46,63] although mechanical factors may play a part [62].

There is disagreement about the mechanism of TLOSRs. Dent and colleagues introduced the term 'inappropriate' TLOSRs to indicate sphincter relaxation occurring independent of swallowing activity. They found these to be the most common events underlying episodes of acid GOR in controls and reflux patients [37,39,51]. These findings are at variance with those of Mittal and McCallum [59,60], who found that the majority of TLOSRs occurred after either oesophageal contractions or recordable mylohyoid muscle electrical activity (Table 1.1). When oesophageal

Table 1.1 Proportions of transient lower oesophageal relaxations accompanied by pharyngeal and oesophageal motor activity (pooled data from normals and reflux patients)

	Mittal and McCallum [60][a]	Dent et al. [39][b]
Submental electromyographic activity (%)	42	Not recorded
Pharyngeal contraction (%)	27	28
Oesophageal contraction (%) (proximal or distal, primary, secondary or tertiary)	64	36

[a] 22 subjects, including 10 healthy controls; 286 transient LOS relaxations accompanied by GOR analysed.
[b] 67 subjects, including 15 judged not to have GOR disease; 644 transient LOS relaxations accompanied by GOR analysed.

contractions preceded TLOSRs, there were either distal spontaneous and simultaneous waves or proximal swallow-related waves failing to conduct to the distal oesophagus [60]. These latter findings are supported by the data from other workers who did not use the Dent sleeve or record from the LOS [65–67]. All of these studies found that the majority of reflux events were accompanied by prior oesophageal motor activity which was frequently abnormal [66,67] and often swallow related [65,66]. In patients with abnormal GOR, an increased proportion of reflux events was accompanied by upper oesophageal motor activity not conducted to the distal oesophagus [67], similar to the findings of Mittal and McCallum [60]. Careful scrutiny of the most recent study of Dent and colleagues, who evaluated 67 patients with suspected GOR, shows that some pharyngeal, upper oesophageal or simultaneous lower oesophageal motor activity preceded 36% of all episodes of TLOSR in all groups of patients [39] (Figure 1.3). Dent's group may have underestimated the proportion of TLOSRs preceded by an aborted swallow because they did not perform electromyographic recordings from the muscles involved in swallowing (Table 1.1).

On the basis that nearly all TLOSRs were preceded by pharyngeal or oesophageal electrical or motor activity, were of long duration and were always terminated by an

6

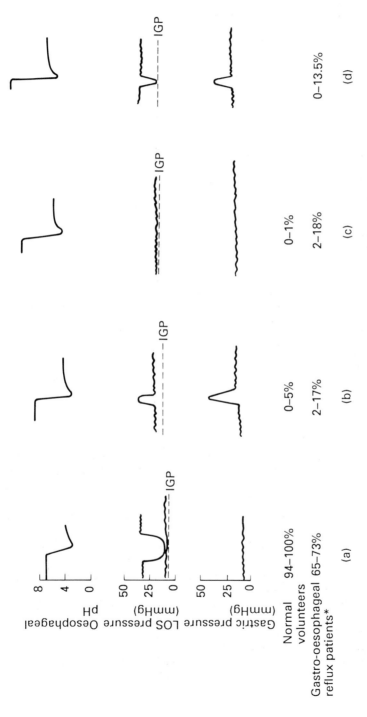

Figure 1.2 Mechanisms of gastro-oesophageal reflux in patients and healthy volunteers. (a) Transient lower oesophageal sphincter relaxation; (b) stress reflux during transient increased intra-abdominal pressure; (c) free reflux across an atonic lower oesophageal sphincter; (d) reflux at the moment of deep inspiration. IGP = intragastric pressure. * Mechanism uncertain in 9.3% of Mittal and McCallum's [60] patients. (Adapted from Dodds *et al.* [59]; figures derived from Dodds *et al.* [51] and Mittal and McCallum [60])

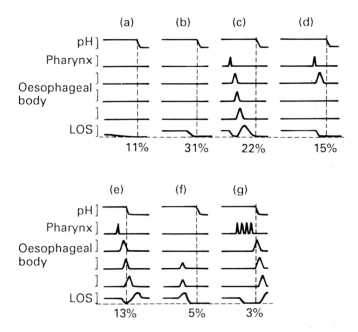

Figure 1.3 Schema showing the different patterns of oesophageal and lower oesophageal sphincter (LOS) motor function associated with acid reflux events. The numbers below each pattern indicate the percentage of total reflux episodes for each pattern for the whole group of 67 patients (53 refluxers). The broken horizontal line indicates intragastric pressure. The vertical broken line indicates the onset of the reflux event. (a) LOS pressure drift; (b) spontaneous transient LOS relaxation (LOSR); (c) LOSR occurring immediately after a normal peristaltic sequence (post-swallow transient LOSR); (d) LOSR associated with a failed primary peristaltic sequence; (e) reflux during a normal peristaltic sequence; (f) LOSR after spontaneous synchronous contractions in the distal oesophagus; (g) LOSR induced by multiple swallows. (Adapted from Dent *et al.* [39])

oesophageal contraction, Mittal and McCallum have proposed that a long train subthreshold vagal stimulus causes the LOS and oesophageal events occurring during a TLOSR [59]. The finding by Dent and colleagues [39] of refractoriness of the smooth muscle oesophagus during a TLOSR suggests neural inhibition and supports the hypothesis put forward by Mittal and McCallum.

The above studies using a Dent sleeve have all been conducted in supine patients. It appears that TLOSRs are relatively suppressed in this position [68,69]. In the sitting position, an increased number of TLOSRs occurs in relation to belching [69] and this can be stimulated by gaseous gastric distension. A similar increase in TLOSRs occurs if the stomach is distended by a balloon, suggesting that gastric distension could mediate the increase in TLOSRs occurring postprandially [70]. In an experimental dog model, gas reflux and TLOSRs are abolished by vagal cooling [71], whilst the finding that TLOSRs do not occur in achalasia provide indirect support for a neural reflex in humans [72].

It has been suggested that the proximal stomach might be able to 'sense' if air or fluid is available to be vented and thus provide a mechanism for control of TLOSRs in the supine patient [68,69]. However, experimental support for this contention is lacking [73].

In summary, transient LOS relation has been shown to be the major mechanism for GOR in controls and patients. In reflux patients, more of the TLOSRs are accompanied by acid GOR than in controls, although it remains unclear whether the actual number of TLOSRs is increased in GOR patients. Transient LOS relaxations are increased after meals or by gastric distension, but suppressed in the supine position. Two mechanisms for TLOSRs have emerged: in relation to incomplete swallows or to a belch reflex mediated by gastric distension. In either case, the vagus nerve is likely to be important. Low basal LOS tone, responsible for some episodes of reflux in GOR patients, is probably due in part to defective extrinsic vagal neural stimulation [68], whilst GOR resulting from failure of LOS adaptation to increased intra-abdominal pressure almost certainly represents a defect in a vagal reflex [63,64]. The unifying thread behind all of these mechanisms is the vagus nerve: failure of vagal reflexes seems likely to be responsible for the failure of LOS barrier function in relation to all these situations.

Oesophageal acid clearance

The acid clearance test

The concept of oesophageal acid clearance, recently well reviewed by Johnson [74], was first proposed by Booth and his colleagues [75], who introduced the standard acid clearance test. As originally described, this test involved instilling 15 ml of 0.1 M hydrochloric acid into the distal oesophagus and requesting the subject to swallow at 30-second intervals. The number of swallows required to raise the intraoesophageal pH to 6 was recorded. In asymptomatic patients with or without a hiatus hernia, 10 swallows or less were required, but in patients with symptomatic GOR with or without a hiatus hernia, this value was exceeded. Their findings have been confirmed by Stanciu and Bennett [76]. However, the test is neither sensitive nor specific for GOR disease; some patients with this condition have a normal test and patients with oesophageal motility disorders but no GOR may have a prolonged result [76]. Kjellen and his co-workers noted that the acid clearance test could be considerably prolonged in normal subjects, and that it was poorly reproducible [77]. Orr and colleagues found that the standard acid clearance test did not discriminate between controls and patients with oesophagitis, although a modified test in which subjects were allowed to swallow at will did so [78]. Furthermore, although 90% of patients with oesophagitis have abnormal acid clearance tests, 60% of symptomatic GOR patients without oesophagitis have an abnormal result, so that the test fails to discriminate between individuals falling into these two categories [79].

Acid clearance and oesophagitis

Despite the shortcomings of this technique as a diagnostic test, the concept has stimulated research and thrown interesting light on the pathophysiology of GOR disease.

Stanciu and Bennett found that the calculated mean duration of reflux episodes during prolonged oesophageal pH monitoring correlated well with the results of standard acid clearance tests [76] and this parameter, as well as the number of reflux episodes lasting longer than 5 minutes, have been used as measures of acid clearance [80]. It has been reported that acid clearance is particularly delayed in recumbent sleeping patients and this factor has been implicated in the development of oesophagitis [11,79,81]. Delayed postprandial oesophageal acid clearance is also highly correlated with oesophagitis [82], although it is uncertain whether true or apparent delayed clearance (the result of multiple superimposed reflux episodes) is being measured.

With regard to the night-time, supine posture results in longer acid clearance times than upright posture, and head-down tilt even more so [77]. This suggests that gravity is important, and has important therapeutic implications, because propping up the head of the bed results in improvement in nocturnal acid clearance [83] and microscopic oesophagitis [76]. Sleep itself is also of importance, as Orr and colleagues have found that acid clearance is greatly prolonged in both normal controls and patients with oesophagitis if the presence of acid in the oesophagus does not result in arousal from sleep [78]. Indeed, hypnotics, by delaying arousal, further prolonged nocturnal acid clearance times [84]. The same group has also found that acid, compared with water, instilled into the oesophagus during sleep is more likely to result in arousal and provokes a higher swallowing rate than water [85]. This suggests the presence of a reflex mechanism mediating arousal and swallowing activity when acid is present in the oesophagus. Interestingly, the only difference this group was able to demonstrate between patients with oesophagitis and controls occurred when, following acid-induced arousal, more than 50% of the time after acid instillation was spent in a wakeful state, in which case the oesophagitis patients had more prolonged acid clearance times [78]. This has led Johnson to suggest that patients with oesophagitis are in 'double jeopardy' at night: poor acid clearance is fostered by lack of arousal from sleep and by a 'pump' failure of the oesophagus when awake [74].

Mechanisms of acid clearance

The mechanisms controlling oesophageal acid clearance are now well understood [68,74]. The importance of primary peristalsis can be deduced from the studies of Orr and colleagues [78]. Secondary peristalsis in the smooth muscle oesophagus is not under voluntary control, and would be expected to come into play during sleep when swallowing rates are reduced [86]. Corazziari and colleagues found that lowering the pH of a fluid bolus delivered into the distal oesophagus resulted in a reduction of the volume necessary to induce secondary peristalsis in normal volunteers [87]. These results could not be reproduced by Thompson and colleagues, who found that similar degrees of oesophageal distension by acid, saline or a balloon resulted in similar stimulation of secondary peristalsis at a given level within the oesophagus [88]. The Italian group repeated their studies in patients with oesophagitis and identified an apparent defect, in that the threshold lowering effect of acid on bolus volume was not observed [89]. These findings, which remain unconfirmed, would be compatible with an afferent defect in patients with oesophagitis which will be further considered later in this section. Overall, secondary peristalsis occurs much less frequently than primary peristalsis during spontaneous GOR [66]. Although it may result in volume clearance of acid [66], it does not result in a rise in intraoesophageal pH; this is exemplified by the failure of oesophageal pH to rise during sleep unless arousal and swallow-induced primary peristalsis occur [78,85].

The reason for the importance of primary peristalsis has been elegantly demonstrated by the studies of Helm and his associates [90–92]. Using concurrent radionuclide oesophageal scintigraphy, oesophageal manometry and pH monitoring during an acid clearance test, they found that more than 95% volume clearance occurred after the first primary or secondary peristaltic wave [90]. Stepwise neutralization

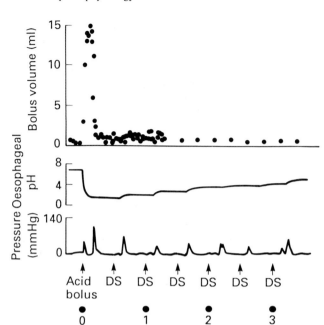

Figure 1.4 Relationships between oesophageal acid clearance, motor activity, and emptying of fluid volume. Only peristaltic pressure complexes from the distal oesophagus are shown. DS denotes dry swallows. Despite clearance of the injected bolus volume to less than 1 ml by the secondary peristaltic sequence, oesophageal pH did not begin to rise until the first dry swallow 30 seconds after bolus injection. Fluid bolus derived from a 15 ml radioisotope-labelled acid bolus delivered into the oesophagus. (From Helm *et al.* [91])

of residual oesophageal acid occurred with each swallow-related peristaltic wave and depended on salivation [90,91]. These features are shown in Figure 1.4. Aspiration of saliva quadrupled acid clearance time, which could be restored to normal by an equivalent amount of sodium bicarbonate but not by an equal volume of water [91]. Measures resulting in an increased salivary secretion of bicarbonate shortened acid clearance times, while abolishing salivary secretion with atropine greatly prolonged it [92]. Stimulated saliva has greater acid neutralizing capacity than resting saliva [92]. No defect in basal or stimulated salivary secretion rates has been found in patients with oesophagitis compared with young healthy volunteers and age-matched controls [93]. Acid perfusion produced a reflex increase in salivary volume and bicarbonate content in volunteers [93,94] and patients with oesophagitis [94], although in one study, neither patients with oesophagitis nor age-matched controls showed an increase in salivation in response to intraoesophageal acid [93]. In the study of Helm and colleagues only subjects developing heartburn showed a salivary response to oesophageal acid [94]. These findings point to a reflex mechanism for increased saliva flow during oesophageal acidification, and a possible age-related loss of this response. However, Helm and his co-workers, in a preliminary report, found increased salivation in response to oesophageal acid perfusion in patients with uncomplicated oesophagitis but not in patients with peptic strictures [95]. This latter group of patients had a normal salivary response to sucking a lozenge, implying a defect in an oesophagosalivary neural reflex arc. It is not known if this is a primary abnormality or secondary to severe oesophageal mucosal damage.

Prolonged acid clearance in patients with GOR disease may result from failed or abnormal primary peristalsis, and this will be further discussed in Chapter 5. Other factors acting to reduce acid clearance include alcohol and smoking [77]. The former has been shown to impair oesophageal function [96], whilst the latter probably results from reduction of salivary flow [97]. The presence of a hiatus hernia appears to affect clearance [98] by a mechanism which is considered later in this chapter.

Mechanical factors

The identification of a physiological LOS in the mid-1950s directed attention away from mechanical influences on gastro-oesophageal competence. However, it is difficult to envisage that success of modern anti-reflux surgery can be attributed to other than mechanical effects, perhaps buttressing the LOS. Although both fundoplication and the insertion of an Angelchik anti-reflux device have been shown to increase basal LOS pressure [4,99–108], there is evidence to suggest that this is not the mechanism of action of these procedures [5,109,110]. This is not surprising, as low basal LOS pressure is itself not the major mechanism for episodes of GOR [39,51,60]. However, transient dysphagia is common after both fundoplication and insertion of the Angelchik prosthesis [4,107] and this suggests that LOS relaxation in response to swallows may be impaired. In fact, there are now data available to show that LOS relaxation is impaired after these operations [108,111,112]. Interestingly, this impairment was found in 87% of patients after fundoplication, despite the fact that 69% did not complain of dysphagia [112]. With regard to the Angelchik device, incomplete LOS relaxation was observed during oesophageal manometry undertaken after the symptom of transient dysphagia had resolved, and it was also noted that only those two patients with a majority of complete post-deglutition LOS relaxations postoperatively showed no decrease (in fact, an increase) in the number of reflux events during oesophageal pH monitoring [108].

A number of mechanisms have been proposed either to act as an external buttress to the LOS or to constitute a mechanical barrier to reflux. These are summarized in Figure 1.5 and include:

1. The pinchcock action of the muscular sling formed by the right crus of the diaphragm surrounding the oesophageal hiatus.
2. A 'flap valve' formed by the acute angle between the oesophagus and the gastric cardia.
3. A 'muscosal choke' formed by folds of the collapsed oesophagus.
4. The overall length of the LOS.
5. The length of the intra-abdominal segment of the oesophagus.

Pinchcock action
With regard to the first factor it is likely that when the LOS lies within the diaphragmatic hiatus (i.e. when there is no sliding hiatus hernia), contraction of the right diaphragmatic crus contributes to the measured LOS pressure. This may account in part for the marked longitudinal and radial asymmetry of the LOS [28]. It may also explain the observations that reflux is more frequent when patients lie on the right side in bed [113] and that consistently lower sphincter pressures have been

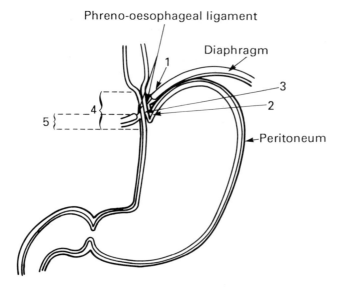

Figure 1.5 Mechanical factors preventing gastro-oesophageal reflux. (1) Pinchcock action of right diaphragmatic crus; (2) flap valve formed by acute angle between oesophagus and gastric cardia; (3) mucosal choke formed by apposed folds of collapsed lower oesophagus; (4) length of lower oesophageal sphincter; (5) length of intra-abdominal portion of lower oesophageal sphincter

noted in subjects lying in the left or right decubitus positions compared with the supine position [114]. In an early study, Atkinson and Sumerling observed the effect of left phrenic nerve paralysis (this nerve supplies the right diaphragmatic crus) and found little evidence of a change in LOS pressures compared to controls, although they used non-perfused, water-filled manometry catheters which underestimate luminal pressure [15]. A recent study in anaesthetized cats found that diaphragmatic paralysis obliterated respiratory oscillations in LOS pressure, and that end-expiratory LOS pressure in non-paralysed animals was identical to basal LOS pressure in the paralysed cats [32]. Artificial ventilation at increasing tidal volumes failed to replicate the magnitude of pressure oscillation recorded during spontaneous respiration, but increasing the concentration of inspired carbon dioxide led to an increased amplitude of respiratory oscillation of sphincter pressure which corresponded to increased amplitudes recorded from the diaphragm by electromyography [32]. A report from McCallum's group has recently confirmed that diaphragmatic contraction in humans augments LOS tone [33]. This enhancing effect was maximal in deep sustained inspiration when the gastro-oesophageal pressure gradient was maximal and would be expected to be most likely to result in GOR. They proposed that diaphragmatic contraction acts as an 'external sphincter' enhancing the effect of the intrinsic LOS [33].

Despite doubts voiced by Dodds and colleagues [115] that respiratory oscillations represent a movement artefact of the LOS over the stationary recording catheter, anchoring the LOS to the catheter does not abolish these movements [32] and it is likely that, in humans, a combination of axial movement of the LOS and diaphragmatic contraction contribute to the respiratory oscillation in recorded pressure [116]. These studies indicate that the diaphragmatic pinchcock effect does exist, and may act as a buttress to the LOS when the greatest gastro-oesophageal pressure gradients exist – during deep inspiration [33] and some manoeuvres increasing intra-abdominal pressure such as straight leg raising [62]. Both these situations have been shown to result in GOR quite frequently in patients with oesophagitis [39,51,60]. Reflux during deep inspiration or increases in intra-abdominal pressure during coughing may be particularly important in patients with chronic obstructive airway disease in whom GOR is common [117]. It may be that, because the diaphragm is flattened in these patients, it is at a mechanical disadvantage and thus less able to function in its role as an 'external sphincter' [32]. To put this in context, by far the largest proportion of reflux events occurs during transient lower oesophageal sphincter relaxation [37,39,51,60] and the presence of a hiatus hernia, with displacement of the LOS out of the diaphragmatic crus, does not necessarily result in GOR disease.

The 'flap valve' mechanism
The 'flap valve' mechanism has some support from cadaver studies. The acute angle between the oesophagus and cardia is probably maintained by the contraction of oblique gastric sling fibres in the muscular coat of the stomach, and disappears in cadavers [15]. However, a similar angle may be recreated in cadavers by applying traction to a loop slung around the anatomical gastro-oesophageal junction, and this manoeuvre provides resistance to the passage of barium from stomach to oesophagus [15]. The occurrence of a sliding hiatus hernia results in loss of this acute angle, but this is not necessarily followed by abnormal amounts of GOR. The role of this mechanism in promoting gastro-oesophageal competence remains uncertain. In total fundoplication, another valve mechanism may operate; the 'spout' of oesophagus surrounded by plicated fundus (well seen on retroflexed views at endoscopy) may act as a one-way 'flutter valve' resisting backward propulsion of gastric contents because increases in gastric pressure will tend to collapse the buried oesophageal spout [5].

'Mucosal choke'
It seems inherently unlikely that folds of mucosa held in apposition by the surface tension forces of the coating fluid will present much of a barrier to GOR when intra-abdominal pressure increases. However, according to Laplace's law, because the pressure within a hollow tube is inversely proportional to its radius, a larger pressure will be required to distend and open the oesophagus than is the case for the stomach [118]. It has to be noted that, in an animal model, excision of the mucosal rosette or elimination of the acute angle of entry of the oesophagus into the stomach did not result in oesophagitis [119].

Length
Lower oesophageal sphincter length and the length of sphincter exposed to intra-abdominal pressure are popular with some groups as an explanation for the prevention of reflux due to increase in intragastric pressure [120]. With regard to the former characteristic, a long overall LOS segment is held to be important because of resistance to opening by distraction [118]. On the basis of animal and in vitro models, Petterson and colleagues propose that increases in intragastric pressure result in distraction of the LOS, thereby decreasing its length, in a manner analogous to the shortening of the neck of a rubber balloon that occurs on blowing it up [118]. This mechanism has been proposed as the mode of action of the Angelchik prosthesis, which appears to act in the same fashion as a ligature placed on the gastric cardia in an experimental animal model [121]. In this respect, it has been shown that overall

oesophageal length [106] and the length of the LOS [108] are increased by insertion of the Angelchik ring.

DeMeester and colleagues have shown, using an in vitro model system, that a short intra-abdominal segment of oesophagus can lead to failure of the sphincter mechanism [122]. This group has proposed that either a low basal LOS pressure (<5 mmHg) or a short intra-abdominal sphincter length (<1 cm) or both are associated with a 90% incidence of abnormal GOR [120,122]. The intra-abdominal segment of the oesophagus is exposed to the same increases in pressure as may occur in the stomach, which results in no net gradient across the gastro-oesophageal junction and prevents GOR. Even in patients with a sliding hiatus hernia, it has been argued that this mechanism may exist, because of the insertion into the oesophageal fascia propria of the phreno-oesophageal ligament. This structure is said to be continuous with the deep fascia covering the undersurface of the diaphragm, and is covered inferiorly by peritoneum continuous with that covering the serosal surface of the stomach [3] as shown in Figure 1.5. Thus, the insertion of this ligament migrates with the LOS into the thorax when a hiatus hernia occurs, and the segment of oesophagus lying below it remains exposed to intra-abdominal pressure. It should be noted that identification of the intra-abdominal LOS depends on the manometric finding of a respiratory inversion point when positive inspiratory pressure deflections on the portions of the viscus exposed to intra-abdominal pressure change to negative deflections in those portions exposed to the intrathoracic environment. Dodds maintains that this is in fact an artefact of manometry, representing the orad and caudad excursions of the LOS over the manometry catheter during respiration [57,115].

There are clearly mechanical factors which support the LOS in its anti-reflux function, but these, in health, are probably subsidiary to the intrinsic sphincter. Joelsson and colleagues have shown that, in a group of patients investigated for GOR, 'functional' (i.e. abnormal GOR by pH monitoring, but LOS pressure >5 mmHg and intra-abdominal LOS length >1 cm) rather than 'mechanical' failures of the cardia are dominant [120]. Mechanical failures seem to respond best to anti-reflux surgery [122], and clearly mechanical factors form the dominant basis for the success of modern anti-reflux surgery.

The role of a sliding hiatus hernia

During the last 20 years, the pendulum has swung away from the thesis that hiatus hernia is an indispensable feature of GOR disease, as early mechanistic theories required [2,3]. This swing was prompted by the identification of a physiological LOS [12] followed by the recognition that sphincteric incompetence was the prime abnormality in GOR disease regardless of the presence of a hiatus hernia [14,40,41]. Now that basal LOS pressure has been found to be of less importance than hitherto believed, there has been a revival of interest in the role of a hiatus hernia. This has been prompted perhaps by the knowledge that, although many patients with hiatus hernia are asymptomatic [123], about 90% of patients with oesophagitis have hiatus hernia as assessed by radiology [124].

Evidence is accumulating that GOR across a relaxed LOS is more likely to occur and that oesophageal clearance mechanisms may be impaired in the presence of a hiatus hernia. Longhi and Jordan, in a study combining barium radiology and

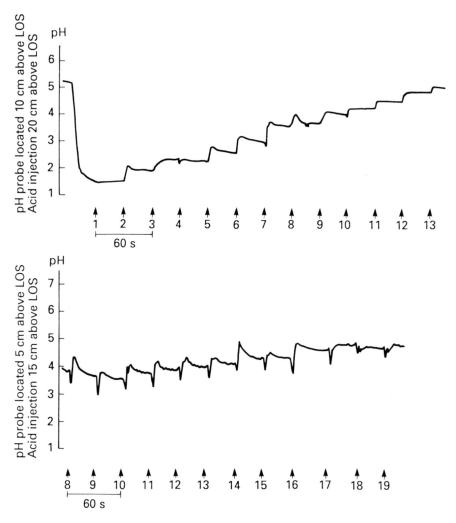

Figure 1.6 An example of a pH record during oesophageal acid clearance in a subject with hiatus hernia. At 5 cm above the LOS, swallows (indicated by arrows) resulted in biphasic pH responses, i.e. an initial fall followed by a rise in pH. However, at 10 cm in the same subject, swallows resulted in monophasic pH response. Also note that acid clearance was faster at 10 cm than at 5 cm above LOS. (From Mittal *et al.* [98])

oesophageal manometry, noted that following a dry swallow, residual barium from a previous barium swallow flowed back from its position within a hiatus hernia into the oesophagus across the relaxed LOS. The barium was then cleared into the hiatus hernia by the on-coming peristaltic stripping wave [125]. Mittal and colleagues have recently confirmed these findings using scintigraphic labelling of a 15 ml bolus of 0.1 M hydrochloric acid instilled into the distal oesophagus and simultaneous pH monitoring [98]. As shown in Figure 1.6, with each dry swallow, both the scintigraphic and pH records demonstrate a biphasic pattern in patients with a hiatus hernia but not those without. They interpreted this as meaning that a small amount of acid becomes trapped in the hernial sac after clearance from the oesophagus, and this is then available for reflux into the oesophagus during a subsequent swallow-related LOS relaxation.

Two previous studies had demonstrated delayed oesophageal acid clearance in patients with hiatus hernia compared to those without [81,126]. In these studies, oesophageal acid clearance was measured by calculating the mean acid clearance time and counting the number of reflux episodes (pH < 4) lasting more than 5 minutes during 24-hour oesophageal pH monitoring. However, measuring clearance in this way does not take account of the possibility of repeated reflux episodes being superimposed and thus simulating delayed clearance. This is because a reflux episode is arbitrarily defined as beginning when the pH falls below a predetermined threshold level, and as ending when the pH rises to that or another predetermined level. This clearly takes no account of what occurs in between. DeMeester's group also carried out radioisotope oesophageal transit studies in some of their patients: four with hiatus hernia and GOR, four with hiatus hernia but no reflux and four controls [126]. They chose to compare the percentage retention of isotope in the oesophagus at 10 seconds as a measure of delayed clearance, which is unacceptable, as normal values for liquid oesophageal transit are up to 15 seconds [127]. Despite the small numbers and the evident overlap between the groups, they claim to gain support for their hypothesis of ineffective oesophageal clearance in patients with hiatus hernia, particularly those with GOR.

Scrutiny of the illustration of the radionuclide transit result in one of the hiatus hernia patients in DeMeester's report appears to highlight the difficulties of measuring oesophageal transit in the presence of a hiatus hernia [128]. In this illustration, most of the isotope has cleared within 12 seconds, leaving a residual level of about 25% of the administered isotope in the oesophagus. This is exactly the pattern that would be expected from failure to exclude the hiatus hernia from the oesophageal area of interest when calculating the oesophageal transit time [128]. Thus, DeMeester's findings do not exclude apparent delay in clearance resulting from the mechanism elegantly described by Mittal and colleagues [98]. Nevertheless, defective oesophageal clearance resulting from a hiatus hernia remains possible, and DeMeester believes this to be due to oesophageal shortening because oesophageal clearance, measured during prolonged oesophageal pH monitoring, can be improved by reducing the hiatus hernia and anchoring the gastro-oesophageal junction within the abdomen by a posterior gastropexy [126]. This finding is supported by the finding of other groups of increased overall oesophageal length related to insertion of the Angelchik device [106] and, perhaps by this mechanism, improvement in oesophageal acid clearance [108]. Two groups have, however, found the standard acid clearance test to be normal in patients with hiatus hernia but no symptoms of GOR disease [75,76], which argues against an effect on acid clearance of hiatus hernia in itself.

Symptomatic hiatus hernias are said to be more likely to be small than large. There are theoretical reasons to explain this [125]. Since, from Laplace's law, the pressure within the gastric pouch is inversely proportional to its radius, a small hiatus hernia may have a mechanical advantage over a large one [129]. When the diameter of the hernia greatly exceeds that of the oesophagus, the advantage is lost and the tendency for reflux reduced. Small hernias are also likely to have a narrower hiatus with a demonstrable zone of high pressure [130,131] resulting from the pinchcock effect of the right diaphragmatic crus. This will tend to retard emptying of a small hernia and to encourage reflux across a relaxed LOS.

Oesophageal mucosal resistance

Relatively little work has been done in this area compared to the gastroduodenal mucosa. However, some interesting work has focused on how oesophageal squamous epithelium resists attack by acid, and the underlying biochemical mechanisms of epithelial disruption are being clarified. In general terms, three lines of defence exist for any gastrointestinal surface, and these have been termed 'pre-epithelial', 'epithelial' and 'post-epithelial' [132].

Pre-epithelial defence mechanisms

Pre-epithelial defences include a mucous layer overlying the mucosa, and an unstirred layer below this, immediately adjacent to the surface. A continuous mucous layer has not been demonstrated in the oesophagus, although an unstirred layer, possibly derived from swallowed saliva and submucosal gland secretions, is said to exist and may have a thickness of about 30 µm [132]. A 30 nm glycocalyx has been demonstrated overlying the effete functionless cells of the stratum corneum of the oesophageal epithelium [133], whilst acid and neutral mucosubstances surround the superficial cells [134]. These cells, which are shed into the lumen, are parakeratinized, a process stimulated by intraluminal acid [135], and may form a physical barrier to attack by refluxed gastroduodenal contents. Hills and colleagues have found that the lining of the upper gastrointestinal tract is hydrophobic and have proposed that this may be a function of a phospholipid monolayer adsorbed into the mucosal surface [136]. This provides a waxy covering to the mucosa tending to resist attack by aqueous solutions of acid. Hills' group also found that the oesophageal mucosa in dogs is hydrophobic to a lesser though similar degree to the stomach, but more so than the distal duodenum and colon which are not exposed to an acid environment. This hydrophobic barrier also exists in humans [137], and preliminary results indicate that hydrophobicity is reduced in patients with oesophagitis compared to those with a normal oesophagus (P. Goggin and J. de Caestecker, unpublished observations). *Campylobacter pylori* infection of the gastric antrum is associated with reduced hydrophobicity of the antral mucosa [138]. It is of interest that one study has reported the frequent finding of colonies of this organism associated with oesophageal ulceration in patients with GOR disease [139]. These observations require confirmation and may open a new avenue of research into the role of epithelial defences in the pathogenesis of oesophagitis.

Epithelial defences

The oesophageal squamous epithelium can be divided into four zones, similar to other squamous epithelia. There is an upper layer of effete cells (stratum corneum) and a thick layer of functional cells (stratum granulosum) containing glycogen [134]. The prickle cell layer (stratum spinosum) and the actively proliferating basal layer form the basal part of the epithelium. The functional layer appears to resist acid and enzyme attack more readily than the prickle cell or basal layers [135]. This reflects the effectiveness of the intercellular junctions of the functional layer [140,141]. The cells of this layer contain membrane coating granules filled with lipid, neutral mucin and lysosomal enzymes, including an acid phosphatase [142,143]. These substances are released into the intercellular spaces by exocytosis in response to acid stimulation [135,141]. The lipid contributes to the lamellated bodies of the intercellular junctions which probably form an important component of the mechanism for resisting penetration by acid. In the inflamed oesophagus, the decrease in acid phosphatase [144] probably reflects decreased numbers of functional cells due to increased cell turnover and loss.

The prickle cell layer underlies the functional layer, and these cells have incorporated in their basolateral membranes the $Na^+/K^+ATPase$ [145,146] which, as will be seen later, plays an important role in maintaining cellular integrity in epithelium exposed to acid.

Cellular turnover is increased in oesophageal mucosal cells exposed to acid [147] and this, together with increased cell loss from the surface, probably accounts for the histological lesion found in the acid-exposed oesophageal mucosa, i.e. basal cell hyperplasia and suprapapillary thinning [148]. This represents another means of epithelial defence. Epithelial restitution, a mechanism for rapid covering of mucosal defects in the stomach [149], has not been demonstrated in the oesophagus, although such a mechanism could be responsible for the colonization of the oesophagus by gastric-type epithelium in Barrett's oesophagus. Histological studies in an experimental model have suggested that cells grow out from the necks of oesophageal submucosal glands in this condition [150].

A growing body of work is shedding light on the biochemical mechanisms controlling the maintenance of mucosal cellular integrity in the face of an acid insult. A negative electrochemical gradient or potential difference (PD) is known to exist between the oesophageal lumen and the body tissues. This PD is reduced in human oesophagitis [151] and in an experimental rabbit model in which the oesophagus was perfused with acid [145].

The transmucosal PD results from sodium (Na^+) transport from mucosa to serosa, and to a smaller degree from chloride (Cl^-) or bicarbonate (HCO_3^-) transport in the opposite direction [146,152]. It is known that prolonged exposure (up to 5 hours) to H^+ concentrations of less than 40 mmol/l produces a delayed increase in PD, while the increase is seen in the early phase (during the first hour) of acid perfusion as the H^+ concentration reaches 80 mmol/l [145,153,154]. Prolonged perfusion with this latter concentration produces a fall in PD after an initial increase, while concentrations in excess of 80 mmol/l lead to an immediate and continued decline in transmucosal PD with time [145]. Addition of pepsin to 80 mM hydrochloric acid increased the rate at which the PD declined [155]. Orlando and colleagues have correlated the changes in PD in vivo with measurements in vitro of electrolyte flux across the epithelium [145] and histological studies [155]. They found that the initial increase in PD was due to both H^+ flux out of the lumen and to H^+-stimulated, amiloride-sensitive Na^+ absorption which continued when the perfusing acid was replaced by saline [145]. When the PD was reduced by 40–50%, a decrease in electrical resistance was found, probably reflecting damage to the intercellular tight junctions, as mannitol flux was also increased [155]. Electron microscopy at this stage revealed dilated intercellular spaces [155]. The third stage, when PD was reduced by 100%, was characterized by swollen and ruptured cells in the mid-zone of the epithelium on microscopy [155], and was thought to be the culmination of H^+-stimulated Na^+ entry coupled with acid inhibition of the $Na^+/K^+ATPase$ activity [145]. This enzyme is located on the basolateral membranes of the cells of the prickle cell layer, accounting for the morphological location of the injury [145]. The activity of the enzyme is markedly pH dependent, with significant inhibition below pH 5 and above pH 8 [145].

One of the attractions of this model is that it requires intermittent exposure of the mucosa to acid alternating with fluid rich in Na$^+$ ions (e.g. saliva) similar to the situation in GOR disease. Orlando and Powell have shown the same changes in PD and Na$^+$ flux during acid perfusion in humans in vivo and in oesophageal specimens examined in vitro [146]. They found that in patients with a positive Bernstein test (all of whom had microscopically verified oesophagitis), the PD did not show the biphasic (increase at first followed by a decrease) change found in healthy controls, but instead fell rapidly, suggesting a functional impairment of the mucosal barrier in these patients [146]. Perhaps the thinning of the functional layer [142,148] allows more rapid access of acid to the prickle cell layer with consequent inhibition of Na$^+$/K$^+$ATPase.

There are two possible routes for H$^+$ penetration into cells: directly across the apical membrane, and by the paracellular route. Hydrogen ions penetrating into cells may threaten cell survival by another mechanism, lowering intracellular pH. This is resisted by active extrusion of H$^+$ in exchange for Na$^+$ across the apical cell membrane (this is the amiloride-sensitive mechanism mentioned above) and by an electroneutral exchange of Cl$^-$ for HCO$_3$$^-$ across the basolateral cell membrane [132]. The HCO$_3$$^-$ is then available to neutralize intracellular H$^+$.

Paracellular penetration of acid is resisted by intercellular junctions [141]. These are lined by negative charges which render them cation selective [156]. As luminal H$^+$ concentration rises, these charges are neutralized to repel cations. Polyvalent cations such as calcium, aluminium and magnesium can also neutralize the negative charges in these intercellular channels, making them less permeable to cations. It is tempting to suppose that this may, in part, explain the effect of antacid preparations.

Post-epithelial defences

The chief mechanism in this category is blood flow. This has been shown to increase early during exposure of the mucosa to luminal acid [157]. It may be that this provides additional HCO$_3$$^-$ buffer, allows more rapid dispersion of H$^+$ from the tissues and delivers more nutrients to the epithelium [156]. Unlike the stomach, it has not been clearly shown that prostaglandins are cytoprotective in the oesophagus. In fact, indomethacin reduces the severity of radiation [158] and acid-induced [159] oesophagitis in experimental animals. The submucosal glands are abundant in humans and the North American opossum, but sparse in the rabbit oesophagus. These have been little studied, but are known to secrete fluid rich in Na$^+$ and Cl$^-$ in response to cholinergic and adrenergic stimulation [160]. Their structure and histochemical characteristics have been reported [161], but their role, if any, in mucosal protection is unknown.

Studies of mucosal defence have enhanced understanding of the pathogenesis of acid-induced oesophageal damage. Further exploration of the possibility of reduced mucosal resistance to refluxed gastroduodenal contents in patients with oesophagitis may shed more light on this complex condition.

Gastric factors: the nature and volume of refluxate

Acid and pepsin

Hydrochloric acid and pepsin are both prime candidates for the production of oesophagitis. This is exemplified by the success of omeprazole in the treatment of oesophagitis [162]. Experimental models have been developed which illustrate this.

Thus, hydrochloric acid alone, at a pH of 1–1.3 induced oesophagitis in a cat model [163], and this model has been used to study the effects of experimental oesophagitis on LOS function [164–166]. Others have shown that hydrogen ion flux across the oesophageal mucosa, a precursor to mucosal damage [153], only occurs when the H^+ concentration is greater than 80 mmol/l [154]. At a lower acid concentration (pH 1.6–2), addition of pepsin is necessary to produce oesophagitis, which may then be severe [163]. Pepsin is denatured at a pH of less than 1, and is inactive against oesophageal epithelial proteins at pH values above 2, although some activity occurs up to pH 4 with other protein substrates such as haemoglobin [163].

It might be expected that patients with GOR disease produce more gastric acid and pepsin than control subjects. However, maximal acid output to histamine [167] or pentagastrin [168,169] is similar in symptomatic GOR patients and asymptomatic controls, unless a duodenal ulcer is present when the acid output is significantly increased [167]. Spencer found a linear relationship between duration of acid GOR during prolonged oesophageal pH monitoring and maximal acid output in duodenal ulcer patients, but no relationship between these measurements on symptomatic patients with hiatus hernia [170]. Boesby confirmed the lack of relationship between maximal acid output and GOR in 108 subjects [171], but he found that basal acid secretion was weakly correlated with GOR. Baldi and colleagues also found that basal acid output and volume were increased in patients with GOR compared to controls [169], possibly implying a difference in fasting gastric emptying.

Flook and Stoddard have reported that many duodenal ulcer patients (who, as a group, tend to have high gastric acid outputs) have oesophagitis and abnormal gastro-oesophageal reflux measured by prolonged pH monitoring, but normal LOS pressures compared to controls [172]. Similar results were obtained after vagotomy, although reflux symptoms were much reduced, implying that high acid output was related to the development of GOR disease in these patients. Perhaps the reduction in acid output after vagotomy explains the reduced symptoms of GOR.

All these results taken together suggest that increased volumes of gastric secretion or high concentrations of acid (and pepsin?) are responsible for GOR and oesophagitis in duodenal ulcer patients, but not in GOR patients without ulcers in whom other factors are presumably more important. These factors may be important in complicated oesophagitis, as one preliminary study has reported significantly higher concentrations of intraoesophageal pepsin in patients with strictures or Barrett's oesophagus compared with controls or patients with uncomplicated oesophagitis [173]. Severe oesophagitis may be a feature of the Zollinger–Ellison syndrome, probably the result of high gastric acid and pepsin concentrations, because LOS basal pressure is higher in these patients than normal [174].

Duodenogastric reflux of bile and pancreatic secretions

Bile is another candidate of potential significance to the development of oesophagitis. Unconjugated bile acids precipitate out of solution at an acid pH, but conjugated bile salts remain in solution. In an experimental rabbit model, H^+ flux across the oesophageal mucosa was increased in the presence of the conjugated bile acids taurocholate and taurodeoxycholate [154]. At neutral pH, unconjugated bile acids also increased H^+ flux across the oesophageal mucosa [154]. However, bile salts in themselves are only capable of causing mild oesophagitis and do not seem to modify or increase the damage caused by pepsin [175]. Nevertheless, bile acids are found in fasting and postprandial gastric juice of patients with oesophagitis, albeit in concentrations lower than those used in the animal model to induce oesophagitis [176].

There has been some debate about whether increased duodenogastric reflux occurs in GOR patients. Several groups of investigators, using intubation to sample gastric or duodenal contents, have found that duodenogastric reflux is increased in GOR patients compared to controls [168,177], while Gillison and colleagues, who used combined pyloric intubation and radiology, found pyloric incompetence to be common in patients with a symptomatic hiatus hernia [178]. These results have not been confirmed in other studies, including two using a radioisotopic technique with ^{99m}Tc-HIDA (hepatoimidoacetic acid) or ^{99m}Tc-diethyl-IDA to label bile [179–181]. However, as some duodenogastric reflux is now considered a normal phenomenon [182], whether it is increased or not in GOR disease is perhaps secondary to the question of whether bile gets into the oesophagus and causes oesophagitis.

Although perfusion and incubation studies in vitro suggest that bile salts are little if at all noxious to the oesophagus [175,183], the findings in a monkey model suggest that bile contamination of gastric juice makes oesophagitis of all grades more likely [184]. At least four groups have now attempted to measure bile concentrations in oesophageal refluxate. Three studies have demonstrated that bile is detectable in the fasting and postprandial periods in patients with oesophagitis, but in much lower concentrations than those shown in experimental models to produce oesophageal damage [168,185,186]. Mittal and colleagues were unable to confirm these findings [187]. They introduced a note of caution, pointing out that certain foods may give rise to falsely high readings by the commonly used hydroxysteroid dehydrogenase assay. Gotley and colleagues, using high performance liquid chromatography, found low concentrations of intraoesophageal bile acids during the day (after or in between meals), but high levels exceeding $200\,\mu mol/l$ in 25% of patients during the night [186]. The relevance of bile salts to the pathogenesis of reflux oesophagitis therefore remains uncertain.

Trypsin has been shown to cause severe oesophagitis when studied (at an alkaline pH) in an animal model [183]. The relevance of these findings to human oesophagitis is unknown, as true alkaline reflux is rare in patients who have not undergone gastric resections. Little and colleagues, finding fewer episodes of alkaline intragastric pH in oesophagitis patients compared to GOR patients without oesophagitis, in fact argue that, in patients with an intact stomach, refluxed alkaline contents may protect against the development of oesophagitis by neutralizing acidic gastric contents and inactivating pepsin [188].

Gastric emptying

An attractive hypothesis proposes that impairment of gastric emptying may promote GOR as a consequence of larger gastric volumes persisting after meals. Unfortunately, the results of studies to investigate this possibility have given conflicting results. This is at least in part attributable to differences in methodology [189]. For instance, the use of ^{99m}Tc-DTPA incorporated into a solid meal to measure solid emptying [179,190] is inappropriate, as DTPA (diethylenetriaminepentaacetic acid) does not adhere firmly to solid particles [189]. Notwithstanding these difficulties, a minority (about 40%) of patients with GOR disease have been demonstrated to show delayed emptying of solids from the stomach [190,191]. This has not been confirmed by other groups [192,193]. Velasco and co-workers [194] found that abnormal gastric empty-ing was not affected by successful anti-reflux surgery, which they interpreted as evidence that these abnormalities were not the result of secondary vagal damage from oesophagitis. Liquid gastric emptying has been reported to be delayed in patients with oesophagitis [169,179,191] but this has not been confirmed by other studies [192,194,195]. No study has specifically examined the early phase of gastric liquid emptying, which would be expected to be unusually rapid if gastric fundal receptive relaxation is impaired [196]. However, the findings of King and colleagues [197] using real time ultrasound in patients with GOR indicate increased gastro-duodenal liquid flow and could be explained by postulating that receptive relaxation is impaired in these patients. If such an abnormality were present, it would be compatible with other evidence that vagal impairment is common in GOR patients [64].

Thus, while gastric emptying abnormalities would form an attractive mechanism for enhancing GOR, their existence in these patients is controversial. At best, current evidence would suggest that they occur only in a minority of patients, and that delayed gastric emptying cannot be predicted on the basis of clinical symptoms [191].

Oesophageal sensation and gastro-oesophageal reflux disease

Heartburn is a symptom that many people have experienced at least occasionally [198]. Its frequent occurrence and relationship to posture and meals forms one of the cardinal clinical features of GOR disease. However, up to 20% of patients with oesophagitis and its complications never experience heartburn [199,200], while patients experiencing severe and frequent heartburn may have neither markedly abnormal amounts of GOR nor endoscopic oesophagitis [80,201]. Two issues need therefore to be addressed: do some reflux patients have a lowered oesophageal sensory threshold (giving rise to acid-induced symptoms) and do those who develop oesophagitis and its complications have impaired oesophageal sensation?

Oesophageal sensory threshold in symptomatic gastro-oesophageal reflux

It is known from several studies that the majority of patients with classic GOR symptoms develop their usual heartburn within 5 minutes of starting an acid perfusion test [42,202,203]. One study has found that the time to pain during oesophageal acid perfusion in such patients was significantly less than in controls and patients with chronic chest pain atypical for GOR [42]. It has been proposed that as GOR induces papillary elongation with thinning of the suprapapillary epithelium in the distal oesophagus [148], this will bring submucosal nerve endings closer to the lumen of the oesophagus and thus more accessible to intraluminal acid [204]. Fine free nerve terminals have been demonstrated ramifying within the oesophageal squamous epithelium [205], so a mechanism of this type is possible. Because of the patchy and variable nature of the oesophageal epithelial change [206], it will be difficult to prove a relationship between histological changes of this sort and oesophageal sensitivity. Johnson and colleagues were unable to demonstrate a relationship between the severity of heartburn and the degree of papillary elongation of the dermal papillae in oesophageal biopsies [81]. A poor relationship exists between symptoms and microscopic oesophagitis [201], although the histological changes referred to above are not in themselves signs of oesophageal inflammation [207].

It is well recognized that, with regard to polymodal cutaneous nociceptors, sensitization to a painful stimulus occurs after repeated noxious stimulation [208]. This possibility has not been addressed in the oesophagus, although it could be proposed that repeated nocturnal exposure to acid without arousal might lead to sensitization of oesophageal pain receptors which subsequently respond to much shorter diurnal episodes of acid reflux. Some support for this idea is provided by the finding that long-term treatment with cimetidine significantly prolonged the time to pain during an acid perfusion test in symptomatic GOR subjects [209]. The time course of this effect has not been documented, but the author noted (and it is a common clinical observation) that symptoms tended to relapse rapidly after stopping treatment. This is an area which warrants further exploration with newer more potent H_2-receptor antagonists and by assessing the effect of, for instance, head-up tilt of the bed at night.

The role of oesophageal sensation in the pathogenesis of oesophagitis

In patients with oesophagitis, there is some evidence for an oesophageal sensory deficit which may have a role in pathogenesis. However, it is always difficult to be sure whether defects of this sort are primary or secondary to oesophageal wall damage. Ogilvie and colleagues have shown that, in patients with oesophagitis, the time to pain during oesophageal acid perfusion was significantly prolonged in those with a subnormal LOS pressure response to increased intra-abdominal pressure compared to those with a normal LOS pressure response [64]. The same group have previously shown that the afferent pathway for the LOS response to increased intra-abdominal pressure is carried in the vagus nerve [63]. These findings indicate a vagal afferent defect in some patients with oesophagitis. Vagal efferent function may also be impaired, and this is not confined to alimentary vagal function [64,210], suggesting that vagal damage is not simply a consequence of oesophageal wall inflammation.

Failure of salivary response to oesophageal acidification has been demonstrated in patients with benign oesophageal strictures [95] and in one study in patients with oesophagitis [93]. In patients with oesophagitis, acidification of an acid bolus does not result in lowering of the threshold volume for secondary peristalsis that is observed in healthy controls [87,89]. These findings can be interpreted as indicating failure of normal reflex mechanisms, and may well be the result of afferent impairment as, in patients with complications of oesophagitis such as benign peptic strictures [95] and Barrett's oesophagus [211], the time to pain during acid perfusion is prolonged. Further support for afferent impairment in patients with Barrett's oesophagus comes from the preliminary findings reported by Schlesinger [212]. In patients with oesophagitis or Barrett's oesophagus studies by prolonged oesophageal pH monitoring, fewer reflux episodes, in particular those of long duration (> 5 minutes) were accompanied by heartburn compared to symptomatic GOR patients without oesophagitis. These findings do not differentiate between a primary or secondary cause for sensory impairment, but do indicate that such a defect may tend to worsen oesophageal clearance and thus increase oesophageal acid exposure.

Gastric acid secretion is stimulated by the presence of acid in the oesophagus [213,214]. It appears that this response is exaggerated in patients with symptomatic hiatus hernia, especially those with oesophagitis [214]. One group found that it was only those patients who developed heartburn during oesophageal acid perfusion who showed an increase in gastric acid output, and that the magnitude of the response was not related to the maximal histamine-stimulated acid output [213]. It would thus appear that this response has a sensory afferent component, but its relevance to the development of oesophagitis is unknown. However, as previously noted, several investigators have found an increase in basal acid output and basal volume of gastric secretion in oesophagitis patients [169,171]. It is possible that this is in part due to stimulation of gastric acid secretion in response to refluxed acid in the oesophagus.

Two other possible effects of sensory impairment may be mentioned. First, if there is decreased oesophageal acid sensitivity, this will tend to lead to failure of arousal and consequent failure of clearance of acid refluxed during sleep [78,85]. Secondly, King and colleagues using real time ultrasound to study antroduodenal motility and fluid movement in patients with GOR disease, found that forward gastroduodenal liquid flow is increased compared to controls [197]. Liquid flow from the stomach is regulated by fundal tone and this in turn is modulated by receptive relaxation in response to food entering the stomach [196]. It is known that vagotomy impairs receptive relaxation [196], so the findings of King's study are compatible with the hypothesis that gastric vagal function (afferent or efferent) may be impaired in reflux oesophagitis. Impaired receptive relaxation leads to increased intragastric pressure and this will tend to increase GOR across a relaxed LOS. Transient LOS relaxations occur most frequently in both normal and GOR subjects in the postprandial period [37,51,58], but only a proportion is accompanied by GOR. This proportion is increased in GOR disease patients [51,60]. The combination of impaired gastric receptive relaxation and frequent postprandial transient LOS relaxations may lead to increased frequency of episodes of GOR in reflux patients after meals.

The development of complications of oesophagitis

It is a common observation that between 25% and 40% of patients with benign peptic stricture have no antecedent history of heartburn [199,200,215]. This is compatible with the findings already discussed, indicating that some of these patients with complications have an afferent oesophageal defect. Helm and colleagues have shown that increased salivation ('waterbrash') occurs in normal subjects and those with oesophagitis in response to oesophageal acidification, as long as heartburn is produced [94]. The same group have found a defective salivary response to oeso- phageal acid perfusion in most patients with benign strictures, and this appears to be due to the fact that few of these patients develop heartburn during the test [95]. A poor salivary response to intraoesophageal acid may be one factor promoting poor acid clearance in such patients [90,91].

Oesophageal acid exposure is greater in patients wth Barrett's oesophagus than in those with uncomplicated oesophagitis and clearance of spontaneously refluxed acid is delayed in such patients [216–218]. In support of these findings, there have been reports of regression of columnar epithelium after successful anti-reflux surgery [219]. In an experimental model, Gillen and co-workers found that pentagastrin-stimulated acid secretion after creation of an incompetent gastro-oesophageal sphincter was the most potent stimulus to the development of columnar epithelialization in areas of the lower oesophagus denuded of squamous epithelium [150]. They also found that columnar epithelium developed in a denuded area not contiguous with the gastric epithelium at the cardia. This supports the contention that columnar epithelialization is a metaplastic process rather than the result of upward migration of gastric epithelium to cover the defect. The same group has presented preliminary histologi- cal evidence that the abnormal epithelium grows out from deep oesophageal mucous glands [150]. The clinical observation of isolated islands of columnar epithelium in the oesophagus of some patients supports this finding [220]. It has been suggested by others that columnar epithelium extends up the oesophagus from the gastric mucosa

[221], and clinical observation of the healing of some cases of linear oesophagitis by streaks of columnar epithelium could favour this [220]. Gillen and colleagues, however, found that the histochemical characteristics of Barrett's epithelium in their experimental model were distinct from that of the gastric cardia [150].

Bile has been implicated in the development of complications (ulcer, stricture or adenocarcinoma) within a Barrett's oesophagus. Thus, Gillen and co-workers found significantly raised intragastric bile acid concentrations for up to 2 hours following a meal in patients with complications of Barrett's oesophagus compared to uncomplicated Barrett's oesophagus, patients with uncomplicated oesophagitis and healthy controls [222]. However, no differences in fasting intragastric bile acid concentrations were found between the groups.

Thus, severe acid reflux (and possibly bile) together with delayed oesophageal acid clearance are implicated in the development of the complications of oesophagitis, but more work needs to be done in this area.

Two other factors may be important with regard to the development of strictures. First, some drugs, in particular non-steroidal anti-inflammatory agents, have been positively associated with the development of strictures in GOR patients [215,223]. This is somewhat surprising, in view of findings that these agents reduce oesophageal damage due to radiation [158] and, in an experimental model, acid perfusion [159] by inhibiting prostaglandin synthesis. A number of other drugs have the potential for causing or exacerbating oesophageal damage [224]. Slow release potassium, emepromium bromide [223], alprenolol, doxycycline, iron and analgesic drugs [225] have been particularly cited in respect of stricture formation.

Secondly, Maxton and colleagues found a significantly higher proportion of those who were either edentulous or had poor dentition among patients with benign strictures than among others undergoing endoscopy [226]. They attributed this finding to either the relative lack of solid food intake in edentulous patients (as solids will tend to dilate the oesophagus more than semisolid or liquid food), or to defective salivation which itself predisposes to dental caries.

Patterns of gastro-oesophageal reflux

Prolonged pH monitoring of the oesophagus has enhanced the understanding of when GOR occurs and of patterns associated with oesophagitis. It has been appreciated for nearly 20 years that some reflux, particularly after meals, is a normal event [11,170]. This corresponds with the findings that basal LOS pressure is lowest and transient LOS relaxation most frequent in the postprandial period in normal and GOR patients [37,51,58]. The incidence and severity of oesophagitis increases with increasing exposure of the distal oesophagus to acid [11,79,82,218], and it has been proposed that certain patterns of GOR are more likely to result in oesophagitis. DeMeester and colleagues defined three patterns seen during prolonged pH monitoring which they termed upright, supine and combined, depending on when, during 24-hour pH monitoring, abnormal GOR was found to occur. The highest incidence of oesophagitis and stricture was found in patients with combined reflux and the lowest in those with 'upright only' reflux [11,79]. This has led to the proposal that night-time reflux, when acid clearance from the oesophagus is particularly prolonged, is the most detrimental [79,81] particularly in respect of the development of complications [218]. However, postprandial reflux is also increased in patients with oesophagitis [82,227–229] and the magnitude of postprandial and daytime reflux is directly related

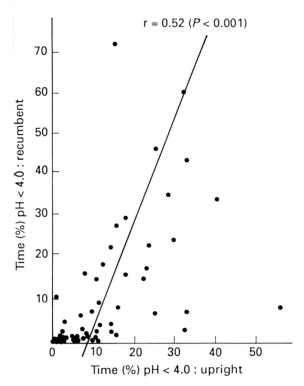

Figure 1.7 Relationship between distal oesophageal acid exposure time during recumbency (y-axis) and the daytime or 'upright' period (x-axis) during 23-hour pH monitoring in 52 patients. The intercept of the regression line with the x-axis at 9% indicates that little or no recumbent reflux occurs with mild degrees of upright reflux. However, it can be calculated that the gradient of the regression line is 4.8, indicating that as upright exposure increases, recumbent acid exposure contributes a progressively larger proportion to the total exposure. (From de Caestecker *et al.* [82])

to that occurring at night [82]. There is evidence that in-patient non-ambulatory monitoring may underestimate the magnitude of daytime reflux [230], which may be the reason for the high proportion of patients (23–37%) in DeMeester's studies who had abnormal reflux only when 'supine' [11,80]. This is in contrast with the lower proportions with 'supine only' reflux, found in patients studied by ambulatory outpatient pH monitoring [82,230]. Rather than there being three distinct patterns of GOR, ambulant studies have shown that as total acid exposure increases, so night-time exposure contributes a progressively larger proportion of the total [82,228]. This is evident from the gradient of the regression line in Figure 1.7, which relates upright and recumbent oesophageal acid exposure. The evening meal is commonly the major meal of the day, and the combination of a late large meal followed by retiring to bed for the night is likely to be particularly hazardous in GOR patients.

Two conclusions follow from these latter observations: first, postprandial monitoring may be a reasonably sensitive test for abnormal GOR [227,229,231–233] and, secondly, treatment should aim to reduce acid reflux whenever it occurs, not only during the night. Robertson and colleagues, using ambulatory 24-hour pH monitoring, observed that patients treated with ranitidine, whose oesophagitis did not heal, were distinguished from those whose oesophagitis did heal by failing to show a reduction in oesophageal acid exposure despite high doses of the drug [234]. Further studies of this type are required to assess the effects of medical anti-reflux therapy on patterns of reflux and the response of oesophagitis to treatment. Studies of prolonged monitoring of intragastric pH and the effect of antisecretory agents are having an important impact on treatment of duodenal ulceration and there is no reason why the same should not hold true for GOR disease [235,236].

Summary

Can an overall unifying hypothesis now be made regarding the pathogenesis of GOR disease? The answer is a qualified 'yes'. Although the pathogenesis of GOR and its complications is multifactorial, the vagus nerve has been implicated in many of the processes which are involved, including those responsible for the reflux of gastric contents (transient LOS relaxations, GOR in response to increased intra-abdominal pressure and free reflux across an atonic sphincter). The clearance mechanisms which may be disordered in those developing complications, involve salivation in response to oesophageal acidification, which itself depends on a vagal reflex. Primary peristalsis is the major mechanism for volume clearance from the oesophagus, although it remains uncertain whether the vagus nerve or the oesophageal intramural nerve plexuses are of primary importance in this respect. Gastric emptying of liquids and solids is dependent on intact vagal pathways.

Mechanical factors such as the pinchcock effect of the diaphragmatic crus and the presence of a hiatus hernia may be contributory factors to GOR, but play a subsidiary role to that of the oesophageal body and LOS. Oesophagitis subsequent to GOR may further impair oesophageal function, leading to a vicious circle of increasing reflux and worsening oesophagitis [76].

Vagus nerve abnormalities have been demonstrated in a large proportion of GOR patients [64]. These are patchy and may involve efferent or afferent pathways or both [64]. Abnormalities of vagal cardiovascular reflexes also occur but there is no evidence of a widespread autonomic defect in GOR patients [64,210]. Afferent fibres form by far the largest proportion of nerve fibres in the vagal nerve trunks [237] and by and large afferent function is more difficult to measure than efferent function, so it is possible that in those patients who have not had a vagal abnormality demonstrated, an as yet undefined afferent defect exists. Vagal abnormalities are not the result of oesophageal wall damage due to oesophagitis and so must be primary [64,210].

The hypothesis is that a primary afferent or efferent vagal defect or defects exist in GOR patients which may affect one or more of the factors described in this chapter involved in the pathogenesis of GOR disease. The exact nature of the vagal defect may differ between individual patients, but all will tend to promote GOR or delayed oesophageal clearance.

References

1. Winkelstein, A. Peptic esophagitis: a new clinical entity. *J. Am. Med. Assoc.* 1935; **104**: 106–108
2. Allison, P. R. Peptic ulcer of the oesophagus. *J. Thorac. Surg.* 1946; **15**: 308–317
3. Allison, P. R. Reflux esophagitis, sliding hiatus hernia and the anatomy of repair. *Surg. Gynecol. Obstet.* 1951; **92**: 419–431
4. DeMeester, T. R., Bonavina, L. and Albertucci, M. Nissen fundoplication for gastroesophageal reflux disease: evaluation of primary repair in 100 consecutive patients. *Ann. Surg.* 1986; **204**: 9–20

5. Jamieson, G. G. Antireflux operations: how do they work? *Br. J. Surg.* 1987; **74**: 155–156
6. Richter, J. E. and Castell, D. Drugs, foods and other substances in the cause and treatment of reflux esophagitis. *Med. Clin. N. Am.* 1981; **65**: 1223–1234
7. Tytgat, G. N. J. Assessment of the efficacy of cimetidine and other drugs in oesophageal reflux disease. In: Baron, J. H., Ed. *Cimetidine in the 80's.* Edinburgh: Churchill Livingstone. 1981: 153–166
8. Pope, C. E. Pathophysiology and diagnosis of reflux esophagistis. *Gastroenterology* 1976; **70**, 445–454
9. Dodds, W. J., Hogan, W. J., Helm, J. F. and Dent, J. Pathogenesis of reflux esophagitis. *Gastroenterology* 1981; **81**: 376–394
10. Anonymous. Gastro-oesophageal reflux (editorial). *Lancet* 1983; **i**: 1081–1082
11. DeMeester, T. R., Johnson, L. R., Joseph, G. J., Toscano, M. S., Hall, A. W. and Skinner, D. B. Patterns of gastroesophageal reflux in health and disease. *Ann. Surg.* 1976; **184**: 459–469
12. Fyke, F. E., Code, C. F. and Schlegel, J. F. The gastroesophageal sphincter in healthy human beings. *Gastroenterologia* 1956; **86**: 135–150
13. Atkinson, M., Edwards, D. A. W., Honour, A. J. and Rowlands, E. N. Comparison of cardiac and pyloric sphincters. *Lancet* 1957; **ii**: 918–922
14. Atkinson, M., Edwards, D. A. W., Honour, A. J. and Rowlands, E. N. The oesophagogastric sphincter in hiatus hernia. *Lancet* 1957; **ii**: 1138–1142
15. Atkinson, M. and Summerling, M. D. The competence of the cardia after cardiomyotomy. *Gastroenterologia* 1954: **92**, 23–134
16. Lind, J. F., Warrian, W. G. and Wankling, W. J. Responses of the gastro-oesophageal junctional zone to increases in abdominal pressure. *Can. J. Surg.* 1960; **9**: 32–38
17. Daniel, E. E., Taylor, G. S. and Holman, M. E. The myogenic bases of active tension in the lower esophageal sphincter (abstract). *Gastroenterology* 1976; **70**: 874
18. Christensen, J., Conklin J. L. and Freeman, B. W. Physiologic specialisation at the esophagogastric junction in three species. *Am. J. Physiol.* 1973; **225**: 1265–1270
19. Christensen, J., Freeman, B. W. and Miller, J. K. Some physiologic characteristics of the esophagogastric junction in the opossum. *Gastroenterology* 1973; **64**: 1119–1125
20. Biancani, P., Goyal, R. K., Phillips, A. and Spiro, H. M. Mechanics of sphincter action: studies on the lower esophageal sphincter. *J. Clin. Invest.* 1973; **52**: 2973–2978
21. Lipshutz, W. and Cohen, S. Physiological determinants of lower esophageal sphincter function. *Gastroenterology* 1971; **61**: 16–24
22. Christensen, J. Pharmacologic identification of the lower esophageal sphincter. *J. Clin. Invest.* 1970; **49**: 681–691
23. Zaninotto, G., Dalla Libera, L., Merigliano, S. and Ancona, E. Is there a biochemical basis for lower oesophageal sphincter (LOS) resting pressure? *Gut* 1986; **27**: 255–259
24. Uddman, R., Alumets, J., Edwinsson, L., Hakanson, R. and Sundler, F. Peptidergic (VIP) innervation of the esophagus. *Gastroenterology* 1978; **75**: 5–8
25. Alumets, J., Fahrenkrug, J., Hakanson, R. Schaffalitzky de Muckadell, O. B., Sundler, F. and Uddman, R. A rich VIP nerve supply is characteristic of sphincters. *Nature* 1979; **280**: 155–156
26. Pope, C. E. A dynamic test of sphincter strength: its application to the LES. *Gastroenterology* 1967; **52**: 779–786
27. Cohen, S. and Harris L. D. Lower esophageal sphincter pressure as an index of lower esophageal sphincter strength. *Gastroenterology* 1970; **58**: 157–162
28. Kaye, M. D. and Showater, J. P. Manometric configuration of the lower esophageal sphincter in normal human subjects. *Gastroenterology* 1971; **61**: 213–223
29. Dent, J. A new technique for continuous sphincter pressure measurement. *Gastroenterology* 1976; **71**: 263–267
30. Dodds, W. J., Hogan, W. J., Stef, J. J., Miller, W. N., Lydon, S. B. and Arndorfer, R. C. A rapid pull through technique for measuring lower esophageal sphincter pressure. *Gastroenterology* 1975; **68**: 437–443
31. Welch, R. W. and Drake, S. T. Normal lower esophageal sphincter pressure: a comparison of rapid vs slow pull through techniques. *Gastroenterology* 1980; **78**: 1446–1451

32. Boyle, J. T., Altschuler, S. M., Nixen, T. E., Tuchman, D. N., Pack, A. I. and Cohen, S. Role of the diaphragm in the genesis of lower esophageal sphincter pressure in the cat. *Gastroenterology* 1985; **88**: 723–730

33. Mittal, R. K., Rochester, D. F. and McCallum, R. W. Effect of diaphragmatic contraction on lower oesophageal sphincter pressure in man. *Gut* 1987; **28**: 1564–1568

34. Richter, J. E., Wu, W. C. Johns, D. N. *et al.* Esophageal manometry in 95 healthy adult volunteers: variability of pressures with age and frequency of "abnormal" contractions. *Dig. Dis. Sci.* 1987; **32**: 583–592

35. Goodall, R. J. R., Hay, D. J. and Temple, J. G. Assessment of the rapid pull through technique in oesophageal manometry. *Gut* 1980; **21**: 169–173

36. Baldi, F., Ferrarini, F., Balestra, R. *et al.* Oesophageal motor events at the occurrence of acid reflux and during endogenous acid exposure in healthy subjects and patients with oesophagitis. *Gut* 1985; **26**: 336–341

37. Dent, J., Dodds, W. J., Friedman, R. H., Sekiguchi, T., Hogan, W. J. and Arndorfer, R. C. Mechanism of gastroesophageal reflux in recumbent asymptomatic subjects. *J. Clin. Invest.* 1980; **65**: 256–267

38. Dent, J., Dodds, W. J., Sekiguchi, T., Hogan, W. J. and Arndorfer, R. C. Interdigestive phasic contractions of the human lower esophageal sphincter. *Gastroenterology* 1983; **84**: 453–460

39. Dent J., Holloway R. H., Toouli, J. and Dodds, W. J. Mechanisms of lower oesphageal sphincter incompetence in patients with symptomatic gastro-oesophageal reflux. *Gut* 1988; **29**: 1020–1028

40. Wankling, W. J., Warrian, W. G. and Lind, J. F. The gastro-oesophageal sphincter in hiatus hernia. *Can. J. Surg.* 1965; **8**: 61–67

41. Cohen, S. and Harris, L. D. Does hiatus hernia affect competence of the gastroesophageal sphincter? *N. Engl. J. Med.* 1971; **289**: 1053–1056

42. Behar, J., Biancani, P. and Sheahan D. G. Evaluation of esophageal tests in the diagnosis of reflux esophagitis. *Gastroenterology* 1976; **71**: 9–15

43. Stanciu, C., Hoare, R. C. and Bennett, J. R. Correlation between manometric and pH tests for gastro-oesophageal reflux. *Gut* 1977; **18**: 536–540

44. Kahrilas, P. J., Dodds, W. J., Hogan, W. J., Kern, R., Arndorfer, R. C. and Reece, A. Esophageal peristaltic dysfunction in peptic esophagitis. *Gastroenterology* 1986; **91**: 897–904

45. Christensen, J. Effect of drugs on esophageal motility. *Arch. Intern. Med.* 1976; **136**: 532–537

46. Lind, J. F., Crispin, J. S. and McIver, D. K. The effect of atropine on the gastro-oesophageal sphincter. *Can. J. Physiol. Pharmacol.* 1968; **46**: 233–238

47. Snape, W. J. and Cohen, S. Hormonal control of esophageal function. *Arch. Intern. Med.* 1976; **136**: 538–542

48. Goyal, R. K. and Cobb, B. W. Motility of the pharynx, esophagus and esophageal sphincter. In: Johnson, L. R., Ed. *Physiology of the Gastrointestinal Tract.* New York: Raven Press. 1981: 359–391

49. Nebel, O. T. and Castell, D. O. Lower esophageal pressure changes after food ingestion. *Gastroenterology* 1972; **63**: 778–783

50. Castell, D. O. and Levine, S. M. Lower esophageal sphincter response to gastric alkalinisation. *Ann. Intern. Med.* 1971; **74**: 223–227

51. Dodds, W. J., Dent, J., Hogan, W. J. *et al.* Mechanisms of gastroesophageal reflux in patients with reflux esophagitis. *N. Engl. J. Med.* 1982; **307**: 1547–1552

52. Babka, J. C. and Castell, D. O. On the genesis of heartburn the effects of specific foods on the lower esophageal sphincter. *Am. J. Dig. Dis.* 1973; **18**, 391–397

53. Dennish, G. W. and Castell, D. O. Caffeine and the lower oesophageal sphincter. *Am. J. Dig. Dis.* 1977; **17**: 993–996

54. Dennish, G. W. and Castell, D. O. Inhibitory effect of smoking on the lower esophageal sphincter. *N. Engl. J. Med.* 1971; **284**: 1136–1137

55. Stanciu, C. and Bennett, J. R. Smoking and gastro-oesophageal reflux. *Br. Med. J.* 1972; **3**: 793–795

56. Hongo, M., Traube, M. and McCallum, R. W. Comparison of effects of nifedepine, propantheline bromide and the combination on esophageal motor function in normal volunteers. *Dig. Dis. Sci.* 1984; **29**: 300–304

57. Dodds, W. J. Current concepts of esophageal motor function: clinical implications for radiology. *Am. J. Roentgenol.* 1977; **129**: 549–561

58. Smout, A. J. P. M., Akkermans, L. M. A., Bogaard, J. W., Ten Thije, O. J. and Wittebol, P. 'Inappropriate' lower esophageal sphincter relaxations in normal subjects (Abstract). *Dig. Dis. Sci.* 1985; **30**: 795

59. Mittal, R. K. and McCallum, R. W. Characteristics of transient lower esophageal sphincter relaxations in humans. *Am. J. Physiol.* 1987; **252**: G636–G641

60. Mittal, R. K. and McCallum, R. W. Characteristics and frequency of transient relaxations of the lower esophageal sphincter in patients with reflux esophagitis. *Gastroenterology* 1988; **95**: 593–599

61. Gill, R. C., Kellow, J. E. and Wingate, D. L. Gastro-oesophageal reflux and the migrating motor complex. *Gut* 1987, **28**: 929–934

62. Dodds, W. J., Hogan, W. J., Miller, W. N., Stef., J. J., Arndorfer, R. C. and Lydon, S. B. Effect of increased intra-abdominal pressure on lower esophageal sphincter pressure. *Dig. Dis.* 1975; **20**: 298–308

63. Ogilvie, A. L. and Atkinson, M. Influence of the vagus nerve upon reflex control of the lower oesophagal sphincter. *Gut* 1984; **25**: 253–258

64. Ogilvie, A. L., James, P. D. and Atkinson, M. Impairment of vagal function in reflux oesophagitis. *Q. J. Med.* 1985; **54**: 61–74

65. Welch, R. W. and Gray, J. E. The quantitation of normal esophageal function: a computerised study (abstract). *Gastroenterology* 1981; **80**: 1313

66. Corazziari, E., Bontempo, I., Anzini, F. and Torsoli, A. Motor activity of the distal oesophagus and gastro-oesophageal reflux. *Gut* 1984; **25**: 7–13

67. Kruse-Anderson, S., Wallin, L. and Madsen, T. Relationship between spontaneous non-propagating pressure activity in the oesophagus and acid gastro-oesophageal reflux in pathological and non-pathological refluxers. *Gut* 1987; **28**: 1478–1483

68. Dent, J. Recent views on the pathogenesis of gastro-oesophageal reflux. In: Tytgat, G. N. J., Ed. *Clinical Gastroenterology: Oesophageal disorders*, Vol. 1. London: Ballière Tindall. 1987: 727–745

69. Wyman, J. D., Dent, J., Heddle, R., Dodds, W. J., Toouli, J. and Lewis, I. Belching: a clue to understanding of pathological gastroesophageal reflux (Abstract). *Gastroenterology* 1984; **86**: 1303

70. Holloway, R. H., Hongo, M., Berger, K. and McCallum, R. W. Gastric distension: a mechanism for postprandial gastroesophageal reflux. *Gastroenterology* 1985; **89**: 779–784

71. Martin, C. J., Patrikios, J. and Dent, J. Abolition of gas reflux and transient lower esophageal sphincter relaxation by vagal blockade in the dog. *Gastroenterology* 1986; **91**: 890–896

72. Holloway, R. H., Dent, J. and Wyman, R. B. Impairment of belch reflex in achalasia: evidence for neural mediation of transient lower esophageal sphincter (LES) relaxation (Abstract). *Gastroenterology* 1986; **91**: 1055

73. Cox, M. R., Martin, C. J. and Dent, J. Postural suppression of transient lower esophageal sphincter relaxation is not mediated by gastric fluid receptors in the dog (Abstract). *Gastroenterology* 1987; **92**: 1357

74. Johnson, L. F. Methods of testing esophageal clearance. In: Dubois, A. and Castell, D. O., Eds. *Esophageal and Gastric Emptying*. Boca Raton, Florida: CRC Press. 1984: 12–27

75. Booth, D. J., Kemmerer, W. T. and Skinner, D. B. Acid clearing from the distal esophagus. *Arch. Surg.* 1968; **96**: 731–734

76. Stanciu, C. and Bennett, J. R. Oesophageal acid clearing: one factor in the production of reflux oesophagitis. *Gut* 1974; **15**: 852–857

77. Kjellen, G. and Tibbling, L. Influence of body position, dry and water swallows, smoking and alcohol on oesophageal acid clearing. *Scand. J. Gastroenterol.* 1978; **13**: 283–288

78. Orr, W. C., Robinson, M. G. and Johnson, L. F. Acid clearance during sleep in the pathogenesis of reflux esophagitis. *Dig. Dis. Sci.* 1981; **26**: 423–427

79. Little, A. G., DeMeester, T. R., Kirchner, P. T., O'Sullivan, G. C. and Skinner, D. B. Pathogenesis of esophagitis in patients with gastroesophageal reflux. *Surgery* 1980; **88**: 101–107

80. DeMeester, T. R., Wang, C. I., Wernly, J. A. *et al.* Technique, indications and clinical use of 24 hour esophageal pH monitoring. *J. Thorac. Cardiovasc. Surg.* 1980; **79**: 656–667

81. Johnson, L. F., DeMeester, T. R. and Haggitt, R. C. Esophageal epithelial response to gastro-esophageal reflux: a quantitative study. *Dig. Dis.* 1978; **23**: 498–509

82. de Caestecker, J. S., Blackwell, J. N., Pryde, A. and Heading, R. C. Daytime gastro-oesophageal reflux is important in oesophagitis. *Gut* 1987; **28**: 519–526

83. Johnson, L. F. and DeMeester, T. R. Evaluation of elevation of the head of the bed, bethanechol and antacid foam tablets on gastroesophageal reflux. *Dig. Dis. Sci* 1981; **26**: 673–680

84. Orr, W. C., Robinson, M. G. and Rundell, O. H. The effect of hypnotic drugs on acid clearance during sleep (Abstract). *Gastroenterology* 1985; **88**: 1526

85. Orr, W. C., Johnson, L. F. and Robinson, M. G. Effect of sleep on swallowing, esophageal peristalsis and acid clearance. *Gastroenterology* 1984; **86**: 814–819

86. Kruse-Anderson, S., Wallin, L. and Madsen, T. Acid gastro-oesophageal reflux and oesophageal pressure activity during postprandial and nocturnal periods. *Scand. J. Gastroenterol.* 1987; **22**: 926–930

87. Corazziari, E., Pozzesere, C., Dani, S., Anzini, F. and Torsoli, A. Intraluminal pH and esophageal motility. *Gastroenterology* 1978; **75**: 275–277

88. Thompson, D. G., Andreollo, N. A., McIntyre, A. S. and Earlam, R. J. Studies of the oesophageal clearance responses of intraluminal acid. *Gut* 1988; **29**: 881–885

89. Corazziari, E., Materia, E., Pozzessere, C., Anzini, F. and Torsoli, A. Intraluminal pH and oesophageal motility in patients with gastro-oesophageal reflux. *Digestion* 1986; **35**: 151–157

90. Helm, J. F., Dodds, W. J., Pele, L. R., Palmer, D. W., Hogan, W. J. and Teeter, B. C. Effect of esophageal emptying and saliva on clearance of acid from the esophagus. *N. Engl. J. Med.* 1984; **310**: 284–288

91. Helm, J. F., Dodds, W. J., Riedel, D. R., Teeter, B. C., Hogan, W. J. and Arndorfer, R. C. Determinants of esophageal acid clearance in normal subjects. *Gastroenterology* 1983; **85**: 607–612

92. Helm, J. F., Dodds, W. J., Hogan, W. J., Soergel, K. H., Egide, M. S. and Lebode, C. M. Acid neutralising capacity of human saliva. *Gastroenterology* 1982; **83**: 69–74

93. Sonnenberg, A., Steinkamp, U., Weise, A. *et al.* Salivary secretion in reflux esophagitis. *Gastroenterology* 182; **83**: 889–895

94. Helm, J. F., Dodds, W. J. and Hogan, W. J. Salivary response to esophageal acid in normal subjects and patients with reflux esophagitis. *Gastroenterology* 1987; **93**: 1393–1397

95. Helm, J. F., Allendorph, M., Dodds, W. J., Hogan, W. J. and Lipman, S. Loss of the salivary response to esophageal acid perfusion in patients with peptic stricture (Abstract). *Gastroenterology* 1986; **90**: 1456

96. Hogan, W. J., Keigos de Andriale, S. R. and Winship, D. H. Ethanol induced acute esophageal motor dysfunction. *J. Appl. Physiol.* 1972; **32**: 755–760

97. Gupta, R. R. and Kahrilas, P. J. The acute effect of smoking on esophageal clearance time and salivation (Abstract). *Gastroenterology* 1988; **94**: A161

98. Mittall, R. K., Lange, R. C. and McCallum, R. W. Identification and mechanism of delayed esophageal acid clearance in subjects with hiatus hernia. *Gastroenterology* 1987; **92**: 130–135

99. DeMeester, T. R., Johnson, L. F. and Kent, A. H. Evaluation of current operations for the prevention of gastroesophageal reflux. *Ann. Surg.* 1974; **180**: 511–523

100. Ellis, F. H., El-Kurd, M. F. A. and Gibbs, S. P. The effect of fundoplication on the lower esophageal sphincter. *Surg. Gynecol. Obstet.* 1976; **143**: 1–5

101. Brand, D. L., Eastwood, I. R., Martin, D., Carter, W. B. and Pope, C. E. Esophageal symptoms, manometry and histology before and after antireflux surgery: a long term follow up study. *Gastroenterology* 1979; **76**: 1393–1401

102. Goodhall, R. J. R. and Temple, J. G. Effect of Nissen fundoplication on competence of the gastro-oesophageal junction. *Gut* 1980; **21**: 607–613

103. Starting, J. R., Reichelderfer, M. O., Pellet, J. R. and Belzer, F. O. Treatment of symptomatic gastroesophageal reflux using the Angelchik prosthesis. *Ann. Surg.* 1982; **195**: 686–690

104. Kozarek, R. A., Phelps, J. E., Sanowski, R. A., Grobe, J. L. and Fredell, C. H. An antireflux prosthesis in the treatment of gastroesophageal reflux. *Ann. Intern. Med.* 1983; **98**: 310–315

105. Kozarek, R. A., Brayko, C. M., Sanowski, H. and Fedell, C. H. Evaluation of Angelchik antireflux prosthesis: long term results. *Dig. Dis. Sci.* 1985; **30**: 723–732

106. Wale, R. J., Royston, C. M. S., Bennett, J. R. and Buckton, G. K. Prospective study of the Angelchik antireflux prosthesis. *Br. J. Surg.* 1985; **72**: 520–524

107. Morris, D. L., Jones, J., Evans, D. F. *et al.* Reflux versus dysphagia: an objective evaluation of the Angelchik prosthesis. *Br. J. Surg.* 1985; **72**: 1017–1020

108. de Caestecker, J. S., McLean-Ross, H., Heading, R. C. and McLeod, I. B. Appraisal of the Angelchik antireflux prosthesis based on clinical and manometric data and pH monitoring. *J. R. Coll. Surg. Edin.* 1989; **34**: 9–12

109. Fisher, R. S., Malmud, L. S., Letis, I. F. and Macer, W. P. Antireflux surgery for symptomatic gastroesophageal reflux: mechanism of action. *Am. J. Dig. Dis.* 1978; **23**: 152–160

110. Bancewicz, J., Mughal, M. and Marples, M. The lower oesophageal sphincter after floppy Nissen fundoplication. *Br. J. Surg.* 1987; **74**: 162–164

111. Kiroff, G. K., Madden, G. J. and Jamieson, G. G. A study of factors responsible for the efficacy of fundoplication in the treatment of gastro-oesophageal reflux. *Aust. N.Z. J. Surg.* 1984; **54**: 109–112

112. Gill, R. C., Bowes, K. L., Murphy, P. D. and Kingman, Y. J. Esophageal motor abnormalities in gastroesophageal reflux and the effects of fundoplication. *Gastroenterology* 1986; **91**: 364–369

113. Pattrick, F. G. Investigation of gastro-oesophageal reflux in various positions with a two-lumen pH electrode. *Gut* 1970; **11**: 659–667

114. Babka, J. C., Hagar, G. W. and Castell, D. O. The effect of body position on lower esophageal sphincter pressure. *Am. J. Dig. Dis.* 1973; **18**: 441–442

115. Dodds, W. J., Stewart, E. T., Hogan, W. J., Stef, J. J. and Arndorfer, R. C. Effect of esophageal movements on intraluminal esophageal pressure recordings. *Gastroenterology* 1974; **67**: 592–600

116. Welch, R. W. and Gray, J. E. Influence of respiration on recording of lower esophageal sphincter pressure in humans. *Gastroenterology* 1982; **83**: 590–594

117. Goldman, J. and Bennett, J. R. Gastro-oesophageal reflux and respiratory disorders in adults. *Lancet* 1988; **ii**: 493–495

118. Petterson, G. B., Bombeck, C. T. and Nyhus, L. M. The lower esophageal sphincter: mechanism of opening and closure. *Surgery* 1980; **88**: 307–314

119. Meiss, J. H., Grindlay, J. H. and Ellis, F. H. The gastroesophageal sphincter mechanism. *J. Thorac. Surg.* 1958; **36**: 156–165

120. Joelsson, B. E., DeMeester, T. R., Skinner, D. B., Lafontaine, E., Waters, P. F. and O'Sullivan, G. C. The role of the esophageal body in the antireflux mechanism. *Surgery* 1982; **92**: 417–423

121. Samelson, S. L., Weiser, H. F., Bombeck, T. *et al.* A new concept in the surgical treatment of gastroesophageal reflux. *Ann. Surg.* 1983; **197**: 254–258

122. DeMeester, T. R., Wernly, J. A., Bryant, G. H., Little, A. G. and Skinner, D. B. Clinical and in vitro analysis of determinants of gastroesophageal competence: a study of the principles of antireflux surgery. *Am. J. Surg.* 1979; **137**: 39–45

123. Dyer, N. H. and Pridie, R. B. Incidence of hiatus hernia in asymptomatic subjects. *Gut* 1968; **9**: 696–699

124. Ott, D. J., Wu, W. C. and Gelfand, D. W. Reflux esophagitis revisited: prospective analysis of radiologic accuracy. *Gastrointest. Radiol.* 1981; **6**: 1–7

125. Longi, E. H. and Jordan, P. H. Pressure relationships responsible for reflux in patients with hiatal hernia. *Surg. Gynecol. Obstet.* 1969; **129**: 734–748

126. DeMeester, T. R., Lafontaine, E., Joelsson, B. E. *et al.* Relationship of a hiatus hernia to the function of the body of the esophagus and the gastroesophageal junction. *J. Thorac. Cardiovasc. Surg.* 1981; **82**: 547–558

127. Blackwell, J. N., Hannan, R. J., Adam, R. D. and Heading, R. C. Radionuclide transit studies in the detection of oesophageal dysmotility. *Gut* 1983; **24**: 421–426

128. Blackwell, J. N., Richter, J. E., Wu, W. C., Cowen, R. J. and Castell, D. O. Esophageal radionuclide transient tests: potential false-positive results. *Clin. Nucl. Med.* 1984; **9**: 674–683

129. McLaurin, C. Intrinsic sphincter in prevention of gastro-oesophageal reflux. *Lancet* 1963; **ii**: 132

130. Habibulla, K. S. The diaphragm as an anti-reflux barrier. A manometric oesophagoscopic and transmucosal potential study. *Thorax* 1972; **27**: 692–701

131. Code, C. F., Kelly, M. L., Schlegel, J. F. and Olsen, A. M. Detection of hiatal hernia during esophageal motility tests. *Gastroenterology* 1962; **43**: 521–531

132. Orlando, R. C. Esophageal epithelial resistance. *J. Clin. Gastroenterol.* 1986; **8** (suppl. 1): 12–16

133. Logan, K. R., Hopwood, D. and Milne, G. Ultrastructural demonstration of cell coat on the cell surface of normal oesophageal epithelium. *Histochem. J.* 1977; **9**: 495–504

134. Hopwood, D., Logan, K. R., Coghill, G. and Bouchier, I. A. D. Histochemical studies of mucosubstances and lipids in normal oesophageal epithelium. *Histochem. J.* 1977; **9**: 153–161

135. Hopwood, D., Milne, G. and Logan, K. R. Electron microscopic changes in human oesophageal epithelium in oesophagitis. *J. Pathol.* 1979; **129**: 161–167

136. Hills, B. A., Butler, B. D. and Lichtenberger, L. M. Gastric mucosal barrier: hydrophobic lining to the lumen of the stomach. *Am. J. Physiol.* 1983; **244**: G561–G568

137. Spychal, R. T., Marrero, J. M., Saverymuttu, S. H. and Northfield, T. C. Measurement of the surface hydrophobicity of human gastrointestinal mucosa. *Gastroenterology* 1989; in press

138. Marrero, J., Spychal, R. T., Goggin, P. M. *et al.* A new angle on *Campylobacter* (Abstract). *Gut* 1989; **30**: A 731–732

139. Borkert, M. V. and Beker, J. A. Treatment of ulcerative reflux oesophagitis with colloidal bismuth subcitrate in combination with cimetidine. *Gut* 1988; **29**: 385–389

140. Logan, K. R., Hopwood, D. and Milne, G. Cellular junctions in human oesophageal epithelium. *J. Pathol.* 1978; **126**: 157–163

141. Bateson, M. C., Hopwood, D., Milne, G. and Bouchier, I. A. D. Oesophageal epithelial ultrastructure after incubation with gastrointestinal fluids and their components. *J. Pathol.* 1981; **133**: 33–51

142. Hopwood, D., Logan, K. R. and Milne, G. Mucosubstances in the normal oesophageal epithelium. *Histochemistry* 1977; **54**: 67–74

143. Hopwood, D., Logan, K. R. and Milne, G. The light and electron microscopic distribution of acid phosphate activity in normal human oesophageal epithelium. *Histochem. J.* 1978; **10**: 159–170

144. Hopwood, D., Ross, P. E., Logan, K. R., Nicholson, G. and Bouchier, I. A. D. Changes in enzyme activity in normal and histologically inflamed oesophageal epithelium. *Gut* 1978; **20**: 769–774

145. Orlando, R. C., Bryson, J. C. and Powell, D. W. Mechanisms of H^+ injury in rabbit esophageal epithelium. *Am. J. Physiol.* 1984; **246**: G718–G724

146. Orlando, R. C. and Powell, D. W. Studies of oesophageal epithelial electrolyte transport and potential difference in man. In: Allen, A., Garner, A., Flemstrom, G., Silen, W. and Turnberg, L. A., Eds. *Mechanisms of Mucosal Protection in the Upper Gastrointestinal Tract.* New York: Raven Press. 1984: 75–78

147. De Baker, A., Haentjens, P. and Willems, G. Hydrochloric acid – a trigger of cell proliferation in the oesophagus of dogs. *Dig. Dis. Sci* 1985; **30**: 884–890

148. Ismail Beigi, F., Horton, P. F. and Pope, C. E. Histological consequences of gastroesophageal reflux in man. *Gastroenterology* 1970; **58**: 163–174

149. Lacey, E. R. Rapid epithelial restitution of the superficially damaged gastric mucosa. In: Rees, W. D. W., Ed. *Advances in Peptic Ulcer Pathogenesis.* Lancaster: MTP Press. 1988: 163–181

150. Gillen, P., Keeling, P., Byrne, P. J., West, A. B. and Hennessy, T. P. J. Experimental columnar metaplasia in the canine oesophagus. *Br. J. Surg* 1988; **75**: 113–115

151. Khani, B., Kennedy, C., Finucane, J. and Doyle, J. S. Transmucosal potential difference: diagnostic value in gastro-oesophageal reflux. *Gut* 1978; **19**: 396–398

152. Powell, D. W., Morris, S. M. and Boyd, D. D. Water and electrolyte transport by rabbit esophagus. *Am. J. Physiol.* 1975; **229**: 438–443

153. Chung, R. S. K., Magri, J. and DenBesten, L. Hydrogen in transport in the rabbit esophagus. *Am. J. Physiol.* 1975; **229**: 496–499

154. Harman, J. W., Johnson, L. F. and Magdonovitch, C. L. Effects of acid and bile salts on rabbit esophageal mucosa. *Dig. Dis. Sci.* 1981; **26**: 65–72

155. Orlando, R. C., Powell, D. W. and Carney, C. N. Pathophysiology of acute acid injury in the rabbit esophageal epithelium. *J. Clin. Invest.* 1981; **68**: 286–293

156. Powell, D. W. Physiological concepts of epithelial barriers. In: Allen, A., Garner, A., Flemstrom, G., Silen, W. and Turnberg, L. A., Eds. *Mechanisms of Mucosal Protection in the Upper Gastrointestinal Tract.* New York: Raven Press. 1984: 1–5

157. Bass, B. L., Schweitzer, E. J. and Harman, J. W. H^+ back diffusion interferes with intrinsic reactive regulation of esophageal mucosal blood flow. *Surgery* 1984; **96**: 404–413

158. Northway, M. G., Libshitz, H. I. and Osborne, B. M. Radiation esophagitis in the opossum: radioprotection with indomethacin. *Gastroenterology* 1980; **78**: 883–892

159. Eastwood, G. L., Beck, D. D., Castell, D. O., Brown, F. L. and Fletcher, J. R. Beneficial effect of indomethacin on acid-induced esophagitis in cats. *Dig. Dis. Sci* 1981; **26**: 601–608

160. Boyd, D. D., Carney, C. N. and Powell, D. W. Neurohumeral control of esophageal epithelial electrolyte transport. *Am. J. Physiol.* 1980; **239**: G5–G11

161. Hopwood, D., Coghill, G. and Sanders, D. S. A. Human oesophageal submucosal glands. Their detection, mucin, enzyme and secretory protein content. *Histochemistry* 1986; **86**: 107–112

162. Hetzel, D. J., Dent, D. J., Reed, W. D. *et al.* Healing and relapse of severe peptic esophagitis after treatment with omepazole. *Gastroenterology* 1988; **95**: 903–912

163. Goldberg, H. I., Dodds, W. J., Gee, S., Montgomery, C. and Zboralske, F. F. Role of acid and pepsin in acute experimental esophagitis. *Gastroenterology* 1969; **56**: 223–230

164. Eastwood, G. L., Castell, D. O. and Higgs, R. H. Experimental esophagitis in cats impairs lower esophageal sphincter pressure. *Gastroenterology* 1975; **69**: 146–153

165. Higgs, R. H., Castell, D. O. and Eastwood, G. L. Studies on the mechanisms of esophagitis-induced lower esophageal sphincter hypotension in cats. *Gastroenterology* 1976; **71**: 51–57

166. Biancani, P., Barwick, K., Selling, J. and McCallum, R. W. Effects of acute experimental esophagitis on mechanical properties of the lower esophageal sphincter. *Gastroenterology* 1984; **87**: 8–16

167. Williams, C. B., Lawrie, J. H. and Forrest, A. P. M. Acid secretion in symptomatic sliding hiatus hernia. *Lancet* 1967; **i**: 184–185

168. Crumplin, M. K. H., Stol, D. W., Murphy, G. M. and Collis, J. L. The pattern of bile salt reflux and acid secretion in sliding hiatus hernia. *Br. J. Surg.* 1974; **61**: 611–616

169. Baldi, F., Corinaldesi, R., Ferrarini, F., Stanghellini, V., Miglioli, M. and Barbara, L. Gastric secretion and emptying of liquids in reflux esophagitis. *Dig. Dis. Sci* 1981; **26**: 886–889

170. Spencer, J. Prolonged pH recording in the study of gastro-oesophageal reflux. *Br. J. Surg.* 1969; **56**: 912–914

171. Boesby, S. Relationship between gastro-oesophageal acid reflux, basal gastro-oesophageal sphincter pressure and gastric acid secretion. *Scand. J. Gastroenterol.* 1977; **12**: 547–551

172. Flook, D. and Stoddard, C. J. Gastro-oesophageal reflux and oesophagitis before and after vagotomy for duodenal ulcer. *Br. J. Surg.* 1985; **72**: 804–807

173. Gotley, D. C., Ball, D. and Copper, M. J. Peptic activity in the refluxate of patients with uncomplicated gastro-oesophageal reflux (GOR) (Abstract). *Gut* 1988; **29**: A1451

174. Isenberg, J., Csendes, A. and Walsh, J. H. Resting and pentagastrin stimulated gastroesophageal sphincter pressure in patients with Zollinger–Ellison syndrome. *Gastroenterology* 1971; **61**: 655–658

175. Gotley, D. C., Flaks, B. and Cooper, M. J. Do bile acids (BA) modify the cytopathic effects of pepsin (P) on oesophageal mucosal cells? (Abstract). *Gut* 1988; **29**: A1451

176. Collins, B. J., Crothers, G., McFarland, R. J. and Love, A. H. G. Bile acid concentrations in the gastric juice of patients with erosive oesophagitis. *Gut* 1985; **26**: 495–499

177. Kaye, M. D. and Showalter, J. P. Pyloric incompetence in patients with symptomatic gastroesophageal reflux. *J. Lab. Clin. Med.* 1974; **83**: 198–206

178. Gillison, E. W., Cooper, W. M., Arith, G. R., Gibson, M. J. and Bradford, I. Hiatus hernia and heartburn. *Gut* 1969; **10**: 609–613

179. Donovan, I. A., Harding, L. K., Keighley, M. R. B., Griffin, D. W. and Collis, J. L. Abnormalities of gastric emptying and pyloric reflux in uncomplicated hiatus hernia. *Br. J. Surg.* 1977; **64**: 847–848

180. Krog, M., Gustavsson, S. and Jung, B. Studies on oesophagitis – no evidence for pyloric incompetence on a primary etiological factor. *Acta Chir. Scand.* 1982; **148**: 439–442

181. Matikainer, M., Taavitsainen, M. and Kalima, T. V. Duodenogastric reflux in patients with heartburn and oesophagitis. *Scand. J. Gastroenterol.* 1981; **16**: 253–255

182. Thompson, D. G. Duodenogastric reflux: is there any progress? *Br. Med. J.* 1982; **284**: 845–846

183. Lillemoe, K. D., Johnson, L. F. and Harman, J. W. Alkaline esophagitis: a comparison of the ability of gastroduodenal contents to injure the rabbit esophagus. *Gastroenterology* 1983; **85**: 621–628

184. Gillison, E. W., de Castro, V. A. M., Nyhus, L. M., Kusakasi, K. and Bombeck, C. T. The significance of bile on reflux esophagitis. *Surg. Gynecol. Obstet. 1972;* **134**: 419–424

185. Smith, M. R., Buckton, G. K. and Bennett, J. R. Bile acid levels in stomach and oesophagus of patients with acid gastro-oesophageal reflux (Abstract). *Gut* 1984; **25**: A556

186. Gotley, D. C., Morgan, A. P. and Cooper, M. J. Bile acid concentrations in the oesophageal refluxate of patients with uncomplicated and complicated gastro-oesophageal reflux (Abstract). *Gastroenterology* 1989; **94**: A151

187. Mittal, R. K., Reuben, A., Whitney, J. O. and McCallum, R. W. Do bile acids reflux into the

esophagus? A study in normal subjects and patients with gastroesophageal reflux disease. *Gastroenterology* 1987; **92**: 371–375

188. Little, A. G., Martinez, E. I., DeMeester, T. R., Blough, R. M. and Skinner, D. B. Duodenogastric reflux and reflux esophagitis. *Surgery* 1984; **96**: 447–454

189. Dubois, A. Clinical relevance of gastroduodenal dysfunction in reflux esophagitis. *J. Clin. Gastroenterol.* 1986; **8** (suppl. 1): 17–25

190. McCallum, R. W., Berkowitz, D. M. and Lerner, E. Gastric emptying in patients with gastroesophageal reflux. *Gastroenterology* 1981; **80**: 285–291

191. Maddern, G. J., Chatterton, B. E., Collins, P. J., Horowitz, M., Shearman, D. J. C. and Jamieson, G. G. Solid and liquid gastric emptying in patients with gastro-oesophageal reflux. *Br. J. Surg.* 1985; **72**: 344–347

192. Coleman, S. L., Rees, W. D. W. and Malagelada, J. R. Normal gastric function in reflux esophagitis (Abstract) *Gastroenterology* 1979; **76**: 1115

193. Shay, S. S., Eggli, D., McDonald, C. and Johnson, L. F. Gastric emptying of solid in patients with gastroesophageal reflux. *Gastroenterology* 1987; **92**: 459–465

194. Velasco, N., Hill, L., Gannar, R. M. and Pope, C. E. Gastric emptying and gastroesophageal reflux: effects of surgery and correlation with esophageal motor function. *Am. J. Surg.* 1982; **144**: 58–61

195. Behar, J. and Ramsby, G. Gastric emptying and antral motility in reflux esophagitis: effect of oral metoclopramide. *Gastroenterology* 1978; **74**: 253–256

196. Heading, R. C. Gastric emptying: a clinical perspective. *Clin. Sci.* 1982; **63**: 231–235

197. King, P. M., Pryde, A. and Heading, R. C. Transpyloric fluid movement and antiduodenal motility in patients with gastro-oesophageal reflux. *Gut* 1987; **28**: 545–548

198. Nebel, O. T., Fornes, M. F. and Castell, D. O. Symptomatic gastroesophageal reflux: incidence and precipitating factors. *Am. J. Dig. Dis.* 1976; **21**: 953–956

199. Palmer, E. D. The hiatus hernia – esophagitis – esophageal stricture complex. *Am. J. Med.* 1968; **44**: 566–579

200. Patterson, D. J., Graham, D. Y., Smith, J. L. *et al.* Natural history of benign esophageal stricture treated by dilatation. *Gastroenterology* 1983; **85**: 846–850

201. Sladen, G. E., Riddell, R. H. and Willoughby, J. M. T. Oesophagoscopy, biopsy and acid perfusion test in diagnosis of 'reflux oesophagitis'. *Br. Med. J.* 1975; **1**: 71–76

202. Hockman, P., Siegel, C. I. and Hendrix, T. R. Failure of oxethazaine to alter acid induced esophageal pain. *Am. J. Dig. Dis.* 1966; **11**: 811–813

203. Winnans, G. R., Meyer, C. T. and McCallum, R. W. Interpretation of the Bernstein test: a reappraisal of criteria. *Ann. Intern. Med.* 1982; **96**: 320–322

204. Schulze-Delrieu, K. Esophageal sensations. *Gastroenterology* 1984; **86**: 767–768

205. Christensen, J. Origin of sensation in the esophagus. *Am. J. Physiol.* 1984; **246**: G221–G225

206. Weinstein, W. M., Bogech, E. R. and Howes, K. L. The normal human esophageal mucosa: a histological reappraisal. *Gastroenterology* 1975; **68**: 40–44

207. Pope, C. E. Mucosal response to esophageal motor disorders. *Arch. Intern. Med.* 1976; **136**: 549–555

208. Witt, I. and Griffin, J. P. Afferent cutaneous C fibre activity to repeated thermal stimuli. *Nature* 1962; **194**: 776–777

209. Behar, J., Brand, L., Brown, F. C. *et al.* Cimetidine in the treatment of symptomatic gastroesophageal reflux: a double blind controlled trial. *Gastroenterology* 1978; **74**: 441–448

210. Chakraborty, T. K., Ogilvie, A. L., Heading, R. C. and Ewing, D. J. Abnormal cardiovascular refluxes in patients with gastro-oesophageal reflux. *Gut* 1989; **30**: 46–49

211. Ball, C. S. and Watson, A. Acid sensitivity in reflux oesophagitis with and without complications (Abstract). *Gut* 1988; **29**: A728

212. Schlesinger, P. K. Diminished esophageal acid sensitivity in patients with advanced esophagitis (Abstract). *Gastroenterology* 1987; **92**: 1622

213. Giles, G. R., Clark, C. G. and Buchan, R. Effect of oesophageal perfusion with acid on basal acid secretion. *Gut* 1968; **9**: 52–56

214. Ward, A. S. Oesophageal reflux and gastric secretion. *Gut* 1970; **11**: 738–742

215. Wilkins, W. E., Ridley, M. G. and Posniak, A. L. Benign stricture of the oesophagus: role of non-steroidal anti-inflammatory drugs. *Gut* 1984; **25**: 478–480

216. Flook, D. and Stoddard, C. J. Gastro-oesophageal reflux (GOR) in patients with oesophagitis or a columnar lined (Barrett's) oesophagus (Abstract). *Gut* 1983; **24**: A1007

217. Gillen, P., Keeling, P., Byrne, P. J. and Hennessy, T. P. J. Barrett's oesophagus: pH profile. *Br. J. Surg.* 1987; **74**: 774–776

218. Robertson, D., Aldersley, M., Shepherd, H. and Smith, C. L. Patterns of reflux in complicated oesophagitis. *Gut* 1987; **28**: 1484–1488

219. Brand, D. L., Ylvisakes, J. T., Gelfound, M. and Pope, C. E. Regression of columnar esophageal (Barrett's) epithelium after anti-reflux surgery. *N. Engl. J. Med.* 1980; **302**: 844–848

220. Monnier, P., Fontolliet, C., Savary, M. and Ollyo, J. B. Barrett's oesophagus or columnar epithelium of the lower oesophagus. *Clin. Gastroenterol.* 1987; **1**: 769–789

221. Bremner, C. G., Lynch, V. P. and Ellis, F. H. Barrett's esophagus: congenital or acquired: An experimental study of esophageal mucosal regeneration in the dog. *Surgery* 1970; **68**: 209–216

222. Gillen, P., Keeling, P., Byrne, P. J., Healy, M., O'Moore, R. R. and Hennessy, T. P. J. Implication of duodenogastric reflux in the pathogenesis of Barrett's oesophagus. *Br. J. Surg.* 1988; **75**: 540–543

223. Heller, S. R., Fellows, I. W., Ogilvie, A. and Atkinson, M. Non-steroidal anti-inflammatory drugs and benign oesophageal strictures. *Br. Med. J.* 1982; **285**: 167–168

224. Kikendell, J. W., Friedman, A. C., Oyewole, M. A., Fleischer, D. and Johnson, L. F. Pill induced esophageal injury: case reports and review of medical literature. *Dig. Dis. Sci.* 1983; **28**: 174–182

225. Carlborg, B., Kumlein, A. and Olsson, H. Medikamentella esofagusstrikturer. *Lökartidningen* 1978; **75**: 4609–4611

226. Maxton, D. G., Ainley, C. C., Grainger, S. L., Morris, R. W. and Thompson, R. P. H. Teeth and benign oesophageal stricture. *Gut* 1987; **28**: 61–63

227. Rokkas, T., Anggiansah, A., Uzdechina, E., Owen, W. J. and Sladen, G. E. The role of shorter than 24-h pH monitoring periods in the diagnosis of gastro-oesophageal reflux. *Scand. J. Gastroenterol.* 1986 **21**: 614–620

228. Kruse-Anderson, S., Wallin, L. and Madsen, T. Acid gastro-oesophageal reflux and oesophageal pressure activity during postprandial and noctural periods: a study in subjects with and without pathological gastro-oesophageal reflux. *Scand. J. Gastroenterol.* 1987; **22**: 926–930

229. Galmiche, J. P., Guillard, J. F., Denis, P., Boussaker, K., Lefrancois, R. and Colin, R. Etude du pH oesophagien en periode post-prandiale chez le sujet normal et au cours du syndrome de reflux gastro-oesphagien: interet diagnostique d'une score de reflux acide. *Gastroenterol. Clin. Biol.* 1980; **4**: 531–539

230. Branicki, F. J., Evans, D. F., Ogilvie, A. L., Atkinson, M. and Hardcastle, J. D. Ambulatory monitoring of oesophageal pH in reflux oesophagitis using a portable radiotelemetry system. *Gut* 1982; **23**: 992–998

231. Fink, S. M. and McCallum, R. W. The role of prolonged esophageal pH monitoring in the diagnosis of gastroesophageal reflux. *J. Am. Med. Assoc.* 1984; **252**: 1160–1164

232. Ottignon, Y., Ampelas, M., Voigt, J. J., Cassigneul, J. and Pascal, J. P. Comparaison de trois methodes d'enregistrement de pH oesophagien dans le diagnostic du reflux gastro-oesophagien acide. *Gastroenterol. Clin. Biol.* 1984; **8**: 609–615

233. Jouin, H., Chamonard, P., Baumann, R., Duclos, B., Meyer, C. and Constantinesco, A. Scintigraphie et pH-metrie oesophagienne chez des adultes ayant un reflux gastro-oesophagien. *Ann. Gastroenterol. Hepatol. (Paris)* 1987; **23**: 239–242

234. Robertson, D. A. F., Aldersley, M. A., Shepherd, H., Lloyd, R. S. and Smith, C. L. H_2 antagonists in the treatment of reflux oesophagitis: can physiological studies predict the response? *Gut* 1987; **28**: 946–949

235. Orr, W. C., Robinson, M. G., Humphries, T. J., Antonello, J. and Cagliola, A. Dose–response effect of famotidine on patterns of gastro-oesophageal reflux. *Aliment. Pharmacol. Therap.* 1988; **2**: 229–235

236. Klinkenberg-Knol, E. C., Festen, H. P. M. and Meuwissen, S. G. M. The effects of omeprazole and ranitidine on 24 hour pH in the distal oesophagus of patients with reflux oesophagitis. *Aliment. Pharmacol. Therap.* 1988; **2**: 221–227

237. Mei, N. La sensibilite viscerale. *J. Physiol. Paris* 1981; **77**: 597–612

Chapter 2

Clinical features of reflux

Thomas P. J. Hennessy

Introduction

The classic symptoms of gastro-oesophageal reflux are heartburn and regurgitation. Heartburn describes a searing or burning pain of variable intensity located behind the sternum and sometimes radiating upwards to the angle of the jaw and down the arm most often on the left (Figure 2.1). Common variants are location of the pain

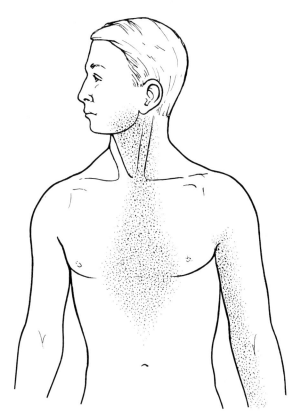

Figure 2.1 Distribution of pain in gastro-oesophageal reflux

principally in the subxyphoid or epigastric region or radiation of the pain into the back. On occasion paraesthesia may be experienced in the arm and hand rather than pain. The retrosternal pain may be accompanied by a feeling of tightness in the chest. The pain may be precipitated by taking food and both the quantity and quality of the food may be implicated. Large meals are particularly prone to initiate symptoms although paradoxically hunger may be the precipitating factor in some cases. Ingestion of alcohol, spicy food, raw fruit or carbonated drinks are frequently followed by typical symptoms of heartburn.

Symptoms are considerably influenced by posture. Stooping or bending commonly causes pain and this may have serious implications where a patient's occupation involves constant activity of this kind. Symptoms are often most severe when the patient lies down and the patient may be unable to sleep. Relief from pain by assuming an erect position or by sleeping propped up or with elevation of the head of the bed is common (Figure 2.2).

Discomfort often described as a raw feeling or pain is sometimes felt mainly in the throat in the region of the pharynx and upper oesophagus. Although generally not severe it may be exacerbated by swallowing food and hot or cold liquids. Odynophagia or painful swallowing is usually a very temporary phenomenon and associated with an acute exacerbation of oesophagitis initiated by excessive intake of alcohol or spicy food.

Regurgitation is a severe problem for many patients. Regurgitation of stomach or oesophageal content should be distinguished from vomiting. The latter is accompanied by nausea and is a forceful ejection of gastric contents. Regurgitation from the oesophagus occurs when oesophageal stricture or spasm is present. It occurs promptly after taking food and does not have a sour or bitter taste. Regurgitation from the stomach may be associated with belching and consists of the effortless return of gastric contents producing a sour or bitter taste.

Nocturnal regurgitation may have serious consequences because of aspiration into the respiratory tract. Bronchitis, asthma, bronchiectasis and pneumonia are likely consequences of aspiration and Paulson [1] reported that 60% of his patients with gastro-oesophageal reflux suffered from these respiratory problems. Iverson et al. [2] recorded a 40% incidence of pulmonary complications. Surgical correction of the reflux brought about cure or improvement in the vast majority of patients with respiratory symptoms according to Lomasney [3]. However, Pellegrini [4] has questioned the frequency of pulmonary problems attributable to reflux. Of 48 patients suspected of aspiration only 8 could be confirmed and 5 were found to have a primary respiratory disorder.

Dysphagia may be experienced without the presence of a stricture. It is usually intermittent and associated with severe oesophagitis and subsides with successful treatment. When a stricture develops dysphagia is more constant and progressive. Gastro-oesophageal reflux has been implicated as a causal factor in patients with cricopharyngeal spasm and dysphagia located in the cervical region. Abnormally high upper sphincter pressures in patients with reflux oesophagitis were reported by Hunt et al. [5]. Belsey [6] noted an improvement in dysphagia after anti-reflux surgery. However, Stanciu and Bennett [7] were unable to detect any changes in upper sphincter pressure in association with gastro-oesophageal reflux.

Significant bleeding may occur when erosive oesophagitis is present. Bleeding may occur in the absence of other symptoms and a profound anaemia may develop with muscular weakness and dyspnoea. Although not a common occurrence, patients may sometimes present with either haematemesis or melaena. Massive haemorrhage is

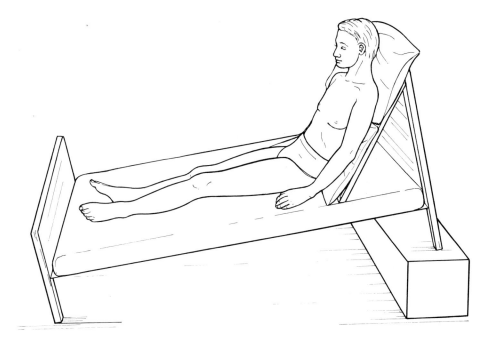

(a)

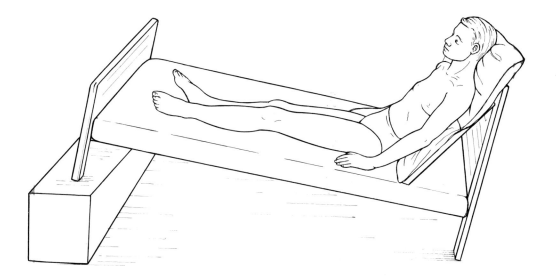

(b)

Figure 2.2 Alternative methods of minimizing nocturnal reflux: (a) with head of bed raised patient tends to slide towards the foot of the bed; (b) with foot of bed raised patient's position is maintained against back-rest

rare and is most likely to be due to a penetrating Barrett's ulcer. Anti-reflux surgery is usually successful in controlling bleeding and resection for bleeding is seldom necessary except in Barrett's ulcer.

Air swallowing and belching are not uncommon symptoms of reflux and may occur with or without heartburn. While not clinically significant these symptoms are a source of considerable embarrassment to patients. The habit of air swallowing may be very difficult to eradicate and may cause considerable discomfort to the patient if it persists after fundoplication when it may exacerbate and prolong 'gas-bloat' symptoms.

Differential diagnosis

Classic symptoms of reflux cannot with certainty be attributed to the presence of acid in the oesophagus. Similar symptoms may be present in patients with cholelithiasis and peptic ulcer, and the coexistence of either or both conditions with sliding hiatus hernia and reflux oesophagitis may make it difficult or impossible to attribute symptoms accurately to the underlying pathology.

Symptoms indistinguishable from acid-peptic reflux oesophagitis may be present after total gastrectomy [8]. O'Sullivan *et al.* [9] studied a group of symptomatic patients who had undergone surgery for peptic ulcer. Acid reflux was present in the majority but pH monitoring showed a mixed acid–alkaline pattern in nine and pure alkaline reflux in four. Goldstein *et al.* [10] found bile reflux in 36 patients without previous gastric surgery 23 of whom had had cholecystectomy. The experiments of Jones [11] have demonstrated that balloon distension of the oesophagus can reproduce the symptoms of heartburn. Distention of the upper oesophagus was accompanied by sensations of choking and fullness but distension of the balloon in the cardia gave rise to a sensation of burning.

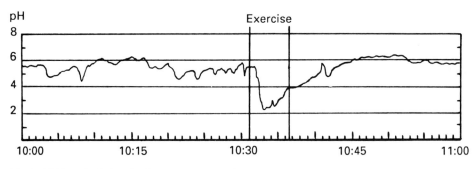

Figure 2.3 Exercise-induced reflux

Symptoms of retrosternal pain exacerbated by large meals and by exercise, while typical of gastro-oesophageal reflux, are also highly suggestive of angina pectoris, particularly when accompanied by radiation into the neck and arms and it can be difficult to differentiate between them (Figure 2.3). If regurgitation is a prominent symptom an oesophageal cause for the symptoms is more likely. Nausea and vomiting may suggest a coexisting peptic ulcer or cholelithiasis. However classic the symptoms, clinical diagnosis is entirely speculative and must be confirmed by objective assessment of oesophageal function.

Provocative tests

In addition to his balloon experiments Jones [11] studied the effect of infusing various liquids into the lower oesophagus by means of a nasogastric tube placed above the cardia. Warm water, cold water, 0.1M NaOH, 0.1 M HCl and gastric juice were infused at different times and at different rates. Heartburn was the symptom most frequently induced and was more likely with rapid rates of infusion and with repetition.

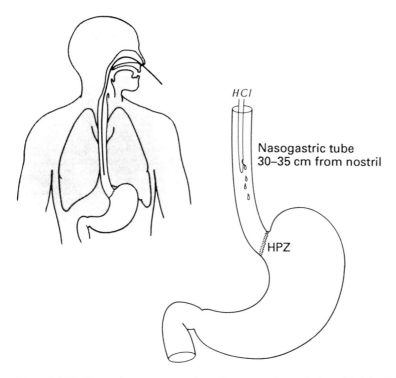

HCl

Nasogastric tube
30–35 cm from nostril

HPZ

Figure 2.4 The Bernstein test: provocation of symptoms by perfusion with 0.1 M HCl

Bernstein and Baker [12] introduced the acid infusion test which was designed to reproduce typical symptoms of heartburn in the presence of oesophagitis. The test is carried out with the patient upright and a nasogastric tube positioned 30/35 cm from the nostrils (Figure 2.4). Infusion with physiological saline is begun initially at a rate of 100 drops/min. The infusate is then changed without the patient's knowledge to 0.1 M HCl and continued for 30 minutes or until typical symptoms appear. If no symptoms appear the test is negative. If symptoms appear perfusion with physiological saline is resumed until they disappear. Although the test produces a 15% false negative result in patients with oesophagitis and a 15% false positive result in normal patients, it remains of value in the investigation of patients with chest pain of uncertain origin. However, it has to some extent been superseded by the availability of 24-hour ambulatory pH monitoring in which reflux events can be correlated with pH changes and with which the frequency and duration of reflux episodes and the ability of the lower oesophagus to clear acid can be evaluated.

Mechanisms of pain

Sensation from the oesophagus is conveyed centrally by afferent fibres in the sympathetic and parasympathetic nerves. Although pain receptors have not been specifically identified in the oesophagus, cold, heat and distension may all give rise to pain [11]. The pain produced by acid or bile reflux has been attributed to chemo-receptors. Pressure receptors may account for the pain produced by balloon distension or muscle spasm. The mucosal inflammation with superficial ulceration caused by severe reflux is commonly associated with pain and it is assumed that exposed nerve endings are stimulated. However, similar symptoms may occur with an intact mucosa. Ismail-Beigi *et al.* [13] have described the changes in oesophageal epithelium induced by reflux. The basal layer, normally less than 15% of the total thickness, becomes thicker and the papillae increase their vascularity and extend more than two-thirds of the distance to the surface. These changes are attributed to increased loss of surface cells due to the reflux and an increased cell turnover in the basal layer. It is suggested that the closer proximity of the papillae to the surface makes stimulation of nerve fibres by luminal contents more likely. In spite of this topical anaesthesia does not abolish pain [14]. Pain perception is also influenced by the type of mucosa present. Patients with Barrett's oesophagus are sometimes entirely symptom free in the presence of significant reflux. The metaplastic columnar epithelium appears to be relatively insensitive [15]. Oesophageal pain may also be influenced by the pH level in the lower oesophagus [16]. Patients who experience pain similar to their reflux symptoms at pH 1–1.5 may be free of symptoms when the oesophagus is perfused with a solution of pH 2.5 or higher. The poor correlation between gastro-oesophageal reflux and symptoms, and motor disorders and symptoms, illustrates the complexity of the mechanism of pain perception in the oesophagus.

Relationship of symptoms to reflux events

An event marker can record the onset and duration of symptoms during the course of a 24-hour pH analysis. Correlation is regarded as positive when a pH of 4 or less coincides with symptoms or when the fall in pH and the symptoms occur wthin 10 minutes of each other (Figure 2.5). The long lag period may be related to the length of time taken for the acid to penetrate surface mucus. Lack of correlation may be due to insensitivity of the oesophageal mucosa in asymptomatic patients or neutral or alkaline reflux in symptomatic patients whose pH level remains static.

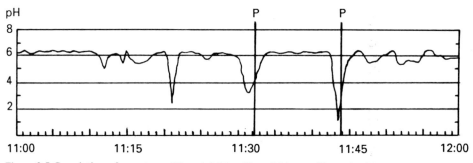

Figure 2.5 Correlation of symptoms (P) and fall in pH on 24-hour pH monitoring

Dysmotility and pain

The observation that symptomatic gastro-oesophageal reflux is frequently accompanied by motility disturbances has led to the hypothesis that the motility disorder is responsible for the pain. Manometry during acid infusion demonstrated simultaneous non-peristaltic contractions in the oesophagus [17]. In another study [18] patients with a positive Bernstein test exhibited increased peristaltic activity, tertiary contractions and increased resting tone in the oesophagus. The studies of Atkinson and Bennett [19] demonstrated two effects arising from the presence of acid in the oesophagus. Pain was produced and non-propulsive motor activity was initiated. They could occur together or separately. When both were present pain could be relieved by infusion of sodium bicarbonate without affecting motility. Conversely, the abnormal motility could be abolished without relief of pain.

Non-cardiac chest pain

Patients with retrosternal pain with or without radiation into the neck and arm are suspected of having ischaemic heart disease and are automatically referred for cardiac investigation. The presence or absence of cardiac disease can usually be determined by electrocardiogram, exercise stress testing, echocardiogram and coronary angiography. If these tests are normal the possibility of microvascular angina, also known as syndrome X, should be considered. According to Cannon et al. [20] this condition occurs in patients with typical angina symptoms and normal coronary epicardial arteries. During atrial pacing with ergonovine testing these patients develop typical chest pain and demonstrate diminished coronary vasodilator reserve, with higher coronary resistance, less lactate consumption and a higher left ventricular end-diastolic pressure. Prinzmetal's variant angina occurs in the absence of coronary artery stenosis and is due to localized or diffuse vasospasm [21]. The chest pain occurs at rest usually at night and is not provoked by day-time exertion. Coronary artery spasm can be induced by administration of ergonovine.

Exclusion of a cardiac cause of the chest pain transfers attention to the oesophagus. The oesophageal abnormalities most frequently associated with angina-like chest pain are motor abnormalities such as achalasia, diffuse spasm and nutcracker oesophagus, and gastro-oesophageal reflux.

In a study involving 200 patients Bennett and Atkinson [22] examined the incidence of different causes of chest pain in patients admitted to hospital and assessed the diagnostic value of various clinical features associated with chest pain. They found that 23% of patients had alimentary tract disease only and most of these were patients with oesophagitis. They also found that while the pain was more likely to be described as gripping, tight or vice-like in patients with ischaemic heart disease and more commonly referred to as burning in patients with reflux, the character of the pain is not a reliable diagnostic factor. Similarly, radiation to the arms, neck or jaw, although more frequently noted in cardiac patients, also occurred in patients with oesophageal disease. Back pain occurred with comparable frequency in both groups of patients. Abdominal pain was more common in oesophagitis but was also found in patients with ischaemic heart disease. Precipitation of the pain occurred more frequently with exercise in cardiac patients and with postural change in oesophagitis. Dyspnoea was much more common in ischaemic heart disease and regurgitation more usually associated with gastro-oesophageal reflux. However,

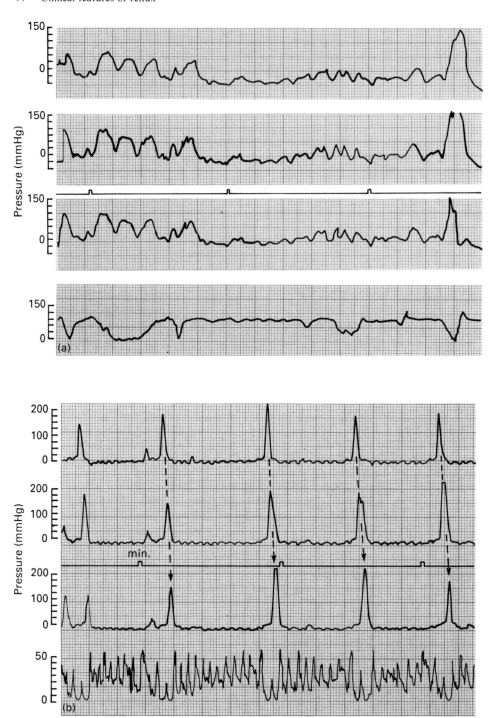

Figure 2.6 (a) Diffuse oesophageal spasm; (b) symptomatic oesophageal peristalsis or 'nutcracker oesophagus'. Both motility disorders may be induced by gastro-oesophageal reflux

chest pain may be the only symptom in gastro-oesophageal disease. According to de Caestecker *et al.* [23] 30% of patients with non-cardiac chest pain suffer from reflux. The Bernstein test may be useful in establishing the diagnosis. Monitoring oesophageal pH over 24 hours may also be of value. The mere presence of an abnormal pH profile is not sufficient to establish the diagnosis. However, good correlation between symptoms and reflux episodes provides strong supportive evidence. If endoscopy reveals oesophagitis the diagnosis is certain.

Motor disorders of the oesophagus are also associated with angina-like chest pain [24–28]. The nutcracker oesophagus, also known as symptomatic oesophageal peristalsis, is characterized by high amplitude (>150 mmHg) peristaltic waves of prolonged duration. The waves may be single or multi-peaked. In diffuse oesophageal spasm simultaneous non-peristaltic contractions occur. These contractions are also of prolonged duration and may be of high, low or normal amplitude.

It has been suggested that these motor abnormalities induce chest pain by restricting oesophageal blood flow and causing local ischaemia in oesophageal muscle [29]. However, these abnormal motility patterns are frequently present without symptoms. Furthermore, although typical symptoms may be precipitated by exercise, our long-term manometric studies have shown that the amplitude of the waves in the nutcracker oesophagus is reduced to normal during exercise [30].

While it is accepted that both the nutcracker oesophagus and diffuse oesophageal spasm exist as primary motility disorders they may also occur in conjunction with gastro-oesophageal reflux and may occur in response to abnormal pH levels in the lower oesophagus (Figure 2.6).

The prevalence of cardiac and oesophageal disease increases with age. Oesophageal disease was found in 50% of patients with coronary artery disease in a study by Svensson *et al.* [31]. In two studies on patients with microvascular angina the prevalence of oesophageal motility disorders was 58% and 75% respectively [32,33]. In patients with coexisting cardiac and oesophageal disease the Bernstein test can induce symptoms indistinguishable from angina and cause typical ischaemic changes in the electrocardiogram [34] (Figure 2.7). Similar symptoms and electrocardiographic changes can be stimulated by oesophageal balloon distension [35].

Using simultaneous pH assessment and manometry Vantrappen *et al.* [36] studied 33 patients with angina-like chest pain of oesophageal origin. In 12 patients the

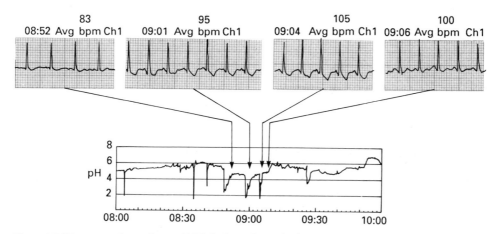

Figure 2.7 ST segment depression on ECG during reflux episode

episodes of pain were accompanied by motor disorders alone. Eleven patients had gastro-oesophageal reflux alone with the pain. In the remaining 10 patients the pain was accompanied by both motor disorders and reflux. In three patients the reflux and dysmotility always occurred simultaneously. In the remaining seven some pain episodes were accompanied by reflux, some by dysmotility and some by both. They also found that acid perfusion of the oesophagus could produce the typical angina-like pain in patients who had a motor disorder alone at the time of the spontaneous pain. They further showed that edrophonium could produce motor disorders and angina-like chest pain in patients who had gastro-oesophageal reflux alone at the time of the spontaneous pain. They suggest that these patients have what is described as 'the irritable oesophagus'. Whilst patients with motor disorders alone may be helped by nitrites and calcium channel blockers, patients with gastro-oesophageal reflux alone may be helped by anti-reflux treatment. Patients suffering from irritable oesophagus may need an entirely different approach such as psychotropic drugs to lower the threshold of visceral pain. In considering treatment it should be borne in mind that these patients sometimes have a tendency to improve with time. Reassurance that the condition is not life threatening may be of great help. It is known that motility disorders such as diffuse oesophageal spasm may be exacerbated by stress [37,38] and an appropriate adjustment in lifestyle may relieve the symptoms. An association between the irritable bowel syndrome and oesophageal motility disorders has also been recognized [39,40]. The basic disorder appears to be a lowered pain threshold and a high proportion of patients have symptoms referable to the lower gastrointestinal tract in addition to their oesophageal symptoms. While calcium channel blockers may have a significant effect on abnormal oesophageal pressures, they may be no more effective than a placebo in relieving pain [41]. If stress is a major provocative factor anxiolytic drugs may give relief [42]. Bougie dilatation may also give relief and small calibre bougies may be as effective as the larger sizes [43]. Despite anecdotal reports of successful surgical treatment, it is believed that myotomy is contraindicated in nutcracker oesophagus and is not always indicated in diffuse spasm.

Recent technological developments in manometric techniques have allowed more precise definition of normal motor activity in the oesophagus. At the same time a group of non-specific motility disorders has been identified some of which are associated with angina-like chest pain. In order to define more clearly motor disturbances which may be of clinical significance Cohen [44] has proposed the following criteria:

1. There must be a major alteration in oesophageal physiology.
2. The abnormality must be temporally associated with oesophageal symptoms.
3. The abnormality must be demonstrable with alternative techniques.
4. Symptoms must be improved when the abnormality is corrected.

Association of oesophageal symptoms and gallbladder disease

Patients suffering from gallstones and chronic cholecystitis often complain of postprandial epigastric discomfort and fullness, heartburn, belching and regurgitation of bitter fluid in the mouth [45]. These oesophageal symptoms have been attributed to duodenal ileus caused by the adjacent inflamed gallbladder with consequent pyloric incompetence and reflux of bile into the stomach and oesophagus

[46]. Such pyloric incompetence and reflux has been demonstrated radiologically by Johnson [47]. The incidence of oesophageal symptoms in gallbladder disease has been estimated at betweeen 47% and 50% [48,49]. In the study carried out by Barker and Alexander-Williams [50] 34% of patients undergoing cholecystectomy for established gallbladder disease had oesophageal symptoms. In patients who had radiological evidence of gastro-oesophageal reflux and/or an enlarged hiatus at operation, the incidence of oesophageal symptoms was 60%. In patients without such objective evidence of reflux 44% were relieved of their oesophageal symptoms by cholecystectomy. More than 80% of patients with an enlarged hiatus or positive barium studies continued to have reflux symptoms after cholecystectomy. More women than men were cured of the oesophageal symptoms by cholecystectomy. The peak incidence of persistent postoperative symptoms was in the 40–59 year age group. The majority of patients with persistent symptoms appear to have concomitant reflux disease while in patients whose symptoms are abolished by cholecystectomy the reflux symptoms are a consequence of cholecystitis.

Oesophageal symptoms and peptic ulcer

Symptoms of duodenal ulcer closely resemble those of gastro-oesophageal reflux particularly when the pain is located mainly in the epigastrium and radiates to the back. Differentiation on clinical grounds may be impossible unless the pain is classically retrosternal and accompanied by regurgitation. The problem may be further exacerbated by the concomitant presence of a duodenal ulcer and gastro-oesophageal reflux. Flook and Stoddard [51] were able to demonstrate abnormal reflux on pH monitoring in 42% of patients with duodenal ulcer. Oesophagitis identified at endoscopy or confirmed microscopically was present in 30%. Lower oesophageal pressures were normal. Earlam et al. [52] found microscopic evidence of oesophagitis in 25 of 36 patients with duodenal ulcer. Wallin [53,54] demonstrated that patients with duodenal ulcer have a higher incidence of gastro-oesophageal reflux. Resting pressure in the lower oesophageal sphincter was reduced and there was poor clearance of acid from the oesophagus. Siewert et al. [55] found that 40% of their patients with duodenal ulcer also suffered from reflux but could not demonstrate disordered sphincter function.

A possible triggering mechanism for the production of gastro-oesophageal reflux in duodenal ulcer patients was proposed by Kruse-Anderson et al. [56]. They found that more than half the ulcer patients in this study had pathological reflux on pH monitoring. When oesophageal pH and pressure studies were monitored simultaneously a significant increase in abnormal contractions (simultaneous reversed and upper segmental contractions) was apparent prior to a reflux episode in ulcer patients with pathological reflux. It may be, therefore, that gastro-oesophageal reflux in duodenal ulcer patients is a secondary phenomenon unrelated to intrinsic lower sphincter dysfunction.

Bile reflux

The injurious effects of bile on the oesophageal mucosa have been demonstrated experimentally [57,58]. The capacity for bile conjugates to induce pain in patients with reflux disease has also been noted [59]. A combination of bile and acid was found to be an even more potent cause of pain. Henderson *et al.* [60] described two effects from the introduction of bile salts and hydrochloric acid into the canine oesophagus. Grade III oesophagitis was produced and a severe motility disorder developed with reduction in lower sphincter pressure and decreased clearance ability in the body of the oesophagus. Kivilaakso *et al.* [61] concluded that in an acid environment pepsin and conjugated bile salts produce the greatest oesophageal damage. When acid is absent trypsin and deconjugated bile salts are the main injurious agents. The occurrence of oesophagitis after total gastrectomy is well recognized [62,63]. Symptoms of reflux and oesophagitis are also found after partial gastrectomy and vagotomy with drainage [9,64].

Reflux of duodenal contents may occur in the intact stomach also. Patients with heartburn or hiatus hernia may have pyloric dysmotility which promotes duodeno-gastric reflux thus providing an opportunity for reflux of duodenal constituents into the oesophagus [65,66].

Crumplin *et al.* [67] found abnormal bile salt concentrations in the stomachs of patients with oesophagitis. They estimated that approximately half the patients with reflux disease had abnormal pyloric function. Gillen *et al.* [68] noted the presence of excess bile acids in the stomachs of patients with Barrett's oesophagus. Patients with duodenal ulcer may also have pyloric dysfunction and in one study duodenogastric reflux was detected in 40% of patients [69].

Pulmonary complications

Pulmonary complications may occur with gastro-oesophageal reflux [70]. These may range from hoarseness and cough to bronchitis, pneumonia and lung abscess. The high incidence of pulmonary complications in patients with reflux-induced strictures is understandable due to the likelihood of aspiration but the incidence of respiratory problems is surprisingly high in uncomplicated reflux and was found to be 40% by Iverson *et al.* [2]. The association between gastro-oesophageal reflux and asthma is well established. The theory that microaspiration of gastric acid into the trachea is the cause of the bronchoconstriction has been elegantly supported by studies in cats [71]. General acceptance of the microaspiration theory is inhibited by conflicting reports from isotope studies. Two groups reviewing between them nearly 4000 scans noted lung activity due to aspiration in less than 2% [72,73]. In contrast, Sandberg *et al.* [74] who instilled isotope into the stomach at night-time and scanned the lungs the next morning demonstrated pulmonary aspiration in 5 of 19 patients with gastro-oesophageal reflux and respiratory symptoms. The interesting observation of posterior laryngitis in patients with gastro-oesophageal reflux offers indirect support to the microaspiration theory [75].

Reflex bronchoconstriction via vagal afferents has also been suggested as a mechanism by which intraoesophageal acid can affect respiratory function. Mansfield and Stein [76] found that oesophageal acid infusion in patients with gastro-oesophageal reflux and asthma produced respiratory symptoms and a significant increase in total respiratory resistance, changes which were rapidly reversed by antacid. A similar response in dogs could be abolished by bilateral vagotomy [77]. Acid infusion into the oesophagus has no effect in asthmatic patients without oesophagitis [78] but increases airway resistance in patients with a positive Bernstein test [79]. Pierry *et al.* [80] found the bronchoconstriction response to acid infusion more marked in patients with asthma and reflux symptoms than in patients with reflux symptoms only.

Wilson *et al.* [81] studied 20 asthmatic children with night-time acid reflux. In eight of the children there was a significant decrease in the concentration of histamine required to produce a 20% fall from baseline in peak expiratory flow rate.

It has also been suggested that respiratory disease could cause gastro-oesophageal reflux. This suggestion is based on the assumption that increased transdiaphragmatic pressure during airflow obstruction could force gastric contents into the oesophagus [82], particularly in patients taking theophyllines which have been shown to decrease lower oesophageal sphincter tone [83]. Allan *et al.* [84] found that maximal inspiratory efforts in normal subjects while inducing a pressure difference of up to $300\,cmH_2O$ between stomach and oesophagus did not provoke gastro-oesophageal reflux. Tibbling and Ekstrom [85] failed to produce gastro-oesophageal reflux in asthmatic patients on theophylline by histamine-induced bronchoconstriction. Thus it seems that airflow obstruction as such is unlikely to produce gastro-oesophageal reflux in the absence of an oesophageal abnormality.

Improvement in associated respiratory symptoms has been noted after both surgical and medical treatment of reflux. Larrain *et al.* [86] noted the ability of cimetidine and anti-reflux surgery to improve respiratory symptoms in patients with asthma and gastro-oesophageal reflux. Both were superior to placebo and anti-reflux surgery appeared more effective than cimetidine. The beneficial effects of surgery have also been noted by other workers in uncontrolled trials [4,87]. Goodall *et al.* [88] in a double-blind placebo-controlled trial in 20 asthmatic patients demonstrated symptomatic and objective improvement after 6 weeks' treatment with cimetidine.

Summary

The majority of patients with gastro-oesophageal reflux present with the classic symptoms of heartburn and regurgitation. Atypical symptoms may give rise to difficulties. It has been noted that in 10% of patients with reflux chest pain is the only symptom. Complete cardiac and oesophageal investigation is necessary to separate cardiac from non-cardiac chest pain and to establish whether the latter is related primarily to dysmotility or reflux. Other upper gastrointestinal disorders such as gallbladder disease and gallstones or peptic ulcer may mimic the symptoms of reflux and to complicate matters still further, may coexist with reflux. The severity of symptoms is not necessarily reflected in the degree of oesophagitis present. Severe symptoms may be present with little evidence of oesophagitis and profound changes such as Barrett's metaplasia may be present with virtually no symptoms. A number of symptom scoring systems exist which may help in the evaluation of symptoms but no evaluation can be considered complete without the objective analysis provided by pH monitoring, manometry, endoscopy and biopsy.

References

1. Paulson, D. L. Gastroesophageal reflux. *Am. J. Surg.* 1973; **39**: 67–71
2. Iverson, L. I. G., May, I. A. and Samson, P. C. Pulmonary complications in benign esophageal disease. *Am. J. Surg.* 1973; **126**: 223–228
3. Lomasney, T. L. Hiatus hernia and the respiratory tract. *Am. Thorac. Surg.* 1977; **24**: 448–450
4. Pellegrini, C. A., DeMeester, T. R., Johnson, L. F. and Skinner, D. B. Gastroesophageal reflux and pulmonary aspiration: incidence, functional abnormality and results of surgical therapy. *Surgery* 1979; **86**: 110–119
5. Hunt, P. S., Connell, A. M. and Smiley, T. B. The cricopharyngeal sphincter in gastric reflux. *Gut* 1970; **11**: 303–306

6. Belsey, R. H. Functional disease of the oesophagus. *J. Thorac. Cardiovasc. Surg.* 1966; **52**: 164–188

7. Stanciu, C. and Bennett, J. R. Upper esophageal sphincter yield pressure in normal subjects and in patients with esophageal reflux. *Thorax* 1974; **29**: 459–462

8. Scott, H. W. Jr and Longmire, W. P. Jr. Total gastrectomy report of 63 cases. *Surgery* 1949; **26**: 488–498

9. O'Sullivan, G. C., DeMeester, T. R., Smith, R. B. *et al.* Twenty four hour pH monitoring of esophageal function: Its use in evaluation in symptomatic patients after truncal vagotomy and gastric resection or drainage. *Arch. Surg.* 1981; **116**: 581–590

10. Goldstein, F., Thornton, J. J. III, Abrahamson, J. *et al.* Bile reflux gastritis and esophagitis in patients without prior gastric surgery. *Am. J. Gastroenterol.* 1981; **76**: 407–411

11. Jones, C. M. and Chapman W. P. Studies on the mechanisms of pain of angina pectoris with particular relation to hiatus hernia. *Trans. Assoc. Am. Phys.* 1942; **57**: 139–151

12. Bernstein, L. M. and Baker, L. A. A clinical test for esophagitis. *Gastroenterology* 1958; **34**: 760–781

13. Ismail-Beigi, F., Horton, P. F. and Pope, C. E. Histological consequences of gastroesophageal reflux in man. *Gastroenterology* 1970; **58**: 163–174

14. Hookman, P., Siegel, C. I. and Hendrix, T. R. Failure of oxethuzine to alter acid induced esophageal pain. *Am. J. Dig. Dis.* 1966; **11**: 811–813

15. Johnson, D. A., Winters, C., Spurling, T. J., Chobanian, S. J. and Cattar, E. L. Jr. Esophageal acid sensitivity in Barrett's esophagus. *J. Clin. Gastroenterol.* 1987; **9**: 23–27

16. Graham, D. Y., Larkai, E., Opekum, A. R. and Smith J. L. Sensitivity of the esophagus to pH in gastroesophageal reflux. *Gastroenterology* 1987; **92**: 1412A

17. Lazar, H. P., Puletti, E. J., Douglas, W. W., Danovitch, S. and Texter, E. C. Non-peristaltic esophageal motility accompanying experimentally induced heartburn. *J. Lab. Clin. Med.* 1959; **59**: 917–918.

18. Siegal, C. I. and Hendrix, T. R. Esophageal motor abnormalities induced by acid perfusion in patients with heartburn. *J. Clin. Invest.* 1963; **42**: 686–695

19. Atkinson, M. and Bennett, J. R. Relationship between motor changes and pain during esophageal acid perfusion. *Am. J. Dig. Dis.* 1968; **13**: 346–350

20. Cannon, R. O. III, Bonor, R. O., Bacharach, S. L. *et al.* Left ventricular dysfunction in patients with angina pectoris, normal epicardial coronary arteries and abnormal vasodilator reserve. *Circulation* 1985; **71**: 218–226

21. Maseri, A., Severi, S., de Nes, M. D. *et al.* 'Variant' angina: one aspect of a continuous spectrum of vasospastic myocardial ischemia. Pathogenic mechanisms, estimated incidence and clinical and coronary arteriographic findings in 138 patients. *Am. J. Cardiol.* 1978; **42**: 1019–1035

22. Bennett, J. R. and Atkinson, M. The differentiation between oesophageal and cardiac pain. *Lancet* 1966; **ii**: 1123–1127

23. de Caestecker, J. S., Blackwell, J. N., Brown, J. and Heading, R. C. The oesophagus as a cause of recurrent chest pain. *Lancet* 1985; **ii**: 1143–1146

24. Richter, J. E. and Castell, D. O. Diffuse esophageal spasm: a reappraisal. *Ann. Intern. Med.* 1984; **100**: 242–245

25. Branch, D. L., Martin, D. and Pope, C. E. Esophageal manometrics in patients with angina-like chest pain. *Am. J. Dig. Dis.* 1977; **22**: 300–305

26. Benjamin, S. B., Gerhardt, D. C. and Castell, D. O. High amplitude peristaltic esophageal contractions associated with chest pain and/or dysphagia. *Gastroenterology* 1979; **77**: 478–483

27. Herrington, J. P., Burns, T. W. and Balcart, L. A. Chest pain and dysphagia in patients with prolonged peristaltic contractile duration of the esophagus. *Dig. Dis. Sci.* 1984; **29**: 134–140

28. Traube, M., Albibi, R. and McCallum, R. W. High amplitude peristaltic oesophageal contractions associated with chest pain *J. Am. Med. Assoc.* 1983; **250**: 2655–2659

29. Mellor, M. Symptomatic diffuse esophageal spasm: manometric follow-up and response to cholinergic stimulation and cholinesterase inhibition. *Gastroenterology* 1977; **73**: 237–240.

30. Stuart, R. C., Stinson, J., Byrne, P. J. *et al.* The influence of exercise on oesophageal pH motility in patients with angina-like non-cardiac chest pain. *Br. J. Surg.* 1988; **75**: 1229A

31. Svensson, O., Stenfort, G., Tibbling, L. and Wranne, B. Oesophageal function and coronary angiogram in patients with disabling chest pain. *Acta Med. Scand.* 1978; **204**: 173–178

32. Ducrotte, P. H., Berland, M. J., Denis, P. H. *et al.* Coronary sinus lactate estimation and esophageal motor anomalies in angina with normal coronary angiograms. *Dig. Dis. Sci.* 1985; **29**: 305–310

33. Cattan, E. L., Hirzel, R., Benjamin, S. B. and Cannon, R. O. Esophageal motility disorders in patients with abnormalities or coronary flow reserve and atypical chest pain. *Gastroenterology* 1987; **92**: 1339

34. Mellor, M. H., Simpson, A. G., Watt, L. Schoolmeester, L. and Haye, O. L. Esophageal acid perfusion in coronary artery disease: induction of myocardial ischemia. *Gastroenterology* 1983; **83**: 306–312

35. Morrison, L. M. and Swalm, W. A. Role of the gastrointestinal tract in production of cardiac symptoms: experimental and clinical observations. *J. Am. Med. Assoc.* 1940; **114**: 217–223

36. Vantrappen, G., Janssens, G. and Ghillebert, G. The irritable oesophagus – a frequent cause of angina-like pain. *Lancet* 1987; **i**: 1232

37. Stacher, G., Schmicerer, C. and Landgraf, M. Tertiary esophageal contractions evoked by acoustical stimuli. *Gastroenterology* 1979; **44**: 49–54

38. Stacher, G., Steinringer, I., Blau, A. and Landgraf, M. Acoustically evoked esophageal contractions and defence reaction. *Psychophysiology* 1979; **16**: 234–241

39. Watson, W. C., Sullivan, S. N., Corbe, M. and Rush, D. Incidence of oesophageal symptoms in patients with irritable bowel syndrome. *Gut* 1976; **17**: 827–829

40. Clouse, R. E. and Eckert, T. C. Gastrointestinal symptoms of patients with esophageal contraction abnormalities. *Dig. Dis. Sci.* 1986; **31**: 236–240

41. Richter, J. E., Dalton, C. B., Bradley, L. A. and Castell, D. O. Oral nifedipine in the treatment of non-cardiac chest pain in patients with the nutcracker esophagus. *Gastroenterology* 1987; **93**: 21–28

42. Clouse, R. E., Lustman, P. J., Eckert, T. C., Ferney, D. M. and Griffith, L. S. Low-dose trazodone for symptomatic patients with oesophageal contraction abnormalities: a double-blind placebo controlled trial. *Gastroenterology* 1987; **92**, 1027–1036

43. Winters, C., Artnak, E. J., Benjamin, S. B. and Castell, D. O. Esophageal bouginage in symptomatic patients with the nutcracker esophagus. *J. Am. Med. Assoc.* 1984; **252**; 363–366

44. Cohen, S. Esophageal motility disorders and their response to calcium channel antagonists: the sphinx revisited. *Gastroenterology* 1987; **93**: 201–203

45. Rhind, J. A. and Watson, L. Gallstone dyspepsia. *Br. Med. J.* 1968; **1**: 32

46. Capper, W. M., Butler, T. J., Kilby, J. O. and Gibson, M. J. Gallstones, gastric secretion and flatulent dyspepsia. *Lancet* 1967; **i**: 413–415

47. Johnson, A. G. Pylorifunction and gallstone dyspepsia. *Br. J. Surg.* 1972; **59**: 449–454

48. Price, W. H. Gallbladder dyspepsia. *Br. Med. J.* 1963; **2**: 138–141

49. Southam, J. A. The effects of cholecystectomy on oesophageal symptoms. *Br. J. Surg.* 1969; **56**: 671–672

50. Barker, J. R. and Alexander-Williams, J. The effect of cholecystectomy on oesophageal symptoms. *Br. J. Surg.* 1974; **61**: 346–348

51. Flook, D. and Stoddard, C. J. Gastro-oesophageal reflux and oesophagitis before and after vagotomy for duodenal ulcer. *Br. J. Surg.*, 1985; **72**: 804–807

52. Earlam, R. J., Amerigo, J., Kakavoulis, T. and Pollock, D. J. Histological appearances of oesophagus, antrum and duodenum and their correlation with symptoms in patients with a duodenal ulcer. *Gut* 1985; **26**: 95–100

53. Wallin, L. Gastro-oesophageal function in duodenal ulcer patients. *Scand. J. Gastroenterol* 1980; **15**: 145–150

54. Wallin, L. Acid gastro-oesophageal reflux pattern in duodenal ulcer patients related to dyspeptic symptoms. *Scand. J. Gastroenterol.* 1980; **15**: 151–155

55. Siewert, R. Dysphagia, achalasia and gastroesophageal reflux. In: Siewert, R., Baron, J. H., Alexander-Williams, J. *et al.*, Eds. *Vagotomy in Modern Surgical Practice*. London: Butterworths. 1982: 267–275.

56. Kruse-Andersen, S., Wallin, L. and Madsen, T. A possible triggering mechanism producing acid gastroesophageal reflux in duodenal ulcer patients and normal volunteers. In: Siewert, J. R. Ed. *Diseases of the Oesophagus*. Berlin: Springer-Verlag. 1988: 1084–1088

57. Cross, F. S. and Wangensteen, O. H. Role of bile and pancreatic juice in the production of esophageal erosions and anaemia. *Proc. Soc. Exp. Biol. Med.* 1961; **77**: 862–866

58. Gillison, E. W., DeCastro, V. A. M., Nyhus, L. M., Kusakari, K. and Bombeck, C. T. The significance of bile in reflux oesophagitis. *Surg. Gynecol. Obstet.* 1972; **134**: 419–424

59. Orlando, R. C. and Bozynski, E. M. Heartburn in pernicious anemia – a consequence of bile reflux. *N. Engl. J. Med.* 1973; **289**: 522–523

60. Henderson, R. D., Mugashe, F., Jeejeebloy, K. N. *et al.* The role of bile and acid in the production of esophagitis and the motor defect of esophagitis. *Ann. Thorac. Surg.* 1972; **14**: 465–473

61. Kivilaakso, E., Fromm, D. and Silen, W. Effect of bile salts and related compounds on isolated esophageal mucosa. *Surgery* 1980; **87**: 280

62. Helsingen, N. Jr. Oesophagitis following total gastrectomy. *Acta Clin. Scand.* 1960; **118**: 190–201

63. Palmer, E. D. Subacute erosive (peptic) esophagitis associated with achlorhydria. *N. Engl. J. Med.* 1960; **262**: 927–929

64. Henderson, R. D. Gastroesophageal reflux following gastric operation. *Ann. Thorac. Surg.* 1978; **26**: 563–573

65. Stol, D. W., Murphy, G. and Collis, J. L. Duodeno-gastric reflux and acid secretion in patients with symptomatic hiatal hernia. *Scand. J. Gastroenterol.* 1974; **9**: 97–101

66. Gillison, E. W., Nyhus, L. M. and Duthie, H. L. Bile reflux, gastric secretion and heartburn. *Br. J. Surg.* 1971; **58**: 864A

67. Crumplin, M. K. H., Stol, D. W., Murphy, G. M. and Colis, J. L. The pattern of bile salt reflux and acid secretion in sliding hiatal hernia. *Br. J. Surg.* 1974; **61**: 611–616

68. Gillen, P., Keeling, P., Byrne, P. J., Healy, M., O'Moore, R. R. and Hennessy, T. P. J. Implications of duodeno-gastric reflux in the pathogenesis of Barrett's oesophagus. *Br. J. Surg.* 1988; **75**: 540–543

69. Sorgi, M., White, C., Donovan, I. A., Poxon, V., Harding, L. K. and Alexander-Williams, J. In: Baron J. H., Alexander-Williams, J., Allgower, M. *et al.*, Eds. *Vagotomy in Modern Surgical Practice.* London: Butterworths. 1982: 283–284

70. Belsey, R. The pulmonary complications of esophageal disease. *Br. J. Dis. Chest* 1960; **54**: 342–348

71. Tuchman, D. N., Boyle, J. T. and Pack, A. I. Comparison of airway responses following tracheal or esophageal acidification in the cat. *Gastroenterology* 1984; **87**: 872–881

72. Piepz, A. Gastroesophageal radionuclide methods. Abstract 07. *First International Symposium on Gastroesophageal Reflux and Respiratory Disorders.* Brussels, 1988

73. Brendel, A. J., Guillet, J. and Guyot, M. Cine-oesophago-gastro scintigraphy: Clinical application in paediatrics and adults. Results of 3354 studies in 3000 patients. Abstract 08. *First International Symposium on Gastroesophageal Reflux and Respiratory Disorders.* Brussels, 1988

74. Sandberg, N., Mansson, I., Ruth, M. and Bengtsson, V. Bronchopulmonary aspiration in adults with respiratory disease and gastroesophageal reflux. Abstract 09. *First International Symposium on Gastroesophageal Reflux and Respiratory Disorders.* Brussels, 1988

75. Larrain, A., Lira, E., Otero, M. and Pope, C. E. Posterior laryngitis: a useful marker of oesophageal reflux. *Gastroenterology* 1981; **80**: 1204

76. Mansfield, L. E. and Stein, M. R. Gastroesophageal reflux and asthma: a possible reflex mechanism. *Ann. Allergy* 1981; **41**: 224–226

77. Mansfield, L. E., Hameister, H. H., Spaulding, H. S., Smith, N. J. and Glab, N. The role of the vagus nerve in airway narrowing caused by intra-oesophageal hydrochloric acid provocation and oesophageal distension. *Ann. Allergy* 1981; **47**: 431–434

78. Jakes, M. E., Agran, P. and Ong, K. S. Does gastroesophageal reflux (GER) or low pH in the lower oesophagus (LE) cause bronchoconstriction? *Chest* 1982; **82**: 246

79. Spaulding, H. S., Mansfield, L. E., Stein, M. R. Sellner, J. C. and Gremillon, D. E. Further investigation of the association between gastroesophageal reflux and bronchoconstriction. *J. Allergy Clin. Immunol.* 1982; **69**: 516–521

80. Pierry, A., Cooper, D. M., Murple, M., Crook, G., Bernstein, A. and Bancewicz, J. Gastro-oesophageal reflux and airways obstruction. *Br. J. Surg.* 1981; **68**: 358

81. Wilson, N. M., Charrette, L., Thomson, A. H. and Silverman, M. Gastroesophageal reflux and childhood asthma. The Acid Test. *Thorax,* 1985; **40**: 592–597

82. Hughes, D. M., Spiers, S., Rivilin, J. and Levison, H. Gastroesophageal reflux during sleep in asthmatic patients. *J. Pediatr.* 1983; **102**: 666–672

83. Berquist, W. E., Rachelefsky, G. S. and Kadden, M. Effect of theophylline on gastroesophageal reflux in normal adults. *J. Allergy. Clin. Immunol.* 1981; **67**: 407–411

84. Allan, C. J., Anvari, M. and Waterfall, W. E. Is gastroesophageal reflux induced by increased respiratory efforts? Abstract P2. *First International Symposium on Gastroesophageal Reflux and Respiratory Disorders.* Brussels, 1988

85. Tibbling, L. and Ekstrom, T. Can bronchospasm induce gastroesophageal reflux? Abstract P11. *First International Symposium on Gastroesophageal Reflux and Respiratory Disorders.* Brussels, 1988

86. Larrain, A., Carrasco, J., Gallequillos, J. and Pope, C. E. Reflux treatment improved lung function in patients with intrinsic asthma. *Gastroenterology* 1981; **80**: 1204

87. Urschel, H. C. and Paulson, D. L. Gastroesophageal reflux and hiatal hernia. Complications and therapy. *J. Thorac. Cardiovasc. Surg.* 1967; **53**: 21–32

88. Goodall, R. J. R., Earis, J. B., Coper, D. N., Bernstein, A. and Temple, J. G. Relationship between asthma and oesophageal reflux. *Thorax* 1981; **36**: 116–121

Chapter 3

Diagnostic tests for gastro-oesophageal reflux disease

Craig A. Eriksen and Alfred Cuschieri

Introduction

Gastro-oesophageal reflux disease occurs when reflux through the gastro-oesophageal junction causes symptoms and physical complications [1]. It accounts for approximately 75% of oesophageal pathology [2], and can present as an enigmatic diagnostic challenge, as no one test has been accepted as the true gold standard for its diagnosis [3]. The most sensitive test currently available is prolonged 24-hour ambulatory oesophageal pH monitoring [4], but there still remain symptomatic patients who demonstrate a normal oesophageal pH profile [5].

Symptoms related to gastro-oesophageal reflux are common in the general population. They have been reported as occurring daily in 7% and monthly in 36% of a large cohort of 'normal' subjects [6]. In addition, it is well recognized that the severity of symptoms does not correlate with the severity of the disease [7,8]. Thus, before embarking upon a set of diagnostic investigations, it is important to have a thorough understanding of the pathophysiology of the condition. This has been the subject of a number of recent reviews [3,7,9–11], and the role of the high pressure zone (lower oesophageal sphincter) has more recently been highlighted [12,13].

The tests that are currently available evaluate four main areas: oesophageal motility, the presence of refluxed gastric content, the presence of oesophageal mucosal damage, and the response of the distal oesophagus to acid. There is, however, overlap of the areas between the tests. Spiro [14] classified these investigations into: radiological, endoscopic, histological/cytological and physiological. The radiological tests include barium studies [15–17] with fluoroscopy, cinefluoroscopy [18] and radioisotope scanning [19–21]. Endoscopy allows for direct visualization of the oesophageal mucosa [22–24] and is indicated for diagnostic and therapeutic purposes [22]. Mucosal specimens obtained via the endoscope are examined histologically, either by light [23,25,26] or electron microscopy [27] for signs of inflammation or malignant change. Tests of a physiological nature include oesophageal manometry [28–30], oesophageal pH monitoring [31–33], the acid perfusion test of Bernstein [34,35], the acid clearance test [36,37] and the standard acid reflux test [10,38]. In children, the same tests are used, with some modifications [39]. As these investigations often give information about more than one area of interest (e.g. barium studies can be used to assess oesophageal motility, oesophageal mucosal integrity and reflux through the gastro-oesophageal junction), the clinician should have a thorough understanding of the specific indications for, and limitations of, each of the standard tests [40]. In addition, as asymptomatic subjects have positive results in some tests, absolute reliance on any single diagnostic parameter is not possible [41].

Objective assessment of symptoms

The clinical presentation of gastro-oesophageal reflux in the adult patient is, for the most part, distinct and unequivocal, as the symptom complex is classic. The principal symptom is heartburn, with which regurgitation and dysphagia may be associated. Heartburn is usually described as a 'burning' or 'gnawing' sensation that occurs most frequently in the retrosternal region, and it may radiate to the epigastrium or upwards into the neck. It is usually 'spontaneous', in that there is no associated emetic effort [42], typically occurs 30–60 minutes postprandially, and is common at night. It is exacerbated by postural changes or manoeuvres which increase the intra-abdominal pressure. Regurgitation describes the effortless reflux of sour-tasting gastric acid into the mouth, and is often posture related, especially occurring on bending, straining or lying down with pillow-staining at night. In some patients, chronic nocturnal cough due to aspiration is associated with regurgitation.

However, the clinical picture can be complicated by the fact that the incidence of these symptoms does not reflect the true incidence of reflux disease itself and, indeed, the severity of symptoms correlates poorly with either the presence or severity of oesophagitis [7,8,43,44]. This is especially evident in a small subgroup of patients who present with the classic symptoms of reflux and yet have a normal upper gastrointestinal endoscopic picture and a normal oesophageal pH profile [5].

A further complicating factor is that other important pathologies, such as oesophageal or gastric carcinoma, coronary artery disease and some abdominal conditions, may also present in a similar fashion. In addition, reflux may masquerade as atypical chest pain [45,46], asthma [42,47,48] or recurrent pneumonia, secondary to aspiration of gastric content [49,50].

In the primary assessment of each patient it is important to identify and grade the severity of each of these symptoms. Although some studies merely report the presence or absence of symptoms [51], other authors have graded each symptom as being mild, moderate or severe [52–54]. This latter method is prone to wide subjective variation and, as a result, a number of symptom-scoring and symptom-grading systems has been described [43,55–58]. Funch-Jensen et al. [56] evaluated 188 symptomatic reflux patients using an elaborate and complex symptom scoring system of general grades 0–5, while an earlier study used a 0–10 scale to grade seven predetermined symptoms [57].

Moran et al. [58] proposed a comprehensive point scoring system in which each symptom grade, on a scale of 0–3, was specifically described. Subjective interpretation of the symptom severity was eliminated with this method. This concept was modified by DeMeester and co-workers [43,59] into a simpler classification which allows easy objective assessment of the patient's condition. This system is currently used in the authors' laboratory and other centres [60]. The symptom grades are shown in Table 3.1. The authors' modification, however, is that each symptom is assessed individually, and the resulting grades are not added together to give a total score as is done elsewhere [43,60]. The reason is that there is a vast difference between a patient with grade 3 heartburn alone (total score 3) and a second patient with grade 1 of each of heartburn, regurgitation and dysphagia (total score 3).

A more complicated assessment has been proposed [61], in which each symptom is

Table 3.1 Scoring system for symptoms of gastro-oesophageal reflux

Symptom	Grade	Description
Heartburn		
None	0	No heartburn
Mild	1	Occasional episodes
Moderate	2	Reason for medical visit
Severe	3	Interference with daily activities
Regurgitation		
None	0	No regurgitation
Mild	1	Occasional episodes
Moderate	2	Predictable on position or straining
Severe	3	Episodes of pulmonary aspiration manifested by chronic nocturnal cough or recurrent pneumonia
Dysphagia		
None	0	No dysphagia
Mild	1	Occasional episodes
Moderate	2	Requires liquids to clear
Severe	3	Episode of oesophageal obstruction requiring medical treatment

From DeMeester *et al.* [59] with permission.

Table 3.2 An alternative symptom scoring of gastro-oesophageal reflux

	One point	Two points	Three points	Four points
I (frequency)	Occasional; not as often as once a month	More often than once a month but not as often as once a week	More often than once a week but not as often as daily	Daily
II (duration)	Less than 6 months	More than 6 months but less than 24 months	More than 24 months but less than 60 months	More than 60 months
III (severity)	Mild; nuisance value only	Moderate; spoils enjoyment of life	Marked; inter- feres with living a normal life	Severe; worst thing ever

Add frequency to duration and multiply by severity
Minimum score: 2; maximum score: 32
All symptoms of reflux can be scored, i.e. heartburn, dysphagia, regurgitation, odynophagia, bleeding, pulmonary problems, oropharyngeal symptoms
However, for classification purposes, only the maximum scoring system is used
Symptoms classified as: mild (1–7), moderate (8–15), marked (16–23), severe (24–32)

From Jamieson and Duranceau [62] with permission.

assigned a point according to severity, and these are multiplied together. Using this method, Jamieson and Duranceau [62] suggested a system as shown in Table 3.2.

Finally, a simple calculated symptom index (SI) has recently been proposed by Castell's group [63] which quantifies the percentage association between the incidence of symptoms and reflux episodes to pH of less than 4. For each symptom in question, the SI was defined as the number of times the symptom occurred when the oesophageal pH was less than 4, divided by the total number of times the symptom was reported. This was then multiplied by 100 to give a percentage of symptom episodes that correlated with gastro-oesophageal reflux as confirmed by oesophageal pH monitoring:

$$SI = \frac{\text{Number of symptoms with pH} < 4}{\text{Total number of symptoms}} \times 100$$

In infants and children, the clinical presentation of gastro-oesophageal reflux is different. Simple regurgitation is common in the first year of life [64,65], and the incidence is inversely proportional to age. The mechanism is thought to be spontaneous relaxation of the lower oesophageal sphincter. The reflux is usually of little clinical significance unless it causes complications [65], but a lack of communication of the symptoms often results in the reflux being missed [39]. In a recent study [66] of 90 children, with a range of ages from 3 months to 7 years, but with 66 children being younger than 2 years, vomiting and regurgitation were the most common presenting complaints, occurring in 53 children. Recurrent pulmonary disease was present in 25/90 children. Other conditions in which gastro-oesophageal reflux has been implicated are the sudden infant death syndrome, failure to thrive, chronic irritability, pulmonary problems of apnoea, recurrent infections, asthma and chronic lung conditions [39,66–68]. The chest signs of recurrent respiratory distress are the same as bronchospasm and bacteriological culture of sputum is usually negative.

Investigations

Radiological assessment

Radiological examination of a patient with symptoms of gastro-oesophageal reflux is often the first investigation performed [7], and it has been reported that 15% of patients with non-specific upper abdominal symptoms have radiologically detectable oesophageal disease, mainly oesophagitis [16]. The plain chest film rarely provides any evidence of reflux or hiatus hernia, except when an air bubble is seen overlying the heart shadow (Figure 3.1). This is dependent, however, on the size of the air–fluid level and the exposure of the film, and therefore can easily be missed.

Various contrast techniques [15–17,69] have been employed in order to assess oesophageal motility [70,71], presence of reflux [17,72,73] and distal oesophageal mucosal damage [15,74]. With the patient in the erect left posterior oblique position, a suspension of barium (170–200% weight/volume) is swallowed. Gravity then allows the barium bolus to distend the oesophagus and reach the gastro-oesophageal junction ahead of the primary peristaltic wave. In the normal oesophagus, the lower oesophageal sphincter relaxes and the entire barium bolus is cleared into the stomach on the arrival of the peristaltic wave [71]. This form of examination allows for qualitative and semiquantitative assessment of oesophageal motility [70]. Two disadvantages are that motor abnormalities are only intermittent and thus can be missed, and prolonged evaluation is limited by radiation time [75]. Fluoroscopic observations and cinefluorography, which allows for evaluation of rapid motor sequences especially in the oropharyngeal region [18], have increased the diagnostic accuracy in assessing the motility [70,76], although there is strong dependence on the examiner for selection of anatomical sites for viewing and interpretation of the pictures [19]. Nevertheless, peristaltic dysfunction in the distal oesophagus can be demonstrated by diminished volume clearance of the barium bolus [71], and this

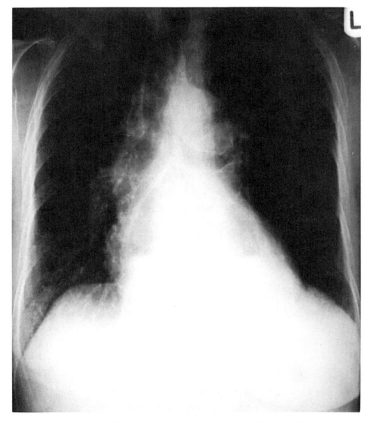

Figure 3.1 Plain chest X-ray showing a gastric air bubble overlying the heart shadow, indicating a large hiatus hernia

motor abnormality has been widely reported in patients with reflux oesophagitis [37,71,77–79].

The acid barium test was introduced in the mid-1960s to elicit motor abnormalities in the distal oesophagus. However, this test produces too many false positives, and is thus not specific enough to be of any appreciable use in the diagnosis of gastro-oesophageal reflux [62].

The diagnostic value of contrast radiology in the assessment of reflux at the gastro-oesophageal junction remains controversial [17,18], as the sensitivity of the test is low, reported values averaging 40% [3,80], but the average specificity is higher, at 85% [3]. Of note was that reflux was demonstrated in 20% of patients with no endoscopic signs of oesophagitis, and was absent in 35% of patients who had moderate and severe grades of oesophagitis [72]. In order to increase the sensitivity of detecting reflux, Christiansen et al. [73] introduced a method which produced reflux by food stimulation. The patient was first positioned in the supine left oblique position and given 300 ml of Mixobar (600 mg/ml) to drink then 20 ml of water to clear the oesophagus. Screening was started and continued after changing the patient to the right anterior oblique position, and giving him bread and paté to eat. Drawing on the concept of the grading of vesicoureteric reflux, they used this type of examination to grade any reflux seen according to the height reached up the oesophagus [73], grade I being to the junction of the middle and distal oesophagus, and grade II up to the cricopharyngeus. Twenty of the 26 patients (77%) demonstrated food-stimulated reflux (grade I: $n = 3$; grade II: $n = 17$), and 23 of the same 26 patients had histologically proven oesophagitis. Reflux and oesophagitis was present in 15 patients (75%). The imporance of this grading has yet to be established. Various postural manoeuvres have also been employed to invoke reflux, but the false positive and false negative rates are up to 50%.

Double-contrast barium techniques have greatly improved visualization of the oesophageal mucosa [17] over single contrast studies, and less barium is used [69]. The technique involves positioning the patient in the erect left posterior oblique (LPO) position and giving him a high density suspension to gulp rapidly [15,17]. This is followed immediately by gaseous distension of the oesophagus either by ingesting effervescent granular powders which produce carbon dioxide [15,17], or by active insufflation via a nasogastric tube as is done in Japan [17]. An alternative method is to swallow air in between sips of barium. Recently, a new method has been proposed which is better tolerated and provides a better view of the distal oesophagus [15]. The

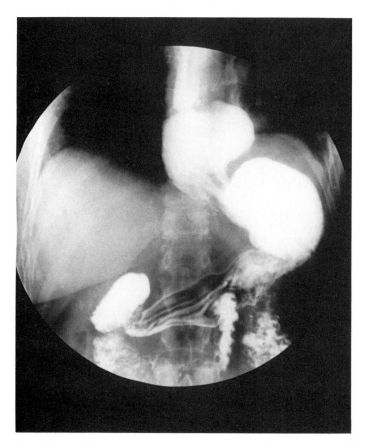

Figure 3.2 Axial or sliding hiatus hernia, as demonstrated by barium studies. (Courtesy of Dr J. D. Begg, Department of Radiology, Ninewells Hospital, Dundee, Scotland)

patient in the LPO position is given 15 ml of an alkaline solution to drink. This is followed immediately by a mixture of 100 ml of high-density barium (250% w/v), 15 ml of an acidic solution and three drops of a bubble breaker containing simethecone.

The mucosal lesions that are detected by these barium techniques are irregular contours caused by an ulcer, thickening of the oesophageal folds and granularity and erosions of the mucosa [16,17,74]. The distensibility of the oesophageal wall and the diameter of the lumen are also assessed. With regard to the latter point, it has been noted that pH-proven reflux was infrequent if the intrahiatal oesophageal diameter was less than two-thirds of the intrathoracic width, whereas pH-proven reflux was more frequent if the width was greater than two-thirds of the intrathoracic diameter [81]. Additionally, widening of the intra-abdominal oesophageal diameter is a reflection of the integrity of the phreno-oesophageal membrane [82].

The axial or sliding hiatus hernia can readily be demonstrated by barium studies (Figure 3.2), and the upward tenting of the stomach and loss of the acute oesophago-gastric angle are seen. The presence of a hiatus hernia is a common finding, but need not be of clinical significance [55,83]. A multicentre study from Italy [84] reported the prevalence of endoscopically diagnosed hiatus hernia as 5.8%, and its presence in 32% of patients with oesophagitis. On the other hand, only 21% of patients with a hiatus hernia were found to have oesophagitis. A second study [85] found reflux oesophagitis to be significantly related to the presence of such a hernia, and the defect was reported to be present in approximately 50% of patients with gastro-oeso-phageal reflux disease [23]. A further study found that only 10% of reflux patients had a hiatus hernia alone, but 50% of patients demonstrated a manometric defect as well as a hernia [86].

In children, the sensitivity of barium studies to detect reflux is less than other investigations and varies from 39% in one study [67], to 76% with symptoms but 37% without symptoms in another study [87]. In a third study, the barium oesophagogram successfully identified reflux in 86% of patients, but also showed a positive result in 31% of non-reflux children [88]. The common causes of false positive results are excessive crying by the patient, excessive pressure on the abdomen, the use of the head-down position (water siphon test), and overzealous reporting by the radiologist [11]. The identifying sign is the 'oesophageal beak' which is an inverted cone with the base on the cardia, and this has been associated with reflux in 95% of episodes [87]. A recent report has named this as the 'trumpeting elephant' sign of reflux in children [89]. The cardia represents the head of the elephant while the wide open hiatus and distal oesophagus correspond to the

Table 3.3 Age-related criteria for diagnosing 'acceptable' gastro-oesophageal reflux by radiological studies in infants and children

Group	'Acceptable' number of reflux episodes in 5 minutes
1 (birth–6 weeks)	3
2 (7 weeks–6 months)	2
3 (7 months–1 year)	2
4 (13–18 months)	1
5 (19 months–6 years)	1
6 (6–18 years)	0–1

From Cleveland et al. [87] with permission.

elephant's face and trunk held in a trumpeting position. As the incidence of reflux is inversely proportional to age, Cleveland and colleagues have suggested age-related criteria for 'acceptable' gastro-oesophageal reflux [87] (Table 3.3). The false positive rate of diagnosis is thus reduced by using these criteria.

Upper gastroinstestinal endoscopy

The advent of the modern flexible endoscope has greatly enhanced not only the diagnostic assessment of the upper gastrointestinal tract but also the therapeutic procedures performed in this region, and its use today is widespread. The rigid oesophagoscope, however, is still preferred for removal of foreign bodies from the oesophagus, some stricture dilatations and when deeper biopsies of the oesophageal wall are required. Nevertheless, the flexible endoscope has advantages of easy passage, ability to be used without requiring a general anaesthetic, a bright and magnified field, a decreased risk of oesophageal perforation, and can easily be used in children [90]. Its diagnostic indications are: evaluation of symptoms, evaluation of oesophageal disease, evaluation of radiological findings, especially in patients who have had previous oesophageal or gastric surgery [91], and postoperative evaluation [22–24]. In addition, the location of the oesophagogastric junction, the 'Z line', relative to the diaphragmatic hiatus can be noted, although this position can vary during the endoscopic examination [91]. The diagnosis of a hiatus hernia can be made if the Z line remains more than 2 cm proximal to the diaphragmatic hiatus [23]. The stomach and duodenum are also inspected for concomitant disease.

Qualitative assessment of the distal oesophageal mucosa has led to controversy, because, although the more severe grades of inflammation are easily recognized and agreed upon, there still remains argument as to what constitutes the early macroscopic appearances of oesophagitis. Indeed, due to the subjective interpretation involved, one study regarded patients with grade I oesophagitis (mucosal erythema) as being normal [37]. Sladen and co-workers [35], in an earlier report, noted mucosal friability in 50% of patients with classic symptoms, and also in 25% of patients who presented with atypical symptoms. There are currently numerous endoscopic classifications of oesophagitis [3,4,17,22–24,32,37,92,93], although most tend to be in general agreement with one another. Grade I describes the mucosal lesions which are the early signs of the inflammatory process, and are generally regarded as being erythema with or without mucosal friability. The normal fine vascular pattern is lost [91]. Monnier and Savary [24] also included into this grade reddish spots, possibly with an exudate. Tytgat [93] modified the original Savary–Miller classification [22] (single/isolated erosion with erythema or exudate, or both) to being 'non-confluent oval patch(es) or streak(s) of reddening, covered by a fine white exudate'. In agreement, however, is the erythematous appearance of the distal oesophageal mucosa, possibly with other signs of mild inflammation. Grade II oesophagitis describes the formation of small superficial ulcers which are linear and non-confluent. These are usually on the crest of the mucosal folds [23]. Friability and a definite exudate indicate surface necrosis. Confluence of these ulcers or more extensive linear lesions with islands of oedematous mucosa between erythematous folds (the 'cobble-stoned' appearance) characterize grade III oesophagitis. No stricture formation is evident at this stage. Grade IV indicates the presence of extensive mucosal damage or chronic lesions such as a symmetrical stricture, shortening or Barrett's oesophagus. In the case of stricture formation, the mucosa immediately proximal may be only minimally inflamed as it is now protected from any reflux [91]. At the end of the day, it is important to use a simple, clear grading system which allows for some subjective interpretation, standardization of examination for prospective work and easy comparison of appearances for follow-up purposes. A plea is made for the standardization of such grading systems, thus making interstudy comparisons more meaningful. The classification and grading system presently in use at our institution is based on the Savary–Miller and DeMeester [37] classifications, and is shown in Table 3.4.

Table 3.4 Endoscopic classification of oesophagitis

Grade I:	Erythema ± mucosal friability
Grade II:	Superficial non-confluent linear ulceration
Grade III:	Confluent or circumferential areas of deeper ulceration ± 'cobble-stoned' mucosa
Grade IV:	Extensive mucosal damage or complications of stricture, shortening or Barrett's oesophagus

From Little *et al.* [37] with permission.

Endoscopic evidence of oesophagitis in patients with reflux symptoms varies considerably between reports: 38% [92], 52% [37], 58% [26], 62% [4], 69% [94], 75% [13] and averages 68% [3]. It has been suggested that this wide variation is due in part to patient selection [26] but, as stated earlier, symptoms correlate badly with endoscopic appearances [8,43]. Baldi and co-workers, in a multicentre study, found that only 46% of oesophagitis patients presented with typical reflux symptoms [95]. Thus, the sensitivity is too low to identify patients with the disease at the clinic [4] and a normal endoscopy does not exclude the presence of reflux. On the other hand, the specificity of endoscopy, i.e. the determination of the number of normal results in patients without the disease, is high, being 96%, although inclusion of grade I oesophagitis lowers this figure [3]. The severity of oesophagitis found at endoscopy has been reported to correlate significantly with the exposure to acid in the distal oesophagus [37,44,92].

Although the diagnostic assessments of endoscopy and histology do not always tally [24,62], the sensitivity of endoscopy can be increased with the concomitant use of histology [96], reported as 82% [26] and 92% [94]. There are, however, certain limitations, such as adequacy of specimen size, orientation and depth, problems in sampling [7,97], and multiple biopsies are preferable. Nevertheless, it has recently been suggested that endoscopy and biopsy is possibly the most important diagnostic test for gastro-oesophageal reflux disease [23] and finding of at least two abnormal biopsies allows for better separation of patients and normal subjects [98]. Histological signs of oesophagitis have also been reported in patients with a normal endoscopic picture [25,26,96,99], but one study [35] reported that these microscopic abnormalities did not relate to the symptom pattern. The requirements for a histological diagnosis of oesophagitis are basal cell hyperplasia, dermal papillary extension, and polymorphonuclear leucocytes and eosinophils in the lamina propria [18,25,26,56]. Frank ulceration is evident in severe cases. The basal cell hyperplasia involves up to 50% of the epithelial thickness in mild oesophagitis and over 50% in more severe cases [44], whilst the dermal papillae should extend at least two-thirds of the epithelial thickness to be of significance [26]. These two criteria were found to be absent in 80–90% of control subjects in whom the biopsies were taken more than 2.5 cm proximal to the lower oesophageal high pressure zone [96]. Within 2.5 cm of this area, up to 60% of controls showed these signs. Neutrophilic infiltration has also been noted in oesophagitis [27,56,96]. Although a recent paper [100] concluded that the presence of intraepithelial eosinophils was an unreliable indicator of oesophagitis as these were found in 31% of their patients and 33% of the controls, these cells are nevertheless useful in the diagnosis [101]. The electron microscope provides a more accurate identification of oesophageal inflammation [27], but its use in this field is not routine. Biopsy is especially indicated for suspicious lesions, and its diagnostic accuracy has been reported as 92% when used in combination with brush cytology [102].

Oesophageal manometry

Oesophageal manometry was first introduced in 1883 by H. Kronecker and S. J. Meltzer (cited in Nelson and Castell [18]), and the modern system was established in 1956 by Code [103]. Today, there are a number of different systems available, with some set-ups more appropriate to specific aspects of the manometric study than others. Broadly speaking, the system can be divided into two parts: (1) the pressure monitoring apparatus and (2) the data recording equipment. The oesophageal pressures are measured by one of two systems which are interchangeable. The first is the standard apparatus which employs a low compliance multilumen nasogastric catheter (three to eight lumens) and a pneumohydraulic infusion pump, interfaced by a set of transducers [28,29] (Figure 3.3). The second system is newer and consists of a solid state recording catheter with built-in minitransducers and this connects directly to the data recording equipment. The latter system has a disadvantage in that the

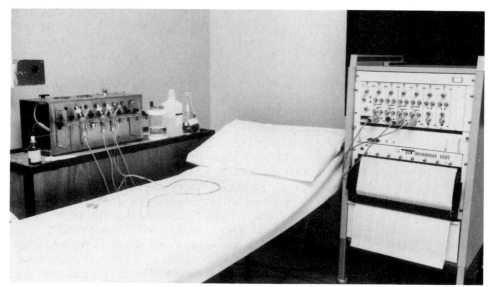

Figure 3.3 The oesophageal manometry laboratory. On the left, is shown the multilumen nasogastric tube, the transducers, pneumohydraulic infusion pump and the water reservoir. On the right, is the multichannel recorder which traces the oesophageal pressures on to a polygraph

whole catheter needs to be replaced or returned to the manufacturer if one transducer is faulty. The data recording apparatus is either a multichannel recorder and amplifier that traces the pressure on heat-sensitive paper (Figure 3.3), or a computerized system in which the pressures are stored on floppy disk.

Manometry is of great value in the diagnosis of oesophageal motility disorders and with advanced technology, the accuracy has been increased [30]. However, it does require expertise in its performance and interpretation [104], and it is difficult to perform in the paediatric patient [105]. There are controversies as to how to measure the high pressure zone (HPZ, lower oesophageal sphincter) pressure, and where the beginning and end of contraction waves are in the body of the oesophagus. The role of oesophageal manometry in the diagnosis of gastro-oesophageal reflux has been questioned [7,28,30,106,107], although it is important to exclude specific motor disorders in those patients in whom surgery is contemplated [7,62]. One study of 102 symptomatic reflux patients showed 6 patients with achalasia, 4 with diffuse oesophageal spasm and 2 with nutcracker oesophagus [28]. In addition, some authors have advocated its use preoperatively to identify those patients who may develop postfundoplication obstructive symptoms [108,109], but this is now disputed [110].

There have been a number of classifications proposed to categorize the specific and non-specific oesophageal motility disorders [106,111,112]. The criterion for diagnosis used in our laboratory is based on that set out by Benjamin *et al.* [111], and is shown in Table 3.5. The mean peristaltic amplitude required for the diagnosis of nutcracker oesophagus has been raised to $\geqslant 180$ mmHg on the recommendation of Castell's group [113].

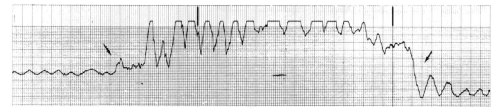

Figure 3.4 Manometry tracing of a normal subject showing the gastric baseline pressure (left), high pressure zone (HPZ, lower oesophageal sphincter) (centre, between the arrows), and intraoesophageal pressure (right)

The HPZ (Figure 3.4), first identified in 1956 by Fyke and co-workers [114], is recorded by withdrawing the catheter by either the slow or rapid pull-through techniques. The former method involves pulling the catheter out of the stomach 1 cm at a time, at 1–2 second intervals, with the patient breathing normally, and it allows measurement of the peak pressure, mean pressure, highest minimum pressure and pressure at the respiratory inversion point. The rapid pull-through technique requires the patient to stop breathing while the HPZ is evaluated. Only the mean pressure is calculated and it is identical to the pressure measured by the slow pull-through technique [115]. Due to the asymmetrical nature of the HPZ and its movement on respiration, Dent [116] designed a 5-cm sleeve which allows for axial displacement during respiration and long-term pressure measurements. A reported problem with the sleeve is that changes in gastric pressures can also be monitored at the same time

Table 3.5 Criteria for manometric diagnosis of oesophageal disease

I. Normal
  1. LES pressure 10–26 mmHg (mean ± 2 s.d.) with normal relaxation
  2. Mean peristaltic amplitude in the distal oesophagus 50–110 mmHg (mean ± 2 s.d.)
  3. Absence of spontaneous, repetitive or simultaneous contractions
  4. Single waveforms (with not more than two peaks)
  5. Mean duration of peristaltic waves in the distal oesophagus 1.9 ± 5.5 s (mean ± 2 s.d.)
II. Primary motility disorders
  1. Achalasia*
     (a) Aperistalsis in oesophageal body
     (b) Incomplete lower oesophageal sphincter (LES) relaxation
     (c) Elevated LES pressure (≥26 mmHg)
     (d) Increased intraoesophageal baseline pressures relative to gastric baseline
  2. Diffuse oesophageal spasm (DES)
     (a) Simultaneous (non-peristaltic) contractions:
         (i) repetitive (at least three peaks) contractions
         (ii) increased duration (>5.5 s)
     (b) Spontaneous contractions
     (c) Periods of normal peristalsis
     (d) Contractions may be of increased amplitude
  3. 'Nutcracker oesophagus,
     (a) Mean peristaltic amplitude (10 'wet' swallows) in the distal oesophagus ≥120 mmHg
     (b) Increased mean duration of contractions (>5.5 s) often found
     (c) Normal peristaltic sequence
  4. Non-specific oesophageal motility disorders (NEMD) – abnormal manometry representing primary oesophageal motor disorders other than achalasia, DES, or 'nutcracker oesophagus'
     (a) Hypertensive LES:
         (i) LES pressure >26 mmHg with normal relaxation
         (ii) normal oesophageal peristalsis
     (b) Decreased or absent amplitude of oesophageal peristalsis:
         (i) normal LESP
         (ii) normal LES relaxation
     (c) Other abnormalities of peristaltic sequence (including any combination of the following):
         (i) abnormal waveforms
         (ii) isolated simultaneous contractions
         (iii) isolated spontaneous contractions
         (iv) normal peristaltic sequence maintained
         (v) LES normal

* a and b required; c usually present; d sometimes present.
From Benjamin *et al.* [111] with permission.

[29]. An alternative to the sleeve is the Kraglund tube/cuff which has an advantage of permitting reliable circumferential recordings [29]. Nelson *et al.* [117] reported the HPZ pressure in a cohort of normal volunteers to be 26.6 ± 10.8 mmHg (mean ± 1 s.d.) with a range of 7.0–58.0 mmHg. More recently, these figures were confirmed by the same unit when they studied an enlarged cohort of 95 control subjects [118]. There has been great interest shown recently in the finding of 'transient lower oesophageal sphincter relaxation' (TLOSR, 'relaxation of HPZ beginning before full submental EMG complex' [13], Figure 3.5) in regard to the pathogenesis of gastro-oesophageal reflux. Dent *et al.* [119] in 1980 first proposed that TLOSR was the mechanism of reflux in normal subjects, and found that such 'inappropriate' relaxations did not occur during steady sleep. Two years later, a report from the same unit [120] demonstrated that TLOSRs were responsible for 94% of reflux episodes in controls, and 65% of episodes in oesophagitis patients. Other factors in the patient group were transient increase in intra-abdominal pressure (17%) and spontaneous

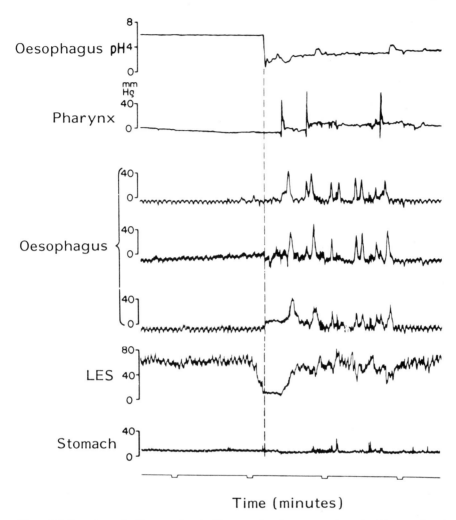

Figure 3.5 Oesophageal reflux associated with a transient lower oesophageal sphincter relaxation (TLOSR), the onset of which is identified by the dotted line. (From Dent *et al.* [119] with permission)

free reflux (18%). The TLOSR is believed to be under vagal control [121]. More recently, Dent *et al.* [12] showed that 82% of reflux episodes in symptomatic patients were due to TLOSR and, with increasing severity of oesophagitis, the mechanism became one of an absence of basal HPZ pressure. This latter finding is a prerequisite for gastro-oesophageal reflux [122]. Of note, is that the patients commonly showed more than one mechanism which invoked a reflux event. These findings have been confirmed by Mittal and McCallum [13], although they studied patients when awake. They also showed that the frequency of TLOSR was the same for controls and patients.

Measurement of the HPZ pressure has been regarded as important in patients with reflux symptoms, although there are opposing camps [7,123,124] and, indeed, DeMeester [4] uses a pressure of less than 6 mmHg as one requirement of a 'mechanically defective sphincter'. A low pressure was recorded in up to 78% of patients [94,107,125], but there was large overlap with normal subjects [107]. The major overlap occurs between controls and mild reflux disease patients [7]. Very recently, a computerized system has been described which uses an eight channel probe to give a computer-generated, cylindrical, three-dimensional model of the HPZ [126]. The clinical application of this needs to be evaluated.

Patients with reflux oesophagitis have significantly decreased contraction amplitude in the distal oesophagus [77,127,128] and this also occurs after exercise [129]. This is a reflection of the decreased clearing mechanism of the oesophagus, and does not improve after treatment [77,125,130], although this is disputed [128]. For adequate assessment of the motor function of the distal oesophagus, it was found that more than five to eight 'wet' swallows are required [131].

The new techniques in manometry have been the Dent sleeve [116], and the development of 24-hour dual manometry and oesophageal pH monitoring equipment [132,133]. Janssens et al. [134] have used their dual system to investigate patients with non-cardiac chest pain, and their positive rate of 48% is higher than previously achieved. Within the last 12 months, a further study described a 24-hour ambulatory oesophageal manometry system [135] and suggested its use in differentiating between psychological and organic motility disorders. This appears to be the direction of future manometry investigations.

In summary, oesophageal manometry is used in the diagnosis of gastro-oesophageal reflux to determine the state and function of the HPZ and the peristaltic ability of the distal oesophagus. A recent study [4] showed that manometric evaluation of the HPZ has a sensitivity of 84% and a specificity of 89%. When these positive findings are combined with oesophageal pH monitoring, the sensitivity remains the same but the specificity rises to 100%.

Provocation tests

The acid perfusion (Bernstein) test

The acid perfusion or Bernstein test was introduced in 1958 by Bernstein and Baker, as a test to show the sensitivity of the distal oesophagus to acid [34]. It is performed with the patient sitting in a chair, with a nasogastric tube placed 30 cm from the nostril. Physiological saline is administered through the nasogastric tube at a rate of 100–120 drops/min for 10–15 minutes. The infusion is changed to 0.1 M hydrochloric acid without the patient's knowledge, and the infusion is continued at the same rate for 30 minutes or until the usual symptoms of heartburn or pain occur. If no symptoms occur, the test is regarded as negative. If symptoms are produced, the drip is changed immediately to physiological saline, and the infusion continued until the symptoms abate. Most patients with reflux oesophagitis obtain relief of symptoms within 20 minutes, but some patients have pain for longer. At the conclusion of the test, antacids are given [14].

The initial report found 19/22 patients had a positive test and 20/21 controls had a negative test. Over the next three decades, the test was widely used with variability in results, but the average sensitivity has been 78% and the specificity 84% [62]. Helm et al. [136] found that the onset of heartburn in such patients was accompanied by an increase in the flow of saliva. Positive tests were found in 38% of patients with no previous symptoms of reflux, and in 26% of patients who demonstrated a normal oesophageal pH profile [137]. Clarke [41] also noted that up to 15% of normal subjects may have a positive test.

Although the test shows the sensitivity of the oesophageal mucosa to acid, it is not a test for oesophagitis [3]. It is most useful in those patients with multiple or atypical symptoms [35], or in patients with chest pain of non-cardiac origin [137,138]. It is not, however, favoured by all authors [139].

Acid clearance test

The acid clearance test was first described in 1968 by Booth *et al.* [36], and it assesses the ability of the distal oesophagus to clear a standardized bolus of acid. It is performed after manometry, with the patient in the sitting position. A pH electrode is introduced into the oesophagus and placed 5 cm proximal to the HPZ. The manometry catheter is withdrawn to the same distance above the HPZ. A 15 ml bolus of 0.1 M hydrochloric acid is introduced through a port on the manometry catheter, 10 cm proximal to the pH electrode. The pH intially drops to pH 1.4, and the patient is asked to swallow at 30-second intervals until the oesophageal pH has risen to above 5. Normal subjects clear the acid in one to three swallows (up to 10), whereas patients with oesophagitis require many more [36,37]. It is, however, not regarded as a useful test due to its low sensitivity [62].

Standard acid reflux test

Tuttle and Grossman [38] introduced the concept of what is known today as the standard acid reflux test, when they tested the competency of the gastro-oesophageal junction by assessing its ability to keep an introduced bolus of acid in the stomach and out of the oesophagus. The stomach was filled with 200 ml of 0.1 M hydrochloric acid (HCl) and a pH electrode passed into it. The electrode was then slowly withdrawn into the oesophagus and the pH rise noted. In normal subjects, the pH was found to rise sharply over a 1 cm distance, while reflux patients demonstrated a slower pH rise over a longer distance. The high false positive and false negative rates necessitated the test being modified to the present day standard acid reflux test. The stomach is now filled with 300 ml of 0.1 M HCl and pH electrode positioned 5 cm above the high pressure zone [10]. Reflux is evaluated at rest, after three coughs, three deep breaths, Valsalva and Müller manoeuvres, in four different positions. A drop in oesophageal pH to less than 4 indicates reflux, and the test is considered positive if reflux occurs more than twice during the 20 manoeuvres. The false positive rate has been reported to be 4–20%, and the false negative rate up to 40% [140]. Recently, Fuchs *et al.* [4], in a study to evaluate the objective diagnosis of gastro-oesophageal reflux disease, calculated the sensitivity to be 59% but the specificity to be 98%. The test has been reported to be very accurate in children [141].

The test is useful in as much as it will identify those patients with significant free reflux, but it can only really be used as a quick screening test [62], or in patients with atypical symptoms [18].

Oesophageal pH monitoring

Intraoesophageal pH measurement was used in 1958 by Tuttle and Grossman [38] as described above. Later, prolonged pH monitoring over an 18-hour period was reported [142], and since then the field of oesophageal pH monitoring has developed dramatically, and is now in worldwide use [4,31,32,92,143,144]; it is regarded as the most suitable gold standard test for the diagnosis of gastro-oesophageal reflux. The two important cornerstones of prolonged pH monitoring are that it allows for determination of the pattern of any acid reflux present, as well as the

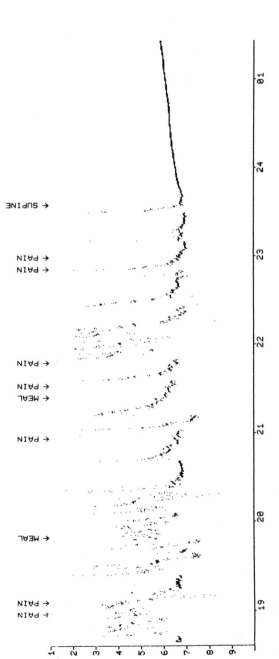

Figure 3.6 Plot of oesophageal pH from a patient with reflux oesophagitis. The pH scale is shown on the y axis and the time of day is along the x axis. Each dot represents a single pH recording, the sampling rate being set at once every 10 seconds. The relationship of the patient's symptoms (pain) to reflux episodes is illustrated

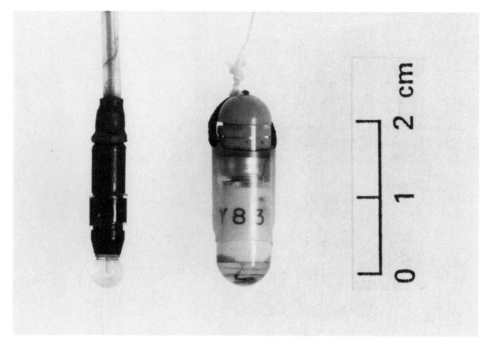

Figure 3.7 Combined pH/reference glass electrode (left) and the radiotelemetry pill (right)

correlation of patient's symptoms to reflux episodes (Figure 3.6). The introduction of microcomputers for data storage and analysis has greatly widened the application of pH monitoring [33,145].

The first prolonged measurements of intraoesophageal pH were by Spencer [145a], Johnson and DeMeester [146] and Pattrick [146a]. A glass pH electrode, passed nasally and positioned 5 cm proximal to the manometrically defined lower oesophageal sphincter, was used in a cohort of hospital inpatients to record the oesophageal pH continuously on to a bedside strip chart recorder. Coffee and smoking were not permitted, but an otherwise normal diet was allowed. A reflux event was defined as a drop in pH to less than 4. Control subjects were noted to experience some reflux, and this 'physiological' reflux was found to occur usually after eating, rarely during sleep and was unaffected by age [43]. Reflux was considered abnormal if the value was more than two standard deviations greater than the mean of the normals. Three patterns of pathological reflux were identified: that occurring while in the erect posture ('upright reflux'), supine reflux, and combined (erect and supine) reflux. Upright refluxers were noted to demonstrate a significantly greater number of reflux events than the controls, and the supine refluxers showed a higher incidence of oesophagitis.

Limitations of this method were requirements for in-hospital monitoring and restriction of normal activities, and this has been confirmed by a recent study [147]. As a consequence, ambulatory systems were developed to allow for home monitoring under normal daily conditions. Currently in use are small glass combined pH electrodes with a built-in reference electrode, finer monocrystalline antimony electrodes [148] and pH-sensitive radiotelemetry pills [149] (Figure 3.7), together with

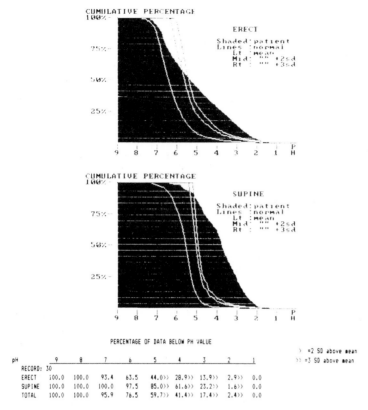

Figure 3.8 Frequency analysis of the oesophageal pH data expressed as the cumulative percentage of the total pH data and stratified into recordings made in the erect (top diagram) and supine (bottom diagram) positions. The shaded area shows the patient's results, and the three lines indicate normal values (from a cohort of 50 asymptomatic volunteers). Left: mean of normals; centre: 2 standard deviations greater than the normal mean; right: 3 standard deviations greater than the normal mean. The figures at the bottom show the actual values obtained, and are expressed as percentages

compact lightweight recorders, the specifications of which have recently been extensively reviewed [150,151]. The reproducibility of such tests using these systems has been confirmed [152,153]. Using a portable radiotelemetry system, the differences between patients in hospital and those ambulatory at home were highlighted by Branicki *et al.* [154]. They found that reflux was more frequent and of longer duration when monitored by the ambulatory system. A further study [155] demonstrated that these differences were due to patients' motility as the recording ability of the stationary pen recorder apparatus was comparable to that of the ambulatory monitor.

It is universally accepted that the pH electrode is placed 5 cm proximal to the high pressure zone (lower oesophageal sphincter). Location of the HPZ is achieved by manometric determination. An alternative method is to insert the electrode into the stomach and slowly withdraw it into the oesophagus. Tuttle and Grossman [38] encountered an abrupt rise in pH as the oesophagus was entered in normal subjects. Rokkas *et al.* [144] found that this method correlated very well with manometric assessment, and it is acceptable to other authors [156] but not all would agree [150,157,158].

Despite the widespread use of pH monitoring, there are differing opinions as to how to define a reflux episode. DeMeester [59,146] defined a reflux event as being when the oesophageal pH decreased to 4 or less, and this has been adopted by other authors [92,148]. Additional criteria used by others relate to duration: 'for at least 5 seconds' [147], and 'at least 20 seconds' [33] (the latter equipment samples the oesophageal pH every 10 seconds). Branicki et al. [154] required a fall in pH of at least 2 units, and other authors defined it as the time spent below a particular cut-off level of pH until the pH returned above that cut-off level [32]. The exact definition is not of prime importance when the oesophageal acid exposure is considered in terms of the percentage of data below a particular pH level (Figure 3.8), but it is of great importance when analysing the frequency and duration of such reflux episodes. With the current computerized data logging systems which sample the pH at a preset rate, it would appear logical that a reflux event be defined as a drop in pH to less than 4 for two or more consecutive sample recordings. Similarly, the pH should remain below 4 for at least two consecutive samples before a new event can begin.

There is additional confusion as to what constitutes abnormal reflux, and which indices of reflux are best used for analysis. It is well recognized that normal asymptomatic subjects experience gastro-oesophageal reflux, and 'normal' values have been published [59]. Abnormal reflux was considered present if values were more than two standard deviations greater than the mean value for the controls. This cut-off point has been adopted by others [156,159,160] although Johnsson et al. [32] have proposed that the 95th percentile should be used as the upper limit of normal due to the data being skewed. DeMeester et al. [43] proposed a composite score, made up of six variables, to discriminate between normal and abnormal reflux, but its value has been questioned [147,150]. The individual variables of greater importance are the number of reflux episodes (per hour) and the mean duration of each reflux event [150]. The duration of reflux episodes reflects the distal clearing mechanism of the oesophagus, both by mechanical emptying and neutralization [161,162], and both of these characteristics are impaired in oesophagitis patients. Reflux events lasting longer than 5 minutes are also an indication of defective clearing [79]. The detailed results of 24-hour pH monitoring in 50 asymptomatic volunteer subjects from our laboratory have been recently published [163], and the normal values for the reflux event analysis are shown in Table 3.6. Very few events were recorded per hour (significantly less in the supine position), and long-lasting (> 5 min) events were very infrequent. The duration per event was similar for both erect and supine postures. The overall reflux experienced in the upright position was

Table 3.6 Reflux event analysis to pH < 4 in 50 asymptomatic normal subjects

pH	Time (min)	Events (n)	Duration per event (min)	Number of events		Longest event (min)
				< 5 min	> 5 min	
< 4						
Erect	1.51 ± 0.26	0.80 ± 0.11	1.79 ± 0.40	0.76 ± 0.11	0.04 ± 0.01	4.35 ± 0.91
Supine	0.47 ± 0.18	0.08 ± 0.02	1.93 ± 0.63	0.05 ± 0.01	0.02 ± 0.01	3.51 ± 1.38
Total	1.04 ± 0.19	0.48 ± 0.07	2.13 ± 0.43	0.45 ± 0.06	0.03 ± 0.01	6.43 ± 1.48

All data have been standardized to 1 hour and results are shown as mean and standard error of the mean.
From Cheadle et al. [163] with permission.

significantly greater than that when supine, and this was mostly due to postprandial reflux, which occurred after the main evening meal, and to a lesser extent after breakfast. Although the percentage of time below pH 4 was two to four times greater than in previous reports [120,146,154,158], this is probably due to the use of an ambulatory system, unrestricted position changes and data being strictly stratified according to position rather than day *vs* night [163].

The authors' results [163] emphasize the need to separate the erect and supine recordings, and are in agreement with the earlier study of DeMeester *et al.* [43] in which refluxers were classified according to posture. Reflux when supine at night was more noxious than daytime reflux [37]. This has recently been disputed by de Caestecker *et al.* [92] who demonstrated that daytime upright reflux (especially postprandially) correlated more closely with the severity of endoscopic oesophagitis than did nocturnal reflux. In addition, these findings were confirmed by Rokkas and Sladen [60] who found that oesophagitis was related to both frequency and duration of reflux episodes, and they concluded that daytime exposure to acid was more important in the development of oesophagitis. Two studies [160,164] concerning patients with Barrett's oesophagus demonstrated that these patients have a greater acid exposure than patients with uncomplicated oesophagitis. A further study [165], documenting the temporal pattern of reflux, showed that the greatest amount of reflux occurred between 17:00 and 24:00 hours, and mostly in patients with oesophagitis. The least amount of reflux was recorded between the hours of 24:00 and 07:00.

Oesophageal pH monitoring over the 24-hour period has been shown to be the most sensitive test available for detecting gastro-oesophageal reflux. The early reported sensitivity was 79% [148], and with more modern equipment varies between 81% and 96% [3,4,31,32,43,156,158,166]. The specificity varies between 96% and 100% [3,4,31,32,146,156,158,166]. Fink and McCallum [167], in 1984, evaluated the roles of shorter monitoring periods of 3 hours postprandially and 12 hours, and they compared the results to those obtained from 24-hour monitoring. The sensitivities were 77% and 94% for the 3- and 12-hour periods respectively, and they concluded that although 24-hour monitoring was the best, the 12-hour record was still highly accurate and the shorter 3-hour postprandial evaluation was practical, less expensive and accurate enough for diagnostic purposes. This has been confirmed more recently [168]. Within the last 12 months, there have been three studies investigating the usefulness of shorter monitoring periods [140,156,169]. The 3-hour postprandial period detected reflux successfully in 70–97% of cases, but the 12-hour period was not as accurate [156]. Although the shorter monitoring period may be more convenient to the patient and laboratory resources, the full 24-hour period remains the most accurate method of detecting reflux and should be the duration used.

As mentioned earlier, one of the cornerstones of prolonged oesophageal pH monitoring is the ability to detect the pattern of reflux under the patient's normal environment, and the ambulatory systems have proved to be extremely useful in this regard. The correlation of pain events to reflux episodes (see Figure 3.6) amounts to an endogenous acid perfusion test, and detailed analysis of the reflux episodes constitutes an assessment of the distal oesophageal clearing mechanism, as well as competence of the gastro-oesophageal junction. However, there remains a small group of patients who demonstrate normal oesophageal pH profiles and yet have the classic symptoms [5]. These patients are thought to have a primary oesophageal motor disorder, or neutral reflux.

In children, oesophageal pH monitoring has yielded the most useful information when assessing the problem of gastro-oesophageal reflux [11,170]. Small 1.6–3.0 mm pH electrodes are now available [150], and the test was shown to detect reflux in 82/ 93 patients in one study [88]. Monitoring periods of 18–24 hours were found to be reliable [171], and shorter periods of measurement are less reliable [11]. It has now become a routine test for apnoea, cases of respiratory distress [36,64,141] and sleep disorders [11], but it is important when investigating infants to remember to position the child correctly (the 'physiological' position is prone) [64]. The test has been shown to be a reliable indicator of the need for surgery in infants [172,173].

Radioisotope scanning

The use of radioisotopes to detect disorders of the oesophagus and stomach is gaining popularity, as the technique is simple, non-invasive and agreeable to the patient. The choice of radionuclide is a gamma-emitting radioisotope with a short half-life and no associated beta emissions [174]. Technetium-99m sulphur colloid (^{99m}Tc) (either ^{99m}Tc-pertechnate or ^{99m}Tc-diethylenetriaminepentaacetate – ^{99m}Tc–DTPA [17]) has these characteristics. It has been the choice of radioisotopes since the 1960s, and it produces a low radiation dose. The scanning techniques are of two types: those evaluating oesophageal transit [20,21,175], and those assessing reflux at the gastro-oesophageal junction [19,26], where it is more accurate than barium studies [17].

Fisher *et al.* [19] were first to use radioisotopes to assess gastro-oesophageal reflux. They studied 30 patients with heartburn and a positive acid reflux test, and 20 normal subjects. The technique involved the instillation of a mixture of ^{99m}Tc (100 Ci), and 300 ml of isotonic saline into the stomach via a nasogastric tube. With the patient lying supine under a gamma camera, a pneumatic abdominal binder was applied to gradually increase the intra-abdominal pressure up to 35 mmHg. Ninety per cent of the patients and only two controls were shown to experience reflux. They proposed a reflux index (RI) to assess the degree of reflux and found that patients had significantly higher RI values than controls. A later paper [52] reported a 70% sensitivity and 87% specificity for this test. There was no relationship found between the severity of symptoms and the volume of reflux, and the conclusion reached was that the test was unreliable as an initial screening test. However, a further study [26], by Kaul *et al.*, recommended its use for this purpose. They found a sensitivity of 86% which was significantly higher than that of either endoscopy of histology. The test does have its criticisms in that it is semiquantitative [62], involves scanning for a short duration [7] and appears to measure oesophageal exposure to the refluxate. More detailed studies, involving greater numbers of patients and controls, are required in order to evaluate fully the clinical usefulness of the technique.

Kazem [176], in 1972, first used ^{99m}Tc (25 µCi) in 10 ml of water to evaluate oesophageal transit in supine subjects. Serial 0.4 second frames were taken by a gamma camera for a total of 50 seconds. Normal subjects were found to clear the radioisotope out of the oesophagus in less than 15 seconds. The first study to quantify oesophageal transit came from Fisher's group [21] in 1979. They identified the proximal, middle and distal portions of the oesophagus and investigated 62 patients with reflux. Those patients with a manometrically identified motility disorder experienced marked hold-up in transit after both single and multiple swallows, whereas those patients, in whom the manometry was normal, demonstrated normal transit after a single swallow but incomplete emptying after multiple swallows. Similar results from 26 symptomatic reflux patients have been reported [51]. This method of dividing the oesophagus into three regions of interest (Figure 3.9) and

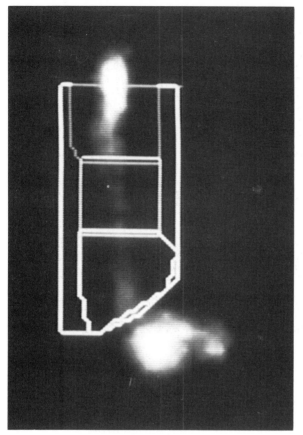

Figure 3.9 Oesophageal scintigram defining the three regions of interest: proximal, middle and distal oesophagus

using a computer for analysis, is widely accepted [20,112], and good correlation between the results from radioisotope scanning and manometry has been reported [175].

Richter *et al.* [177] investigated the relationship of liquid bolus transit to oeso-phageal manometry. They showed that only non-peristaltic contractions and waves of less than 30 mmHg resulted in a delay in transit as shown by scintigraphy. Diffuse oesophageal spasm and non-specific disorders showed an 'incoordinate pattern' and patients with achalasia showed an 'adynamic pattern' [18]. The sensitivity is compar-able to manometry [18]. Doubt as to the test's usefulness as a screening test for oesophageal motor disorders has been raised [178,179].

Liquid bolus transit studies performed in the supine position (to offset the effect of gravity) do not physiologically relate to the real-life situation in the patient's own environment. In order to remedy this problem, the solid bolus oesophageal egg transit (OET) test was developed [20] as a more physiological test. The test is performed with the patient in the erect posture and a 10 ml bolus of poached egg white, labelled with 15–20 MBq of technetium-99m–sodium pertechnetate, is used. The patient is asked to chew the egg and then to swallow it as a single bolus and

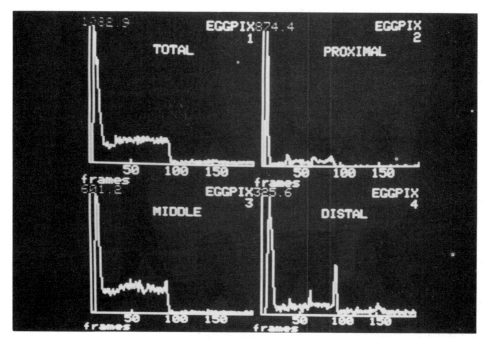

Figure 3.10 Oesophageal egg transit test: activity *vs* time curves for the total, proximal, middle and distal oesophagus. Time is shown on the x axis, and concentration of radioisotope (activity) on the y axis. The delay in transit in the middle third is shown on the horizontal part of the tracing

subsequent swallows are made every 20 seconds. Serial 1-second frames are taken by a gamma camera for a total of 240 seconds (4 minutes), and the data are stored in an on-line computer. Two forms of analyses are generated. First, activity *vs* time curves (Figure 3.10) allow for quantitation of transit times and secondly, the computer, by condensing the serial 1-second frames by row summation, generates an image showing the parameters of time, distance travelled and concentration of radioisotope. This 'condensed image' (Figure 3.11) gives a qualitative and semi-quantitative evaluation of the transit. The total transit time from a cohort of 16 asymptomatic normal subjects was shown to be up to 15 seconds [79], whereas the 55 reflux patients studied experienced a significantly longer transit time (Table 3.7). This test has been compared to oesophageal manometry in a group of 102 reflux patients [28]. There was a significant association between the results of a normal OET and normal manometry on one hand, and abnormal OET and abnormal manometry on the other hand. The predictive value of a positive OET (abnormal) test in detecting abnormal motility was 73% (51/70), and in detecting the specific motor disorders was 100% (10/10). The predictive value of a negative OET (normal) test in detecting normal motility was 69% (22/32), and excluding the specific disorders was 94% (30/32).

Due to the fact that the activity *vs* time curves become extremely complicated with multiple initial swallows and quantitation becomes practically impossible (intricate mathematics [180] makes it theoretically possible), emphasis was laid on the condensed image. Five distinct patterns of transit from the 102 patients were encountered: *normal*; *oscillatory* (propulsion and retropulsion of the egg bolus is seen); *non-*

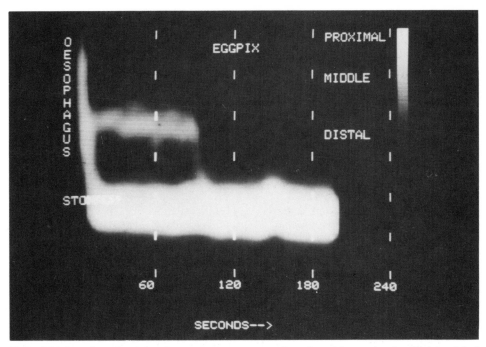

Figure 3.11 Oesophageal egg transit test: computer-generated condensed image showing the 'step-delay' pattern of transit. The segmental hold-up in transit can readily be seen, and this is followed by clearance of the egg bolus into the stomach. (From Eriksen *et al.* [28] with permission)

Table 3.7 Oesophageal egg transit times for patients with reflux oesophagitis and asymptomatic normal subjects

	Oesophageal transit (seconds) in				
	Patients with reflux disease		*Normal subjects*		*P value (Mann–Whitney U-test)*
	Median	*(Range)*	*Median*	*(Range)*	
Total	50.0	(10–240)	9.5	(8–15.7)	<0.001
Proximal third	12.0	(3–240)	4.2	(3–7.5)	<0.001
Middle third	38.0	(6–240)	6.5	(4–9.5)	<0.001
Distal third	35.0	(6–240)	8.2	(6–13.0)	<0.001

From Eriksen *et al.* [79] with permission.

clearance (bolus remains wholly within the oesophagus by the end of 240 seconds of the test's duration); *step-delay* (segmental hold-up in transit is evident in the mid or distal oesophagus); and the *non-specific* pattern [28]. The oscillatory pattern correlated significantly with low amplitude waves (<25 mmHg) and tertiary contractions and identified all six patients with achalasia. The OET test is a useful non-invasive investigation of oesophageal motility, and the authors have advocated its use as a screening test prior to investigation with manometry.

Radioisotope scanning is particularly useful in children, because of the physiological nature of the test, the low radiation dose and convenience [181,182]. Using ^{99m}Tc-labelled fruit juice, and scanning for 30–60 minutes, the test has a sensitivity of 75%. A recent report confirmed these figures [67]. The 'milk scan' [182] allows for prolonged visualization of the oesophagus, and has an advantage of utilizing normally refluxed material (milk). It may also be used to assess any degree of aspiration. In a large study [66] of 90 children, the sensitivity was shown to be 92%. Fisher's reflux index (RI) was used and a positive result was defined as having an RI greater than 2.5%. These authors advocated its use as a screening test for gastro-oesophageal reflux in the paediatric patient.

References

1. Dent, J. Recent views on the pathogenesis of gastro-oesophageal reflux disease. *Baillière's Clin. Gastroenterol.* 1987; **1**: 727–745

2. Zaninotto, G. and DeMeester, T. R. Oesophagus: gastro-oesophageal reflux disease. In: Kumar D., and Gustavsson, S., Eds. *An Illustrated Guide to Gastrointestinal Motility.* Chichester: John Wiley & Sons. 1988: 324–334

3. Richter, J. E. and Castell, D. O. Gastroesophageal reflux. Pathogenesis, diagnosis, and therapy. *Ann. Intern. Med.* 1982; **97**: 93–103

4. Fuchs, K. H., DeMeester, T. R. and Albertucci, M. Specificity and sensitivity of objective diagnosis of gastroesophageal reflux disease. *Surgery* 1987; **102**: 575–580

5. Eriksen, C. A., Cullen, P. T., Sutton, D., Kennedy, N. and Cuschieri, A. Oesophageal dysmotility in symptomatic reflux patients with normal endoscopic and pH profile (Abstract). *Br. J. Surg.* 1989; **76**: 640

6. Nebel, O. T., Fornes, M. F. and Castell, D. O. Symptomatic gastroesophageal reflux: incidence and precipitating factors. *Am. J. Dig. Dis.* 1976; **21**: 953–956

7. Wesdorp, I. C. E. Reflux oesophagitis: a review. *Postgrad. Med. J.* 1986; **62** (Suppl. 2): 43–55

8. Edwards, D. A. W. The anti-reflux mechanism, its disorders and their consequences. *Clin. Gastroenterol.* 1982; **11**: 479–496

9. Dodds, W. J., Hogan, W. T., Helm, J. F. and Dent, J. Pathogenesis of reflux oesophagitis. *Gastroenterology* 1981; **81**: 376–394

10. Nelson, J. B. and Castell, D. O. Reflux oesophagitis: an update. *South. Med. J.* 1985; **78**: 452–457

11. Sondheimer, J. M. Gastroesophageal reflux: update on pathogenesis and diagnosis. *Pediatr. Clin. N. Am.* 1988; **35**: 103–116

12. Dent, J., Holloway, R. H., Toouli, J. and Dodds, W. J. Mechanisms of lower oesophageal sphincter incompetence in patients with symptomatic gastrooesophageal reflux. *Gut* 1988; **29**: 1020–1028

13. Mittal, R. K. and McCallum, R. W. Characteristics and frequency of transient relaxations of the lower oesophageal sphincter in patients with reflux oesophagitis. *Gastroenterology* 1988; **95**: 593–599

14. Spiro, H. M. Esophageal disorders: general considerations. In: Spiro, H. M. Ed. *Clinical Gastroenterology.* New York: Macmillan. 1983: 10–39

15. Young, P. M. F. A simple technique for double-contrast oesophagograms. *Br. J. Radiol.* 1987; **60**: 1021–1022

16. Trenkner, S. W. and Laufer, I. Double-contrast examination: oesophagus, stomach and duodenum. *Clin. Gastroenterol.* 1984; **13**: 41–73

17. De Maria, M., Lagalla, R., Di Gesu, G., Foe, M., Salerno, G. and Guarino, A. Current trends in radiological diagnosis for gastroesophageal reflux. *Rays* 1986: **11**: 81–90

18. Nelson, J. B. and Castell, D. O. Esophageal motility disorders. *Dis. a Month* 1988; **34**: 301–389

19. Fisher, R. S., Malmud, L. S., Roberts, G. S. and Lobis, I. F. Gastroesophageal (GE) scintiscanning to detect and quantitate GE reflux. *Gastroenterology* 1976; **70**: 301–308

20. Cranford, C. A., Sutton, D., Sadek, S. A., Kennedy, N. and Cuschieri, A. A new physiological method of evaluating oesophageal transit. *Br. J. Surg.* 1987; **74**: 411–415

21. Tolin, R. D., Malmud, L. S., Reilley, J. and Fisher, R. S. Esophageal scintigraphy to quantitate esophageal transit time (quantitation of esophageal transit). *Gastroenterology* 1979; **76**: 1402–1408

22. Beauchamp, G. and Duranceau, A. C. Diagnostic and therapeutic esophagoscopy. Indications, contraindications, and complications. *Surg. Clin. N. Am.* 1983; **63**: 801–813

23. Branicki, F. J., Fok, P. J., Choi, T. K. and Wong, J. Benign esophageal disease: diagnostic and therapeutic endoscopy. *Dis. Esophagus* 1988; **1**: 87–102

24. Monnier, P. and Savary, M. Contribution of endoscopy to gastro-oesophageal reflux disease. *Scand. J. Gastroenterol.* 1984; **19** (suppl. 106): 26–44

25. Ismail-Beigi, F., Horton, P. F. and Pope, C. E. Histological consequences of gastroesophageal reflux in man. *Gastroenterology* 1970; **58**: 163–174

26. Kaul, B., Halvorsen, T., Petersen, H., Grette, K. and Myrvold, H. E. Gastroesophageal reflux disease. Scintigraphic, endoscopic, and histologic considerations. *Scand. J. Gastroenterol.* 1986; **21**: 134–138

27. Hopwood, D., Milne, G. and Logan, K. R. Electron microscopic changes in human oesophageal epithelium in oesophagitis. *J. Pathol.* 1979; **129**: 161–166

28. Eriksen, C. A., Holdsworth, R. J., Sutton, D., Kennedy, N. and Cuschieri, A. The solid bolus oesophageal egg transit test: its manometric interpretation and usefulness as a screening test. *Br. J. Surg.* 1987; **74**: 1130–1133

29. Gustavsson, S. and Tucker, R. Manometry. In: Kumar, D. and Gustavsson, S., Eds. *An Illustrated Guide to Gastrointestinal Motility*. Chichester: John Wiley & Sons. 1988: 49–65

30. Castell, D. O. Clinical applications of esophageal manometry. *Dig. Dis. Sci.* 1982; **27**: 769–771

31. Schindlbeck, N. E., Heinrick, G. and Konig, A. Optimal thresholds, sensitivity, and specificity of long-term pH-metry for the detection of gastroesophageal reflux disease. *Gastroenterology* 1987; **93**: 85–90

32. Johnsson, F., Joelsson, B. and Isberg, P-E. Ambulatory 24 hour intraesophageal pH-monitoring in the diagnosis of gastroesophageal reflux disease. *Gut* 1987; **28**: 1145–1150

33. Vitale, G. C., Sadek, S. A., Tulley, F. M. *et al.* Computerised 24-hour esophageal pH monitoring: a new ambulatory technique using radiotelemetry. *J. Lab. Clin. Med.* 1985; **105**: 686–693

34. Bernstein, L. M. and Baker, L. A. A clinical test for esophagitis. *Gastroenterology* 1958; **34**: 760–781

35. Sladen, G. E., Riddell, R. H. and Willoughby, J. M. T. Oesophagoscopy, biopsy, and acid perfusion test in diagnosis of 'reflux oesophagitis'. *Br. Med. J.* 1975; **1**: 71–76

36. Booth, D. J., Kemmerer, W. T. and Skinner, D. B. Acid clearing from the distal oesophagus. *Arch. Surg.* 1968; **96**: 731–734

37. Little, A. G., DeMeester, T. R., Kirchner, P. T., O'Sullivan, G. C. and Skinner, D. B. Pathogenesis of esophagitis in patients with gastroesophageal reflux. *Surgery* 1980; **88**: 101–107

38. Tuttle, S. G. and Grossman, M. I. Detection of gastroesophageal reflux by simultaneous measurement of intraluminal pressure and pH. *Proc. Soc. Exp. Biol. Med.* 1958; **98**: 225–227

39. MacFadyen, U. M. Gastro-oesophageal reflux and chronic bronchopulmonary disease in infancy. In: Milla, P. J. Ed. *Disorders of Gastrointestinal Motility in Childhood*. Chichester: John Wiley & Sons. 1988: 65–70

40. Moosa, A. R. and Skinner, D. B. Gastro-oesophageal reflux and hiatal hernia: a re-evaluation of current data and dogma. *Ann. R. Coll. Surg.* 1976; **58**: 126–132

41. Clarke, J. The lower oesophageal closure mechanism. In: Russel, R. C. G., Ed. *Recent Advances in Surgery*. Edinburgh: Churchill-Livingstone. 1982: 153–168

42. Payne, W. S., Trastek, V. F. and Pairolero, P. C. Reflux esophagitis. *Surg. Clin. N. Am.* 1987; **67**: 443–454

43. DeMeester, T. R., Johnson, L. F., Joseph, G. J., Toscano, M. S., Hall, A. W. and Skinner, D. B. Patterns of gastroesophageal reflux in health and disease. *Ann. Surg.* 1976; **184**: 459–470

44. Johansson, K-E., Ask, P., Boeryd, B., Fransson, S-G. and Tibbling, L. Oesophagitis, signs of reflux, and gastric acid secretion in patients with symptoms of gastro-oesophageal reflux disease. *Scand. J. Gastroenterol.* 1986; **21**: 837–847

45. de Caestecker, J. S., Blackwell, J. N., Brown, J. and Heading, R. C. The oesophagus as a cause of recurrent chest pain: which patients should be investigated and which tests should be used? *Lancet* 1985; **ii**: 1143–1146

46. Anon. Angina and oesophageal disease. *Lancet* 1986; **i**: 191–192

47. Sontag, S. J., Skorodin, M., O'Connell, S. *et al.* Ambulatory 24 hour esophageal pH monitoring in patients with asthma. *Gastroenterology* 1984; **86**: 1261

48. Goodall, R. J. R., Earis, J. E., Cooper, D. N., Berstein, A. and Temple, J. G. Relationship between asthma and gastro-oesophageal reflux. *Thorax* 1981; **36**: 116–121

49. Pellegrini, C., DeMeester, T. R., Johnson, L. and Skinner, D. B. Gastroesophageal reflux and pulmonary aspiration: incidence, functional abnormality, and results of surgical therapy. *Surgery* 1979; **86**: 110–119

50. Wynne, J. W., Ramphal, R. and Hood, C. I. Tracheal mucosal damage after aspiration. A scanning electron microscope study. *Am. Rev. Respir. Dis.* 1981; **124**: 728–732

51. Ferguson, M. K., Ryan, J. W., Little, A. G. and Skinner, D. B. Esophageal emptying and acid neutralization in patients with symptoms of esophageal reflux. *Ann. Surg.* 1985; **201**: 728–734

52. Styles, C. B., Holt, S., Bowes, K. L., Jewell, L. and Hooper, H. R. Gastroesophageal reflux and transit scintigraphy: a comparison with oesophageal biopsy in patients with heartburn. *J. Assoc. Can. Radiol.* 1984; **35**: 124–127

53. Vogten, A. J. M., Jebbink, H. J. A. and Kolkman, J. J. Clinical relevance of ambulatory 24-hour pH-monitoring: Correlation with reflux symptoms and endoscopic abnormalities. *Neth. J. Med.* 1987; **30**: 21–31

54. Csendes, A., Braghetto, I. and Velasco, N. A comparison of three surgical techniques for the treatment of reflux esophagitis: A prospective study. In: DeMeester, T. R. and Skinner, D. B., Eds. *Esophageal disorders: Pathophysiology and Therapy*. New York: Raven Press. 1985: 177–181

55. Henderson, R. D. *The Esophagus: Reflux and primary motor disorders*. Baltimore: Williams & Wilkins. 1980

56. Funch-Jensen, P., Kock, K., Christensen, L. A. *et al.* Microscopic appearance of the esophageal mucosa in a consecutive series of patients submitted to upper endoscopy. Correlation with gastroesophageal reflux symptoms and macroscopic findings. *Scand. J. Gastroenerol.* 1986; **21**: 65–69

57. Jonsell, G. and DeMeester, T. R. Comparison of diagnostic methods for selection of patients for antireflux operations. *Surgery* 1984; **95**: 2–5

58. Moran, J. M., Pihl, C. O., Norton, R. A. and Rheinlander, H. F. The hiatal hernia-reflux complex. Current approaches to correction and evaluation of results. *Am. J. Surg.* 1971; **121**: 403–411

59. DeMeester, T. R., Wang, C-I., Wernley, J. A. *et al.* Technique, indications, and clinical use of 24 hour esophageal pH monitoring. *J. Thorac. Cardiovasc. Surg.* 1980; **79**: 656–670

60. Rokkas, T. and Sladen, G. E. Ambulatory esophageal pH recording in gastroesophageal reflux: relevance to the development of esophagitis. *Am. J. Gastroenterol.* 1988; **83**: 629–632

61. DeDombal, F. T. and Hall, R. The evaluation of medical care from the clinician's point of view: what should we measure and how can we trust our measurements? In: Alperovitch, A., DeDombal, F. T. and Gremy, F., Eds. *The Evaluation of Efficacy of Medical Action*. Amsterdam: North Holland. 1979; 13–29

62. Jamieson, G. G. and Duranceau, A. C. The investigation and classification of reflux disease. In: Jamieson, G. G., Ed. *Surgery of the Oesophagus*. Edinburgh: Churchill Livingstone. 1988: 201–211

63. Wiener, G. J., Richter, J. E., Copper, J. B., Wu, W. C. and Castell, D. O. The symptom index: a clinically important parameter of ambulatory 24-hour esophageal pH monitoring. *Am. J. Gastroenterol.* 1988; **83**: 358–361

64. Vandenplas, Y. and Sacre-Smits, L. Continuous 24-hour esophageal pH monitoring in 285 asymptomatic infants 0–15 months old. *J. Pediatr. Gastroenterol. Nutr.* 1987; **6**: 220–224

65. Brueton, M. J., Clarke, G. S. and Sandhu, B. K. Gastro-oesophageal reflux in infancy. In: Milla, P. J. Ed. *Disorders of Gastrointestinal Motility in Childhood*. Chichester: John Wiley & Sons. 1988: 53–64

66. Gonzalez Fernandez, F., Arguelles Martin, F., Rodriguez de Quesada, B. *et al.* Gastroesophageal scintigraphy: a useful screening test for gastroesophageal reflux. *J. Pediatr. Gastroenterol. Nutr.* 1987; **6**: 217–219

67. Davies, R. P., Morris, L. L. Savage, J. P., Davidson, G. P. and Freeman, J. R. Gastro-oesophageal reflux: the role of imaging in diagnosis and management. *Aust. Radiol.* 1987; **31**: 157–163

68. Berquist, W. E., Rachelefsky, G. S., Kadden, M. *et al.* Gastroesophageal reflux-associated recurrent pneumonia and chronic asthma in children. *Pediatrics* 1981; **68**: 29–35

69. Cotton, P. B. and Shorvon, P. J. Analysis of endoscopy and radiology in the diagnosis, follow-up and treatment of peptic ulcer disease. *Clin. Gastroenterol.* 1984; **13**: 383–403

70. Corazziari, E. and Torsoli, A. Radiology. In: Kumar, D. and Gustavsson, S., Eds. *An Illustrated Guide to Gastrointestinal Motility*. Chichester: John Wiley & Sons. 1988: 49–65

71. Kahrilas, P. J., Dodds, W. J. and Hogan, W. J. Effect of peristaltic dysfunction on esophageal volume clearance. *Gastroenterology* 1988; **94**: 73–80

72. Ott, D. J., Gelfand, D. W. and Wu, W. C. Reflux esophagitis: radiologic and endoscopic correlation. *Radiology* 1979; **130**: 583–588

73. Christiansen, T., Funch-Jensen, P., Jacobsen, N. O. and Thommesen, P. Radiologic quantitation of gastro-oesophageal reflux. *Acta Radiol.* 1987; **28**: 731–734

74. Dodds, W. J. The pathogenesis of gastroesophageal reflux disease. *Am. J. Roentgenol.* 1988; **151**: 49–56

75. Silverstein, B. D. and Pope, C. E. Role of diagnostic tests in esophageal evaluation. *Am. J. Surg.* 1980; **139**: 744–748

76. Dodds, W. J. Current concepts of esophageal motor function: clinical implications for radiology. *Am. J. Roentgenol.* 1977; **128**: 549–561.

77. Eckardt, V. F. Does healing of esophagitis improve esophageal motor function? *Dig. Dis. Sci.* 1988; **33**: 161–165

78. Kahrilas, P. J., Dodds, W. J., Hogan, W. J., Kern, M., Arndorfer, R. C. and Reece, A. Esophageal peristaltic dysfunction in peptic esophagitis. *Gastroenterology* 1986; **91**: 897–904

79. Eriksen, C. A., Sadek, S. A., Cranford, C., Sutton, D., Kennedy, N. and Cuschieri, A. Reflux oesophagitis and oesophageal transit: evidence for a primary oesophageal motor disorder. *Gut* 1988; **29**: 448–452

80. O'Connor, K. W. Diagnosis and treatment of gastroesophageal reflux, or reflux revisited. *Comprehen. Ther.* 1985; **11**: 6–13

81. Lewicki, A. M., Brooks, J. R., Meguid, M., Membreno, A. and Kia, D. pH-tested reflux without hiatus hernia. *Am. J. Roentgenol.* 1978; **130**: 43–45

82. Wolf, B. S. Sliding hiatus hernia: the need for redefinition. *Am. J. Roentgenol.* 1973; **117**: 231–247

83. Condon, R. E. Hiatus hernia and reflux esophagitis. *Clin. Ther.* 1987; **9**: 439–441

84. Baldi, F., Ferrarini, F., Labate, A. M. M. and Barbara, L. Prevalence of esophagitis in patients undergoing routine upper endoscopy: A multicenter survey in Italy. In: DeMeester, T. R. and Skinner, D. B., Eds. *Esophageal Disorders: Pathophysiology and therapy*. New York: Raven Press. 1985: 213–219

85. Berstad, A., Werberg, R., Froyshov Larsen, I., Hoel, B. and Hauer-Jensen, M. Relationship of hiatus hernia to reflux oesophagitis. A prospective study of coincidence, using endoscopy. *Scand. J. Gastroenterol.* 1986; **21**: 55–58

86. Jenkinson, L. R., Norris, T. L. and Watson, A. The manometric features of the lower oesophageal sphincter and oesophageal body, their interaction and relationship to hiatal hernia. *Br. J. Surg.* 1988; **75**: 1241–1242

87. Cleveland, R. H., Kushner, D. C. and Schwartz, A. N. Gastroesophageal reflux in children: results of a standardized fluoroscopic approach. *Am. J. Roentgenol.* 1983; **141**: 53–56

88. Meyers, W. F., Roberts, C. C., Johnson, D. G. and Herbst, J. J. Value of tests for evaluation of gastroesophageal reflux in children. *J. Pediatr. Surg.* 1985; **20**: 515–520

89. Rowen, S. J. and Gyepes, M. T. The 'trumpeting elephant' sign of gastroesophageal reflux. *Radiology* 1988; **167**: 138.

90. Forget, P. P. and Meradsi, M. Contribution of fibreoptic endoscopy to diagnosis and management of children with gastro-oesophageal reflux. *Arch. Dis. Child.* 1987; **57**: 60–68

91. Cotton, P. B. and Williams, C. B. *Practical Gastrointestinal Endoscopy*. Oxford: Blackwell Scientific. 1982

92. de Caestecker, J. S., Blackwell, J. N., Pryde, A. and Heading, R. C. Daytime gastro-oesophageal reflux is important in oesophagitis. *Gut* 1987; **28**: 519–526

93. Tytgat, G. N. J. Non-radiological investigation of the oesophagus. In: Watson, A. and Celestin, C. R., Eds. *Disorders of the Oesophagus: Advances and controversies*, Vol. 3. London: Pitman. 1984: 24–36

94. Brand, D. L., Eastwood, I. R., Martin, D., Carter, W. B. and Pope, C. E. Esophageal symptoms, manometry, and histology before and after antireflux surgery. A long-term follow-up study. *Gastroenterology* 1979; **76**: 1393–1401

95. Baldi, F., Ferrarini, F., Labate, A. M. M. and Barbara, L. Prevalence of esophagitis in patients undergoing routine upper endoscopy: A multicenter survey in Italy. In: DeMeester, T. R. and Skinner, D. B., Eds. *Esophageal Disorders: Pathophysiology and therapy.* New York: Raven Press. 1985: 213–219

96. Weinstein, W. M., Bogoch, E. R. and Bowes, K. L. The normal human esophageal mucosa: a histological reappraisal. *Gastroenterology* 1975; **68**: 40–44

97. Komorowski, R. A. and Leinicke, J. A. Comparison of fibreoptic endoscopy and Quinton tube esophageal biopsy in esophagitis. *Gastrointest. Endosc.* 1978; **24**: 154–155

98. Leape, L. L., Bhan, I. and Ramenofsky, M. L. Esophageal biopsy in the diagnosis of reflux esophagitis. *J. Pediatr. Surg.* 1981; **16**: 379–384

99. Johansson, K-E., Boeryd, B., Fransson, S-G. and Tibbling, L. Oesophageal reflux tests, manometry, endoscopy, biopsy, and radiology in healthy subjects. *Scand. J. Gastroenterol.* 1986; **21**: 399–406

100. Tummala, V., Barwick. K. W., Sontag, S. J., Vlahcevic, R. Z. and McCallum, R. W. The significance of intraepithelial eosinophils in the histologic diagnosis of gastroesophageal reflux. *Am. J. Clin. Pathol.* 1987; **87**: 43–48

101. Schultz, E., Schned, A. R. and Rothstein, R. I. Sensitivity, specificity and bias (letter). *Am. J. Clin. Pathol.* 1988; **89**: 137

102. Mortensen, N. J. McC. and Mackenzie, E. F. D. Accuracy of oesophageal brush cytology: results of a prospective study and multicentre slide exchange. *Br. J. Surg.* 1981; **68**: 513–515

103. Earlam, R. *Clinical Tests of Oesophageal Function.* London: Crosby Lockwood Staples. 1975

104. Duranceau, A. C., Devroede, C., Lafontaine, E. and Jamieson, G. G. Esophageal motility in asymptomatic volunteers. *Surg. Clin. N. Am.* 1983; **63**: 777–786

105. Euler, A. R. and Ament, M. E. Value of esophageal manometric studies in the gastroesophageal reflux of infancy. *Pediatrics* 1977; **59**: 58–61

106. Clouse, R. E. and Staiano, A. Contraction abnormalities of the esophageal body in patients referred for manometry. A new approach to manometric classification. *Dig. Dis. Sci.* 1983; **28**: 784–791

107. Meshkinpour, H., Glick, M. E., Snachez, P. and Tarvin, J. Esophageal manometry. A benefit and cost analysis. *Dig. Dis. Sci.* 1982; **27**: 772–775

108. Pope, C. E. Esophageal motility – who needs it? *Gastroenterology* 1978; **74**: 1337–1338

109. DeMeester, T. R. Surgical management of gastroesophageal reflux. In: Castell, D. O., Wu, W. C. and Ott, D. J., Eds. *Gastroesophageal Reflux Disease.* London: Futura. 1985: 243–280

110. Bancewicz, J., Osugi, H. and Marples, M. Clinical implications of abnormal oesophageal manometry. *Br. J. Surg.* 1987; **74**: 416–419

111. Benjamin, S. B., Richter, J. E., Cordorva, C. M., Knuff, T. E. and Castell, D. O. Prospective manometric evaluation with pharmacologic provocation of patients with suspected esophageal motility dysfunction. *Gastroenterology* 1983; **84**: 893–901

112. Russell, C. O. H., Hill, L. D., Holmes, E. R., Hull, D. A., Gannon, R. and Pope, C. E. Radionuclide transit: A sensitive screening test for esophageal dysfuntion. *Gastroenterology* 1981; **80**: 887–892

113. Castell D. O. The nutcracker esophagus and other primary esophageal motility disorders. In: Castell, D. O., Richter, J. E. and Dalton, C. B., Eds., *Esophageal Motility Testing.* New York: Elsevier. 1987: 130–142

114. Fyke, F. E., Code, C. F. and Schlegel, J. F. The gastroesophageal sphincter in healthy human beings. *Gastroenterologia* 1956; **86**: 135–150

115. Welch, R. W. and Drake, S. T. Normal lower esophageal sphincter pressure: A comparison of rapid v. slow pull through techniques. *Gastroenterology* 1980; **78**: 1446–1451

116. Dent, J. A new technique for continuous sphincter pressure measurement. *Gastroenterology* 1976; **71**: 263–267

117. Nelson, J. L., Wu, W. C., Richter, J. E., Blackwell, J. N., Jones, D. N. and Castell, D. O. What is normal esophageal motility? (Abstract). *Gastroenterology* 1983; **84**; 1258

118. Richter, J. E. Normal values for esophageal manometry. In: Castell, D. O., Richter, J. E. and Dalton, C. B., Eds. *Esophageal Motility Testing.* New York: Elsevier. 1987: 79–90

119. Dent, J., Dodds, W. J., Friedman, R. H. *et al.* Mechanism of gastroesophageal reflux in recumbent asymptomatic human subjects. *J. Clin. Invest.* 1980; **65**: 256–267

120. Dodds, W. J., Dent, J., Hogan, W. T. *et al.* Mechanisms of gastroesophageal reflux in patients with reflux esophagitis. *N. Engl. J. Med.* 1982; **307**: 1547–1552

121. Martin, C. J., Patrikios, J. and Dent, J. Abolition of gas reflux across the canine lower esophageal sphincter (LES) by vagal blockade (Abstract). *Gastroenterology* 1985; **88**: 1491

122. Dent, J., Dodds, W. J., Hogan, W. J. and Toouli, J. Factors that influence induction of gastroesophageal reflux in normal human subjects. *Dig. Dis. Sci.* 1988; **33**: 270–275

123. Meyer, G. W. and Castell, D. O. In support of the clinical usefulness of lower esophageal sphincter pressure determination. *Dig. Dis. Sci.* 1981; **26**: 1028–1031

124. Pope, C. E. Is determination of LES pressure clinically useful? *Dig. Dis. Sci.* 1981; **26**: 1025–1027

125. Ahtaridis, G., Snape, W. J. and Cohen, S. Clinical and manometric findings in benign peptic strictures of the esophagus. *Dig. Dis. Sci.* 1979; **24**: 858–861

126. Klopper, P. J., Bemelman, W. A., van der Hulst, V. P. M. and Dijkhuis, Th. Computerized imaging of gastrointestinal sphincters using eight-channel pressure profiles. *Br. J. Surg.* 1988; **75**: 1234

127. Katz, P. O., Knuff, T. E., Benjamin, S. B. and Castell, D. O. Abnormal esophageal pressures in reflux esophagitis: cause or effect? *Am. J. Gastroenterol.* 1986; **81**: 744–746

128. Barlow, A. P., DeMeester, T. R., Blair, E., Smyrk, T. C., Eypasch, E. P. and Hinder, R. A. The relationship between gastro-oesophageal reflux and oesophageal motility disorders. *Br. J. Surg.* 1988; **75**: 1240–1241

129. Stuart, R. C., Stinson, J., Byrne, P. J. *et al.* The influence of exercise on oesophageal pH and motility in patients with angina-like non-cardiac chest pain. *Br. J. Surg.* 1988; **75**: 1229

130. Baldi, F., Ferrarini, F., Longanesi, A. *et al.* Oesophageal function before, during, and after healing of erosive oesophagitis. *Gut* 1988; **29**: 157–160

131. DeVault, K., Castell, J. and Castell, D. O. How many swallows are required to establish reliable esophageal peristaltic parameters in normal subjects? An on-line computer analysis. *Am. J. Gastroenterol.* 1987; **82**: 754–757

132. Vantrappen, G., Servaes, J., Janssens, J. and Peeters, T. Twenty-four hour esophageal pH- and pressure recording in outpatients. In: Wienbeck, M., *Motility of the Digestive Tract*. New York: Raven Press. 1982: 293–297

133. Peters, L., Maas, L., Petty, D. *et al.* Spontaneous noncardiac chest pain. Evaluation by 24-hour ambulatory esophageal motility and pH monitoring. *Gastroenterology* 1988; **94**: 878–889

134. Janssens, J., Vantrappen, G. and Ghillebert, G. 24-hour recording of esophageal pressure and pH in patients with noncardiac chest pain. *Gastroenterology* 1986; **90**: 1978–1984

135. Eypasch, E. P., DeMeester, T. R., Johansson, K-E., Haplin, M. G. and Hinder, R. A. A new perspective in oesophageal motility: 24-h ambulatory oesophageal manometry. *Br. J. Surg.* 1988; **75**: 1240

136. Helm, J. F., Dodds, W. J. and Hogan, W. T. Salivary responses to esophageal acid in normal subjects and patients with reflux esophagitis. *Gastroenterology* 1987; **93**: 1393–1397

137. de Caestecker, J. S., Pryde, A., and Heading, R. C. Comparison of intravenous edrophonium and oesophageal acid perfusion during oesophageal manometry in patients with non-cardiac chest pain. *Gut* 1988; **29**: 1029–1034

138. Janssens, J. and Vantrappen, G. Angina-like chest pain of oesophageal origin. *Baillière's Clin. Gastroenterol.* 1987; **1**: 843–855

139. Kaul, B., Petersen, H., Grette, K., Myrvold, H. E. and Halvorsen, T. The acid perfusion test in gastroesophageal reflux disease. *Scand. J. Gastroenterol.* 1986; **21**: 93–96

140. Grande, L., Pujol, A., Garcia-Valdecasas, J. C., Fuster, J., Visa, J. and Pera, C. Intraesophageal pH monitoring after breakfast and lunch in gastroesophageal reflux. *J. Clin. Gastroenterol.* 1988; **10**: 373–376

141. Jolley, S. G., Herbst, J. J., Johnson, D. G., Matlak, M. E. and Book, L. S. Esophageal pH monitoring during sleep identifies children with respiratory symptoms from gastroesophageal reflux. *Gastroenterology* 1981; **80**: 1501–1506

142. Spencer, J. Prolonged pH recording in the study of gastro-oesophageal reflux. *Br. J. Surg.* 1969; **56**: 912–914

143. Andreoli, F., Pernice, L. M., Lombardi, P. and Bigiotti, A. 24 hour eosophageal pH-monitoring: recent advances. *Florence J. Surg.* 1983; **1**: 20–24

144. Rokkas, T., Anggiansah, A., Dorrington, L., Owen, W. J. and Sladen, G. E. Accurate positioning of the pH probe in the oesophagus without manometry. *Ital. J. Gastroenterol.* 1987; **19**: 176–178

145. Summers, R. W. The role of computers in the analysis of gut motility. In: Kumar, D. and Gustavsson, S., Eds. *An Illustrated Guide to Gastrointestinal Motility.* Chichester: John Wiley & Sons. 1988: 131–141

145a. Spencer, J. Prolonged pH recording in the study of gastro-oesophageal reflux. *Br. J. Surg.* 1969; **56**: 912–915

146. Johnson, L. F. and DeMeester, T. R. Twenty-four-hour pH monitoring of the distal esophagus: A quantitative measure of gastroesophageal reflux. *Am. J. Gastroenterol.* 1974; **62**: 325–331

146a. Pattrick, F. G. Investigation of gastro-oesophageal reflux in various positions with a two-line pH electrode. *Gut* 1970; **11**: 659–667

147. Schlesinger, P. K., Donahue, P. E., Schmid, B. and Layden, T. J. Limitations of 24-hour intraesophageal pH monitoring in the hospital setting. *Gastroenterology* 1985; **89**: 797–804

148. Ask, P., Edwall, G. and Johansson, K-E. Accuracy and choice of procedures in 24-hour oesophageal pH monitoring with monocrystalline antimony electrodes. *Med. Biol. Eng. Comput.* 1986; **24**: 602–608

149. Colson, R. H., Watson, B. W., Fairclough, P. D. *et al.* An accurate, longterm, pH-sensitive radiopill for ingestion and implantation. *Biotelem. Patient Monit.* 1981; **8**: 213–227

150. Bennett, J. R. pH measurement in the oesophagus. *Baillière's Clin. Gastroenterol.* 1987; **1**: 747–767

151. Evans, D. F. Twenty-four hour ambulatory oesophageal pH monitoring: an update. *Br. J. Surg.* 1987; **74**: 157–161

152. Walker, S. J., Holt, S., Hartley, M. N., Sanderson, C. J. and Stoddart, C. J. The reproducibility of ambulatory pH monitoring. *Br. J. Surg.* 1988; **75**: 1240

153. Johnsson, F. and Joelsson, B. O. Reproducibility of ambulatory oesophageal pH monitoring. *Gut* 1988; **29**: 886–889

154. Branicki, F. J., Evans, D. F., Ogilvie, A. L., Atkinson, M. and Hardcastle, J. D. Ambulatory monitoring of oesophageal pH in reflux oesophagitis using a portable radiotelemetry system. *Gut* 1982; **23**: 992–998

155. Herrera, J. L., Simpson, J. K., Maydonovitch, C. L. and Wong, R. K. H. Comparison of stationary vs ambulatory 24 hr pH monitoring recording systems. *Dig. Dis. Sci.* 1988; **33**: 385–388

156. Bianchi Porro, G. and Pace, F. Comparison of three methods of intraesophageal pH recordings in the diagnosis of gastroesophageal reflux. *Scand. J. Gastroenterol.* 1988; **23**: 743–750

157. Rudolph, I., Herrera, A. F., Stein, G. N. and Roth, J. L. A. Mechanisms of pyrosis. *Am. J. Dig. Dis.* 1971; **16**, 577–588

158. Stanciu, C., Hoare, R. C. and Bennett, J. R. Correlation between manometric and pH tests for gastro-oesophageal reflux. *Gut* 1977; **18**: 536–540

159. Vitale, G. C., Cheadle, W. G., Sadek, S. A., Michel, M. E. and Cuschieri, A. Computerized 24-hour pH monitoring and esophagogastroduodenoscopy in the reflux patient: A comparative study. *Ann. Surg.* 1984; 200: 724–728

160. Sontag, S., Schnell, T., O'Connell, S., Serlovsky, R., Dorociak, P. and Nemchausky, B. Ambulatory 24 hour esophageal pH monitoring in symptomatic gastroesophageal reflux (GER) and Barrett's esophagus (BE) (Abstract). *Gastroenterology* 1985; **88**: 1594

161. Helm, J. F., Dodds, W. J., Riedel, D. R., Teeter, B. C., Hogan, W. J. and Arndorfer, R. C. Determinants of esophageal acid clearance in normal subjects. *Gastroenterology* 1983; **85**: 607–612

162. Helm, J. F., Dodds, W. J., Pelc, L. R., Palmer, D. W., Hogan, W. J. and Teeter, B. C. Effect of esophageal emptying and saliva on clearance of acid from esophagus. *N. Engl. J. Med.* 1984; **310**: 284–288

163. Cheadle, W. G., Vitale, G. C., Sadek, S. A. and Cuschieri, A. Computerized ambulatory esophageal pH monitoring in 50 asymptomatic volunteer subjects. Results and clinical implications. *Am. J. Surg.* 1988; **155**: 503–508

164. Gillen, P., Keeling, P., Byrne, P. J. and Hennessy, T. P. J. Barrett's oesophagus: pH profile. *Br. J. Surg.* 1987; **84**: 774–776

165. Gudmundsson, K., Johnsson, F. and Joelson, B. The time pattern of gastroesophageal reflux. *Scand. J. Gastroenterol.* 1988; **23**: 75–79

166. Lieberman, D. A. 24 hour esophageal pH monitoring before and after medical therapy for reflux esophagitis. *Dig. Dis. Sci.* 1988; **33**: 166–171
167. Fink, S. M. and McCallum, R. W. The role of prolonged esophageal pH monitoring in the diagnosis of gastroesophageal reflux. *J. Am. Med. Assoc.* 1984; **252**: 1160–1164
168. Rokkas, T., Anggiansah, A., Uzoechina, E., Owen, W. J. and Sladen, G. E. The role of shorter than 24-h pH monitoring periods in the diagnosis of gastroesophageal reflux. *Scand. J. Gastroenterol.* 1986; **21**: 614–620
169. Jorgensen, F., Elsborg, L. and Hesse, B. The diagnostic value of computerized short-term oesophageal pH-monitoring in suspected gastro-oesophageal reflux. *Scand. J. Gastroenterol.* 1988; **23**: 363–368
170. Ramenofsky, M. L. and Leape, L. L. Continuous upper oesophageal pH monitoring in infants and children with gastroesophageal reflux. *J. Pediatr. Surg.* 1981; **16**: 374–378
171. Jolley, S. G., Herbst, J. J., Johnson, D. G., Book, L. S. and Matlak, M. E. Patterns for postcibal gastroesophageal reflux in symptomatic infants. *Am. J. Surg.* 1979; **138**: 946–950
172. Evans, D. F., Haynes, J., Jones, J. A., Stower, M. J. and Kapila, L. Ambulatory esophageal pH monitoring in children as an indicator for surgery. *J. Pediatr. Surg.* 1986; **21**: 221–223
173. Ramenofsky, M. L., Powell, R. W. and Curreri, P. W. Gastroesophageal reflux: pH probe-directed therapy. *Ann. Surg.* 1986; **203**: 531–536
174. Gustavsson S. Scintigraphy. In: Kumur, D. and Gustavsson, S., Eds. *An Illustrated Guide to Gastrointestinal Motility.* Chichester: John Wiley & Sons. 1988: 49–65
175. Blackwell, J. N., Hannan, W. J., Adam, R. D. and Heading, R. C. Radionuclide transit studies in the detection of oesophageal dysmotility. *Gut* 1983; **24**: 421–426
176. Kazem, I. A new scintigraphic technique for the study of the esophagus. *Am. J. Roentgenol.* 1972; **115**: 681–688
177. Richter, J. E., Blackwell, J. N., Wu, W. C., Johns, D. N., Cowan, R. J. and Castell, D. O. Relationship of radionuclide liquid bolus transport and oesophageal manometry. *J. Lab. Clin. Med.* 1987; **109**: 217–224
178. Mughal, M. M. M., Marples, M. and Bancewicz, J. Scintigraphic assessment of oesophageal motility: what does it show and how reliable is it? *Gut* 1986; **27**: 946–953
179. Gilchrist, A. M., Laird, J. D. and Ferguson, W. R. What is the significance of the abnormal oesophageal scintigram? *Clin. Radiol.* 1987; **38**: 509–511
180. Nimon, C. C., Lee, T. Y., Britton, K. E., Granowska, M. and Grunewald, S. Practical application of deconvolutional techniques to dynamic studies. In: *Medical Radionuclide Imaging.* International symposium, Heidelberg, 1980. Vienna: I.A.E.A. 1981: 367–388
181. Blumhagen, J. D., Rudd, T. G. and Christine, D. L. Gastroesophageal reflux in children: Radionuclide gastroesophagography. *Am. J. Roentgenol.* 1980; **135**: 1001–1004
182. Heyman, S., Kirkpatrick, J. A., Winter, H. S. and Trevis, S. An improved radionuclide method for the diagnosis of gastroesophageal reflux and aspiration in children (milk scan). *Radiology* 1979; **131**: 479–482

Chapter 4

Barrett's oesophagus

Peter Gillen and Thomas P. J. Hennessy

Introduction

The eponymous term 'Barrett's oesophagus' describes a condition in which a variable portion of the lower oesophagus is lined by columnar epithelium. The condition owes its name to Norman Barrett, the London surgeon who first described it.

When Barrett made his initial observations in 1950 [1], identifying peptic ulceration in columnar epithelium above a hiatus hernia, he drew the wrong conclusions and believed that the condition he described was ulceration in a tubular intrathoracic stomach associated with a congenital short oesophagus. Allison and Johnstone [2] pointed out that the columnar epithelial lining was proximal to the lower oesophageal sphincter, that the musculature was typically oesophageal without peritoneal covering, and that oesophageal mucosal glands could be identified beneath the columnar epithelium. Barrett revised his opinion [3] noting that the segment lined by columnar epithelium exhibited normal oesophageal anatomy in its blood supply and musculature and in its relationship to other mediastinal structures, the only abnormal feature being the unbroken sheets of columnar epithelium. He suggested that the condition should be called 'lower oesophagus lined by columnar epithelium'. More recently an island type of aberrant mucosa has been described [4] in which patches of columnar epithelium can be seen in the distal oesophagus surrounded by squamous epithelium or, alternatively and more frequently, islands of squamous epithelium within areas of aberrant columnar epithelium. Both conditions are correctly described as Barrett's oesophagus. The term 'endobrachyoesophagus' is ponderous, unwieldy and ugly and is best discarded.

The presence of areas of columnar epithelium within the normal squamous mucosa of the proximal oesophagus is a fairly common finding originally described by Schridde in 1904 [5]. These areas are sometimes large enough to be seen by the naked eye. They are usually located in the upper two-thirds of the oesophagus and are often seen in young children. It is likely that such islands of ectopic columnar epithelium are congenital in origin. The oesophagus of the 34 mm embryo is lined by columnar epithelium but by the time the embryo has reached a length of 130 mm, squamous epithelium spreading proximally and distally has replaced the original columnar lining [6]. It has been suggested that premature arrest of this process may cause areas of columnar epithelium to persist. However, these islands are quite unlike Barrett's epithelium which invariably occurs in the distal oesophagus and is associated with inflammatory changes. The occurrence of Barrett's oesophagus in children [7] and in members of the same family [8], including twins [9], and a description of columnar epithelium lining the entire oesophagus [10] are all cited in support of the congenital theory, but in almost all instances a history of heartburn and evidence of reflux was present prior to diagnosis. It is, therefore, now rarely suggested that Barrett's oesophagus might be of congenital origin and the evidence is overwhelming that it is an acquired condition.

Pathogenesis

Acid reflux

The presence of Barrett's epithelium in the lower oesophagus is almost invariably associated with significant gastro-oesophageal reflux [11,12]. On the other hand severe reflux may be present without the development of Barrett's epithelium. In a comparative study of patients with Barrett's oesophagus, oesophagitis without Barrett's epithelium and normal subjects, Iascone *et al.* [13] demonstrated by means of 24-hour pH studies and manometric assessment that patients with Barrett's mucosa had greater acid exposure in the oesophagus than those with oesophagitis only, and both had greater acid exposure in the oesophagus than normal subjects. Similarly, patients with Barrett's mucosa had poorer acid clearance from the oesophagus than patients with oesophagitis or normal subjects. They also found that lower oesophageal sphincter pressure was highest in normal subjects and lowest in patients with Barrett's oesophagus. These authors further demonstrated that the extent of the Barrett's mucosa was inversely related to the lower oesophageal sphincter pressure. Flook and Stoddard [14] also noted that patients with Barrett's oesophagus had hypotensive lower sphincter pressures and had increased acid exposure and poorer clearance than patients with oesophagitis only. Gillen *et al.* [15] studied three groups of patients. One group had oesophagitis, a second group had Barrett's oesophagus and a third group had Barrett's oesophagus with complications such as stricture or ulcer. Both Barrett's groups had greater exposure to acid and poorer clearance than the patients with oesophagitis but there was no significant difference in acid exposure between patients with uncomplicated and complicated Barrett's oesophagus. Lower oesophageal sphincter pressures were not significantly different in the three groups in this study.

Secondary reflux

Patients with scleroderma have severe reflux and poor clearance and the effect of this combination has been demonstrated by Katzha *et al.* In a study involving 24 patients with scleroderma 9 were found to have Barrett's oesophagus [16].

The incidence of gastro-oesophageal reflux after transthoracic myotomy for achalasia has been estimated at 7.7% [17]. The addition of an anti-reflux procedure does not alter the incidence significantly. When myotomy is performed through the abdomen the incidence of reflux is doubled but can be reduced to the same level as transthoracic myotomy by including an anti-reflux procedure. Persistent reflux in combination with the poor clearance associated with achalasia may lead to the development of Barrett's oesophagus [18,19].

Iascone noted that Barrett's patients on the whole were older than patients with oesophagitis and a similar observation was made by Gillen. This suggests the possibility that Barrett's oesophagus might be an end-stage of reflux disease.

There have been several reports of sequential biopsies which have demonstrated proximal extension of columnar epithelium in the oesophagus indicating progression with time [20–22]. This is in accord with Hayward's suggestion [23] that reflux destroys squamous epithelium which is then replaced by columnar cells. Creamer *et al.* [24] have demonstrated that gastric mucosa regenerates at five times the rate of squamous epithelium. This lends some support to the theory that the more rapidly regenerating gastric mucosa might replace the damaged squamous epithelium by a process of 'creeping substitution'.

Borrie and Goldwater [25] had previously observed that the age distribution in Barrett's oesophagus had two peaks, one in a paediatric age group and the other in adults. This finding led them to suggest that the ectopic epithelium in children was congenital in origin and that the adult aberrant mucosa was acquired. The subsequent demonstration of oesophagitis consequent upon reflux in children offers the alternative of an acquired aetiology. Of particular interest is the study by Dahms and Rothstein [11] of 103 children with gastro-oesophageal reflux. Thirteen of these children developed a columnar lining in the lower oesophagus providing strong evidence that, in children as well as adults, Barrett's oesophagus is an aquired condition. The fact that many Barrett's patients have a short history and few symptoms of heartburn or regurgitation does not invalidate the hypothesis that Barrett's oesophagus is an end-stage of reflux disease as the columnar lining of the oesophagus seems to be less sensitive than normal mucosa in its subjective response to acid. Johnson *et al.* [26] used the acid perfusion (Bernstein) test to compare mucosal sensitivity in 15 patients with Barrett's oesophagus and 15 patients with oesophagitis only. All patients with oesophagitis only had a positive test but only 10 of the 15 patients with Barrett's oesophagus experienced pain.

Bile reflux

Duodenogastric reflux of bile has been implicated in the development of oesophagitis. Bremner [27] has postulated that bile reflux may be involved in the development of Barrett's ulcer. In support of this hypothesis he noted the inflammatory response in the lamina propria, the presence of gastritis and the presence of bile in gastric aspirates. Hamilton and Yardley [22] noted that after oesophagogastric anastomoses columnar epithelium covered the anastomosis frequently and in some instances extended proximally beyond the anastomosis. In the cases with proximal extension of columnar epithelium severe reflux was present and the fact that these patients had undergone pyloroplasty made it likely that bile and duodenal secretions were present in the refluxed material.

The importance of acid reflux in the development of Barrett's metaplasia has been clearly shown. It would seem logical to expect that patients with Barrett's oesophagus and severe acid reflux would develop such complications as ulcers and strictures. That this is not always so has been demonstrated in comparative studies of patients with Barrett's oesophagus with and without complications. Arguing that since the columnar epithelium appears to have occurred as a protective event in the face of continuous reflux, Bremner put forward the hypothesis that a further insult other than acid is a necessary stimulus to the development of ulceration. The implication of bile in the pathogenesis of complications of Barrett's oesophagus was reported in a study of complicated and uncomplicated Barrett's patients [28] in which postprandial gastric aspirates from patients with complicated Barrett's oesophagus contained more bile than those with uncomplicated Barrett's oesophagus. These aspirates, despite containing significant concentrations of bile acids on occasions, still possessed a pH of less than 4 – a level which would have recorded such a refluxate as acid on pH monitoring.

Campylobacter pylori in Barrett's oesophagus

Infection with *Campylobacter pylori* may be of significance in gastritis and peptic ulcer disease. The organism is found in the columnar cell lining of the stomach and in areas of gastric metaplasia in the duodenum. While its clinical significance is not clear there is evidence that eradication of the organism lowers the relapse rate in duodenal ulcer patients. *Campylobacter pylori* was found with comparable frequency in the stomachs of patients with Barrett's oesophagus and control subjects by Paull and Yardley [29]. The presence of organisms was associated with active gastritis. The organism was also detected in the columnar cells of the oesophagus in some patients with Barrett's oesophagus but only when present in the stomach. It is not found in the oesophagus of patients with gastro-oesophageal reflux but without Barrett's metaplasia. Patients with *Campylobacter pylori* in the Barrett's epithelium have acute inflammation in the metaplastic epithelium also. However, acute inflammation in Barrett's is regularly observed without the presence of *Campylobacter pylori*. The clinical significance of infection by *Campylobacter pylori* in Barrett's oesophagus is at present unknown.

Experimental studies

Several investigators have examined the pattern of oesophageal mucosal regeneration in canine models. In the experiments of van de Kerckhof and Gahagan [30], healing of artificially created mucosal defects was invariably by squamous epithelium. Hennessy *et al.* [31] studied the effect of free reflux on mucosal repair by establishing a fixed hiatus hernia and ablating the lower oesophageal sphincter by a Wendel cardioplasty. Repair was always by squamous epithelium. In a similar reflux model, Bremner *et al.* [32] stimulated acid secretion by the administration of histamine. Under these conditions of more severe reflux the squamous mucosal defects were replaced by columnar epithelium, thus providing good experimental evidence that the columnar cell-lined oesophagus was an acquired condition. In view of the continuity between gastric mucosa and the new columnar lining of the lower oesophagus, Bremner suggested that proximal migration of columnar epithelium from the stomach to cover squamous defects in the oesophagus created by the injurious effects of reflux might account for the clinical entity of Barrett's oesophagus.

The derivation of the metaplastic epithelium remained speculative, however. Allison and Johnstone [33] had also suggested that it developed from proximal extension of the columnar epithelium lining the gastro-oesophageal junction and the cardia. Alternative suggestions by Trier [34] were an origin from oesophageal mucosal glands or from embryonic remnants of gastric-like columnar cells. Meyer *et al.* [35] noted that, of the different epithelial types found in Barrett's oesophagus, gastric fundus-like epithelium usually lay more distally than the specialized columnar epithelium and postulated that it was derived from the stomach, but that the specialized epithelium arose from the basal cells of the oesophageal squamous epithelium. A possible answer to these speculations has been provided by the canine experiments of Gillen *et al.* [36].

In these studies a fixed hiatus hernia and a Wendel cardioplasty were established in

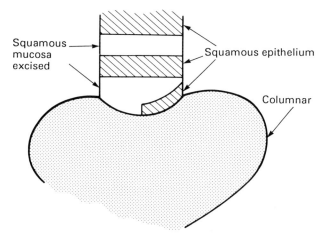

Figure 4.1 Upper and lower circumferential mucosal defects created in the canine oesophagus with a squamous barrier between them. Regeneration by columnar epithelium occurred in a reflux model

three groups of dogs and two circumferential mucosal defects were created in the lower oesophagus with an intervening intact ring of squamous mucosa (Figure 4.1). Acid secretion was stimulated by pentagastrin in one group. The other two groups each had a cholecystogastrostomy so that the refluxate would contain both acid and bile but one was given cimetidine so that bile would be the main constituent of the refluxed material. Regeneration by columnar epithelium occurred above (Plate 1) and below the squamous barrier in the stimulated acid group and below the squamous barrier in the acid and bile group. The columnar epithelium appeared to develop from cuboidal cells lining oesophageal gland ducts. Oesophageal gland ducts possess a squamocuboidal junction at varying levels within the ducts and squamous mucosal injury created by acid or bile reflux may expose these cuboidal and multipotential stem cells to the refluxate in the oesophageal lumen, and establish the milieu for metaplastic regeneration (Plates 2a and 2b). It has been postulated that stem cells in the oesophagus may have the ability to differentiate into a wide variety of cell types in response to the stimulus of luminal reflux and these experiments support this concept. The absence of columnar regeneration with bile reflux alone in these experiments is inconsistent with the clinical reports of Barrett's epithelium developing after total gastrectomy, but in that clinical situation the refluxate contains other constituents of duodenal juice in addition to bile.

Histology

Barrett's mucosa is notable for the variety of epithelial types present. An orderly zonal distribution is often seen. A common pattern displays a distal zone of gastric fundus-like epithelium containing pits, mucous glands, parietal cells and chief cells. More proximally located is a junctional zone with mucous glands and pits but without parietal or chief cells. Most proximally is a zone of specialized columnar epithelium with a villous structure possessing mucous glands, goblet cells and Paneth cells. Above the squamocolumnar junction is normal squamous epithelium. Inflammatory cells are, invariably, present in the columnar epithelium. All three zones described above may be present but sometimes only one or two appear. Specialized

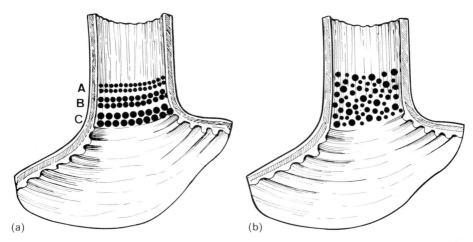

(a)   (b)

Figure 4.2 (a) Zonal distribution of epithelial types in Barrett's oesophagus (A) specialized epithelium, (B) functional epithelium, (C) gastric-type epithelium. (b) Mosaic distribution of epithelial types

epithelium is the most common variety found in adults but a predominance of one epithelial type is not seen in children. Thompson *et al.* [37] have described an epithelium devoid of zonal pattern in which a mosaic of cell gland and architectural types appear (Figure 4.2). There is no correlation between epithelial type and degree of inflammation [38]. Patches of squamous epithelium may be seen within the columnar epithelium. The specialized epithelium was the most prevalent type in the studies reported by Paull *et al.* [39] and was always the most proximally situated. The gastric fundus type was always located most distally. There is usually marked atrophy of this epithelium with fewer and shorter glands. The degree of inflammation present in the columnar epithelium varies from a moderate increase in mononuclear cells and polymorphonuclear cells to the presence of numerous polymorphonuclear cells and mononuclear cells with pit and gland abscesses. Inflammatory changes may occur in the proximal squamous epithelium also with increased thickness of the basal layer and infiltration with polymorphonuclear cells.

Despite the presence of a brush border and microvilli resembling intestinal epithelium, the columnar epithelium of Barrett's oesophagus has little or no absorptive capacity. After perfusion with a micellar lipid, Trier [40] found no evidence of absorption. Some secretory activity is present, although acid secretion by parietal cells is minimal. The goblet cells secrete mucus. The enzymes pepsin and pepsinogen are secreted by chief cells in Barrett's mucosa but, although earlier reports suggested the production of gastrin [41,42], subsequent studies did not confirm this [43,44]. The activity of the enzyme β-glucuronidase in Barrett's epithelium is similar to that of intestinal mucosa, a finding similar to neoplastic epithelium. β-Galactosidase activity is less than that found in intestinal epithelium [45]. This dissimilarity between the enzyme activity of Barrett's mucosa and fundic and intestinal mucosa supports the metaplastic nature of Barrett's epithelium. A wide variety of mucins has been identified including gastric-type neutral mucins, small, intestinal-type, acid, non-sulphated mucins and colonic-type, acid, sulphated mucins. Attempts to link a preponderance of one type of mucin to the development of adenocarcinoma have been described recently by other workers [46–48].

Endoscopic appearance

The endoscopic appearances of Barrett's mucosa are distinctive and have been well described by Savary and Miller [49]. The columnar lining in the oesophagus has a tubular structure with an absence of the folds characteristic of the intrathoracic

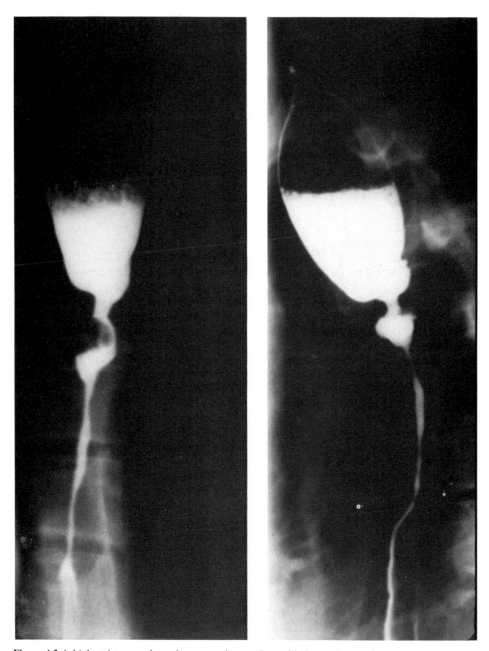

Figure 4.3 A high stricture and an ulcer crater in a patient with Barrett's oesophagus

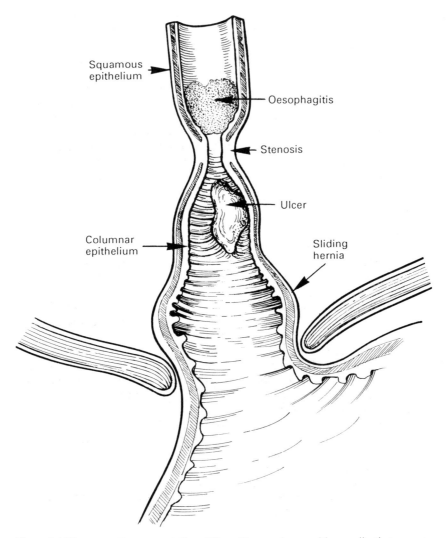

Figure 4.4 Diagrammatic representation of Barrett's oesophagus with complications

stomach. The red colour of the mucosa is in marked contrast to the pale appearance of the squamous epithelium above and is a deeper red than that seen in the lining of the stomach. The mucosa is sufficiently transparent for the submucous vessels to be detected underneath. Patches of squamous epithelium may sometimes be scattered throughout the ectopic epithelium. While the transition from squamous to columnar epithelium is easily identified the line of junction may be quite irregular with tongues of ectopic mucosa extending upwards. Where doubt exists as to which type of epithelium is present a spray of Lugol's iodine solution can resolve the issue [50]. The glycogen in squamous epithelium stains black with Lugol's solution but the columnar epithelium is unaffected. The iodine solution can be applied to the mucosa via a sprayer passed down the biopsy channel of the endoscope [51].

Inflammatory changes may be seen above the squamocolumnar junction. The mucosa is reddened and oedematous and shallow and superficial linear ulcers may be seen. The inflamed mucosa may be covered with patches of necrotic pseudo-membrane which on removal leaves a raw bleeding surface.

A Barrett's ulcer is a deep crater of varying size often lying posteriorly in the columnar lined segment of the oesophagus (Plate 3). The configuration of the ulcer is longitudinal and it may be 3 or 4 cm in diameter. Varying degrees of narrowing may be detected at the squamocolumnar junction. These strictures are usually short but some are several centimetres in vertical height (Figure 4.3). The squamocolumnar junction is located at the distal end of the stricture (Figure 4.4). The cardia can be identified endoscopically and is located above the diaphragm when a sliding hernia is present. However, for accurate diagnosis of Barrett's oesophagus the high pressure zone should be identified manometrically. Distal to the cardia the tubular outline of the oesophagus disappears and gastric folds can be seen.

Clinical features

The presence of Barrett's epithelium does not give rise to symptoms as such and so patients with Barrett's mucosa without complications may be entirely symptom free. The majority, however, are likely to present with symptoms of gastro-oesophageal reflux such as heartburn or regurgitation. If a stricture develops at the squamocolumnar junction dysphagia may occur. Regurgitation of bitter tasting gastric secretions may be a prominent feature. The characteristic ulcer described by Barrett occurs in the columnar epithelium and may give rise to a severe boring pain radiating to the back. These ulcers exhibit all the features of a gastric ulcer and may penetrate through the wall of the oesophagus or perforate into the mediastinum with cata-strophic consequences. The patient becomes shocked with rapid pulse, hypotension and dyspnoea. Severe life-threatening haemorrhage may also occur in Barrett's ulcer. Perforation into the aorta with uncontrollable and rapidly fatal haemorrhage has also been described. It has been suggested that Barrett's ulcer, although identified in the portion of the oesophagus lined by columnar epithelium, actually develops by erosion of a patch of squamous epithelium. In support of this contention clumps of squamous cells have been demonstrated in and around the ulcer. It is significant, however, that such ulcers are not seen above the squamocolumnar junction.

Diagnosis

Radiological

The classic radiological description of Barrett's oesophagus includes a highly placed stricture with or without an ulcer distal to it and a sliding hiatus hernia. Robbins *et al.* [52] have pointed out that Barrett's strictures are more common in the distal oesophagus. Fluoroscopic evidence of gastro-oesophageal reflux can be demon-strated in 50% of patients. Using a double contrast technique Levine *et al.* [53] identified a reticular pattern in the mucosa distal to the stricture. They suggest that the barium-filled grooves and crevices forming this reticular pattern correspond to the villous structure of the specialized metaplastic epithelium of Barrett's oeso-phagus. Although not invariably present, Levine believes that when this pattern can be identified in the mucosa it is pathognomonic of Barrett's oesophagus.

Barrett [54] described a variety of strictures ranging from a narrow submucous band of fibrous tissue to an invasive transmural type which destroys the muscle coat and becomes adherent to other structures in the mediastinum. Pierce and Creamer [55] noted that in five out of nine patients examined radiologically variations in the calibre of the constricting ring occurred during swallowing. However, despite these changes in dimension there was no corresponding change in intraluminal pressure. Nevertheless, they concluded that some of the strictures represented muscular spasm rather than fibrous constriction. The reversible nature of such spastic strictures was demonstrated by Pierce who found complete disappearance of one stricture and considerable improvement in another after surgical correction of the reflux. Similar satisfactory results were reported by Seaman and Wylie [56]. Although most strictures, fibrous or otherwise, are short they can be several centimetres in length.

Manometry

Peristalsis is usually normal in Barrett's oesophagus. Distal oesophageal sphincter pressures are low and there is an inverse relationship between the lower sphincter pressure and the extent of the columnar epithelium. When a hiatus hernia is present two pressure peaks and an intervening plateau may be observed with double respiratory reversal. Although there is no characteristic dysmotility pattern reflux may be accompanied by simultaneous repetitive contractions, tertiary contractions, failed peristaltic waves and complete aperistalsis. As stated above, Iascone et al. [13] claimed that there was a linear relationship between the extent of the columnar epithelium and the amount of reduction of lower sphincter pressure. The authors' own investigations did not confirm this relationship. However, the presence of a hypotensive sphincter has been confirmed by several other authors. Flook and Stoddart [14] noted hypotensive lower sphincters in patients with Barrett's oeso-phagus. Wesdorp et al. [57] failed to detect a lower sphincter in eight of nine patients with a columnar lined oesophagus and in half of the cases of Heitmann et al. [58] the sphincter could not be identified. On the other hand, Gillen et al. [15] found no significant difference between lower oesophageal sphincter pressures measured in patients with oesophagitis, uncomplicated Barrett's oesophagus and complicated Barrett's oesophagus. The findings of Patel et al. [59] were similar. There is considerable overlap between sphincter pressures in normal subjects and patients with reflux and it is likely that similar overlap exists between normal subjects and patients with Barrett's oesophagus. This variation and the short duration of the recordings probably accounts for the disparate results reported and it seems that, while the sphincter pressure is likely to be low, it can be normal in many patients.

pH profile of Barrett's oesophagus

While there is no characteristic reflux pattern in Barrett's oesophagus these patients tend to have poorer clearance and more prolonged exposure to acid than patients with oesophagitis. Although the total number of reflux episodes may be similar in both groups the percentage time during which the pH in the lower oesophagus is less than 4 is greater in patients with Barrett's oesophagus as is the number of reflux episodes which last longer than 5 minutes. It is noteworthy that DeMeester et al. [60] have demonstrated prolonged oesophageal transit times in patients with hiatal hernia although no motility disorder in the oesophageal body could be demonstrated. This observation may be significant in patients with Barrett's oesophagus most of whom have a coexisting hiatus hernia. However, patients with benign oesophageal stricture

Table 4.1 Difference between the pH profiles of patients with oesophagitis and those with either complicated or uncomplicated Barrett's oesophagitis*

	Complicated Barrett's	Uncomplicated Barrett's	Oesophagitis
Total number of reflux episodes	53(5–195)	44(8–133)	20[†] (1–62)
Percentage time pH ≤ 4	30.3(6.4–75.2)	32.3(2.8–73.8)	7.1[‡] (1.0–16.8)
Number of reflux episodes lasting > 5 min	9(3–24)	11(0–25)	4[†] (0–8)

* There is a significant difference between patients with oesophagitis and with Barrett's oesophagitis; there is no significant difference between complicated and uncomplicated Barrett's oesophagitis.
The median and range values are given. Wilcoxon rank sum test: [†] $P < 0.01$; [‡] $P < 0.001$.

but without Barrett's epithelium may have a pattern of prolonged exposure and poor clearance similar to that of Barrett's oesophagus. This reflux pattern was demonstrated by Iascone et al. [13] and confirmed by Gillen et al. [15] who also found that there was no significant difference between reflux patterns in uncomplicated and complicated Barrett's suggesting the possibility of some further mucosal injury to account for the latter (Table 4.1).

Potential difference

Transmural potential difference has been used to identify Barrett's mucosa [61]. Normal squamous epithelium has a potential difference (PD) of -15 ± 5 MV [62]. Columnar epithelium has a PD of greater than -25 MV. However, the ability of this technique to identify accurately the squamocolumnar junction is confounded in the presence of specialized Barrett's epithelium which possesses the same functional properties as squamous epithelium. Thus only the level of junctional or fundic epithelium can be defined clearly. A further complication is the presence of oesophagitis which lowers the PD to -5 MV because of increased mucosal permeability and impaired sodium transport [63].

Scintigraphy
Sodium pertechnetate is actively concentrated by gastric mucosa wherever located. Selective uptake of ^{99m}Tc-pertechnetate by gastric-like mucosa has been used to identify ectopic columnar epithelium in Barrett's oesophagus as well as in Meckel's diverticulum. The fasting patient is given 5 mCi ^{99m}Tc-pertechnetate intravenously. As salivary glands secrete technetium the patient is instructed not to swallow and any secretion of saliva is aspirated using a dental aspirator. The isotope is visualized by scintigraphy. In a normal scan the isotope is concentrated in the stomach and does not appear above the oesophagogastric junction. When a columnar-lined lower oesophagus is present there is significant concentration of isotope in the lower oesophagus. The position of the oesophagogastric junction is confirmed by barium swallow. The technique is performed with the patient upright to minimize reflux. Berquist et al. [64] claimed that the technique was sufficiently reliable to eliminate the need for biopsy confirmation of ectopic mucosa. This view would not be shared by the majority of investigators and Bremner [65] has reported disappointing results.

Endoscopy
The appearance of the ectopic mucosa at endoscopy has been described above. The deep red colour of the columnar epithelium may be seen as an unbroken circumferential lining of the lower oesophagus, as flame-shaped or tongue-shaped upward

extensions from the cardia, or as a patchy change interspersed with fragments of squamous epithelium (Plate 4). Inflammatory changes may be present giving rise to a congested oedematous mucosa with erosions and necrotic areas. Such inflammatory changes may create diagnostic confusion and in these circumstances Lugol's solution may help to differentiate darkly staining squamous epithelium from the unstained columnar mucosa. Toluidine blue may also be used to improve the detection of Barrett's oesophagus. The dye stains the columnar epithelium dark blue and Chobanian *et al.* [66] obtained a higher diagnostic yield with toluidine blue than could be established by endoscopy alone. Biopsy is essential for accurate diagnosis and several specimens should be obtained at varying levels above the lower oesophageal sphincter. The sphincter may be identifiable endoscopically but ideally its level should be established by manometry. The presence of columnar epithelium to a level at least 3 cm above the oesophagogastric junction should be identified in order to establish the diagnosis of Barrett's oesophagus. If the specialized intestinal type columnar epithelium can be identified the diagnosis is unequivocal. Barrett's ulcer is usually found just proximal to the squamocolumnar junction and commonly high in the oesophagus although sometimes they are present in the distal few centimetres. Occasionally there may be more than one ulcer. Strictures are found at the squamocolumnar junction and are infiltrated with inflammatory cells. The squamous epithelium located proximally is of the normal grey appearance, but may exhibit the superficial erosions of oesophagitis.

There are two main pitfalls in endoscopic diagnosis. The normal gastro-oesophageal junction may have a somewhat irregular outline referred to as the Z-line. Small papillary projections measuring 1–1.5 cm may extend upwards from this line into the oesophagus and do not constitute Barrett's epithelium. Hence the emphasis by Skinner *et al.* [67] on the need for a 3 cm projection of columnar epithelium into the oesophagus to establish the diagnosis.

The presence of a hiatus hernia may also cause confusion and a biopsy from fundic epithelium may precipitate a diagnostic error. The appearance of rugal folds in the herniated gastric pouch is quite different from the tubular appearance of true oesophagus and the hernia will slide back and forth across the diaphragm with respiration making recognition easy [68].

Epidemiology

The incidence of Barrett's oesophagus in the general population is not known with certainty as many patients are asymptomatic. A diagnosis of Barrett's oesophagus was made in 4.5% of symptomatic patients by Borrie and Goldwater [25]. Other series record a similar incidence. Age distribution is wide ranging from the neonatal age group to the ninth decade. The condition has not been identified in the fetus. The existence of a bimodal age incidence has already been mentioned; peak age distributions are from 0 to 15 years and from 48 to 80 years. The condition occurs most frequently in males with a male:female ratio of 3:1. A familial incidence was reported by Everhart *et al.* [8] in which a father aged 41 and his two sons aged 14 and 16 had a columnar epithelium lining in the lower oesophagus suggesting an autosomal dominant inheritance pattern. There are reports of the condition affecting twins [9], one of whom presented with an adenocarcinoma. The incidence of Barrett's oesophagus in any particular series will vary with the care and thoroughness employed in seeking the diagnosis, particularly in the island type of Barrett's which may be so easily overlooked and also with the criteria used for diagnosis such as the presence of specialized epithelium and the extent of columnar epithelium proximal to the gastro-oesophageal junction which should be at least 3 cm.

Neoplastic potential

The clinical importance of Barrett's oesophagus is related not only to its association with ulceration and stricture formation but also to its established malignant potential. Dysplastic change is common. The dysplasia may be slight or marked and carcinoma *in situ* may be present. While dysplastic change is indicative of high malignant potential the natural history of its progression to frank malignancy is not known [69]. Endoscopic surveillance in patients with dysplasia is warranted and should be accompanied by biopsy and brush cytology. Other methods of monitoring malignant potential which may be clinically useful are labelling of columnar cells with tritiated thymidine [70] and estimation of the size of the proliferative zone [71]. Estimation of the lysozomal enzyme β-glucuronidase which demonstrates increased activity in neoplastic tissues may also be useful [45].

The development of a squamous cell carcinoma in association with Barrett's oesophagus has been described [72]. The authors suggest that this polypoid tumour may have been responsible for the ectopic epithelial change by mechanical irritation, and erosion of the normal mucosa and subsequent replacement by columnar epithelium. They acknowledge the contributory effect of reflux from the associated hiatus hernia. Polyp formation has also been reported. Mucosal projections are sometimes seen at the squamocolumnar junction in patients with ectopic oesophageal mucosa. The polyp reported by Eller *et al.* [73] was attached by a stalk to the squamocolumnar junction which was located at 26 cm from the incisor teeth. The development of such tumours, however, is rare and coincidental and the real risk is the development of adenocarcinoma. This risk is difficult to estimate. A tendency to confuse prevalence with incidence makes quantitation more difficult. In a review of the Mayo Clinic records of patients with Barrett's oesophagus, Cameron *et al.* [74] found that of the 122 patients in the series 15% had a simultaneous diagnosis of adenocarcinoma and Barrett's oesophagus. Of the remaining 104 patients only two developed an adenocarcinoma during an 8.5 year follow-up. In the series of Spechler *et al.* [75] 2 patients out of 105 developed an adenocarcinoma over a mean follow-up period of 3.3 years. The total length of follow-up for these 105 patients was 350 person-years. Thus the incidence of adenocarcinoma was 1 per 175 person-years. The expected incidence of carcinoma in these patients was 0.13 cases per 1000 person-years so there was a 42.5-fold increase in the incidence of adenocarcinoma in patients with Barrett's oesophagus. However, the authors consider that this represents a low risk in absolute terms. They further suggest that the risk from Barrett's oesophagus alone may be even less because 85% of their patients gave a history of cigarette smoking and 76% were addicted to alcohol. However, while both of these are known risk factors for squamous carcinoma of the oesophagus, their relevance to adeno-carcinoma is less certain.

Primary adenocarcinoma of the oesophagus is a rare tumour. Three different types have been described: adenocarcinoma type ordinaire, adenoacanthoma and adenoid cystic carcinoma sometimes found in the mid-oesophagus. These tumours arise in an otherwise normal oesophagus and are surrounded by normal squamous epithelium. Adenocarcinoma of the cardia extending into the lower oesophagus is relatively common. The distinction between such a tumour and one arising in Barrett's epithelium may be difficult or impossible to make. Kalich *et al.* [76] in a comparative study between the two concluded that tumours of the cardia had a higher male : female ratio and were associated with a higher consumption of tobacco and alcohol whereas Barrett's tumours had a higher frequency of associated hiatus hernia. However, in many series of Barrett's oesophagus consumption of tobacco and alcohol is also high. Griffin and Sweeney [77] found an association between the presence of serotonin in biopsy specimens and adenocarcinoma arising in Barrett's oesophagus. Serotonin was found in the endocrine cells of Barrett's adenocarcinoma in 31% of cases but in only 3.8% of patients with non-Barrett's tumours. Identification of a Barrett's tumour depends on evidence of Barrett's epithelium adjacent to the tumour. With progression of the neoplasm such evidence may be obliterated. Consequently, the findings of Smith *et al.* [78] who reported 58% of adenocarcinomas of the lower oesophagus as showing evidence of Barrett's mucosa and Thompson *et al.* [37] who identified 44% of gastro-oesophageal junction tumours as having arisen in Barrett's epithelium is probably an underestimate.

Adenocarcinoma arising in Barrett's epithelium is usually a large flat ulcerated, often poorly differentiated, deeply infiltrating tumour. A papillary structure is fairly common. Signet ring and mucinous types have also been described. The tumour predominantly occurs in white male patients in their sixth or seventh decade. Many patients give no history of pre-existing reflux symptoms. Survival following resection in Smith's series was 23 months ± 5 but only 3 of his 26 patients had a disease-free interval greater than 2 years.

The development of a tumour in a patient with Barrett's oesophagus is accompanied by the symptoms of weight loss and dysphagia. The mean duration of symptoms referable to the tumour was 5.3 ± 3 (s.d.) months in Smith's series. Haggitt *et al.* [79] reported that 10 of 12 patients with Barrett's carcinoma had symptoms of reflux oesophagitis. Skinner *et al.* [80] found that patients with Barrett's carcinoma had a lower frequency of reflux symptons than patients with Barrett's mucosa who did not have a tumour. The presence of columnar metaplasia in the lower oesophagus appears in many instances to render the oesophagus insensitive to acid so that symptoms are minimal or absent. It has been suggested that such insensitivity may predispose to stricture formation. Perhaps it may also allow asymptomatic progression to carcinoma.

Dysplasia

The development of dysplasia in association with Barrett's epithelium is considered to be of ominous significance and in need of careful evaluation. Dysplasia can be defined as an unequivocal neoplastic alteration in the columnar epithelium. The dysplastic change is graded from negative, through low grade and high grade, the latter including carcinoma *in situ*. In the classification of Skinner *et al.* [80] actively regenerating epithelium was regarded as negative for dysplasia. Changes probably arising from active inflammation were classified as indefinite, probably negative. Enlarged hyperchromatic nuclei with mucin depletion are considered unequivocally dysplastic. In low grade dysplasia these abnormal nuclei are confined to the base of the cell. Cells exhibiting high grade dysplasia have abnormal nuclei in their upper poles. Dysplasia is particularly associated with specialized intestinal-type epithelium (Plate 5).

In the series of patients of Spechler *et al.* [75], two patients with Barrett's oesophagus developed carcinoma during their period of follow-up and eight had a simultaneous diagnosis of Barrett's oesophagus and adenocarcinoma. Seven of these ten patients had high-grade dysplasia. The two patients who developed carcinoma during follow-up were cigarette smokers and alcoholics. One progressed from low grade to high grade dysplasia over a period of 2 years.

Skinner et al. [80] noted regression or absence of progression of dysplasia in eight patients who had successful anti-reflux surgery. On the other hand they associated persistence of or progression of dysplasia with failed anti-reflux surgery and continuation of smoking. He advocated regular endoscopic monitoring with biopsy and suggests that resection should be considered for patients with high-grade dysplasia. Even in these circumstances operative intervention may be too late and many patients who have undergone resection because of high-grade dysplasia found on biopsy already had invasive carcinoma. The presence of high-grade dysplasia unquestionably places the patient in a high-risk category but direct progression from low-grade dysplasia or from ectopic epithelium without dysplasia to invasive cancer may also occur. At present there is no mechanism by which the degree of risk may be quantified.

The interpretation of dysplastic change depends greatly on subjective analysis and biopsy material may not be representative. Determination of cellular DNA content by flow cytometry may provide more objective assessment. Recent flow cytometry studies of biopsy specimens from patients with adenocarcinoma in Barrett's oesophagus and patients with and without dysplasia have been reported [81,82]. A high proportion but not all patients with invasive tumour or dysplasia had aneuploidy. On the other hand a number of patients with aneuploidy had neither a tumour nor dysplasia. However, these latter patients may represent a subject in which DNA abnormalities may be a useful marker for the development of malignancy. Further studies in flow cytometry are needed to establish its usefulness.

Mucin histochemistry

In the stomach incomplete metaplasia with a predominance of sulphomucin is strongly associated with carcinoma. Jass [48] found sulphomucin staining in Barrett's oesophagus more frequently in well differentiated but not in poorly differentiated carcinomas. Peuchmaur [83] noted a predominance of sulphated mucin in 35% of patients and considered it a form of low-grade dysplasia. Haggitt et al. [84], however, were unable to show a correlation between either the presence or predominance of sulphomucin and dysplasia or carcinoma. Rothery et al. [38] found that incomplete intestinal metaplasia and sulphomucin secretion are common features of the columnar-lined oesophagus but not sufficiently discriminating to detect a subgroup of patients at risk of malignant change.

Another approach showing some promise is the measurement of ornithine decarboxylase levels in Barrett's mucosa. Ornithine decarboxylase is the first enzyme in polyamine synthesis. Polyamines have an essential role in cell proliferation and differentiation. Garewal et al. [85] have shown that ornithine decarboxylase activity is increased in Barrett's epithelium when compared to other upper gastrointestinal columnar epithelia. Garewal et al. [86] have demonstrated increased activity of the enzyme in dysplastic Barrett's epithelium when compard with non-dysplastic Barrett's epithelium. Of even greater interest is the fact that growth of cells derived from Barrett's epithelium is inhibited by the enzyme inhibitor difluoromethylornithine [87].

Colorectal neoplasms and Barrett's oesophagus

It has been suggested that patients with Barrett's oesophagus have an increased risk of developing a colonic carcinoma [88]. Tripp *et al.* [89], in a prospective colonoscopic study of 36 patients with Barrett's oesophagus, were unable to find a malignant tumour. Adenomas were found in 33% of patients but this was comparable to the 38% yield of adenomas in a series of colonoscopies undertaken for routine clinical reasons. Ramage [90] and Cooper and Babazet [91] found patients with colon cancer in association with Barrett's oesophagus but concluded that the risk was not great enough to warrant automatic colonoscopic screening of all patients with Barrett's oesophagus.

Treatment of Barrett's oesophagus

The objective in treating Barrett's oesophagus is to alleviate reflux symptoms, if present, to prevent the development of complications such as ulcer or stricture and to minimize the risk of malignant change. A further aim is to induce regression of the metaplastic epithelium.

General measures appropriate to the treatment of any patient with gastro-oesophageal reflux are indicated. They include weight reduction in the overweight individual, abstinence from tobacco and alcohol and the exclusion from the diet of substances inhibitory to lower sphincter tone such as chocolate.

Successful medical treatment has been reported following the use of carbenoxolone, cimetidine and bethanechol. Symptoms were relieved and ulcers healed. The patient reported by Thompson and Barr [92] had a Barrett's ulcer which healed with carbenoxolone but recurred with cessation of treatment. Cimetidine was then substituted with greater effect.

Kothari *et al.* [93] treated patients with complicated Barrett's oesophagus with cimetidine. Healing of Barrett's ulcers occurred. Wesdorp *et al.* [57] maintained nine patients on cimetidine for 2 years. Symptoms were relieved within a few months in five patients and ulcers healed in two. Two-thirds of ulcers will usually heal with standard doses of H_2-receptor antagonists, and others with higher doses [93a]. If H_2-receptor antagonists are ineffective, omeprazole will often induce satisfactory healing [93a, 93b]. These patients with hypotensive lower oesophageal sphincters were treated with bethanechol by Everhart and Humphries [94]. In two patients Barrett's ulcers healed completely and partial healing was achieved in one. The long duration of medical treatment may compromise patient compliance particularly when symptoms have been relieved. Ulceration tends to recur when treatment is discontinued. Strictures are not affected by medical treatment and bougienage must be added. However, medical management may be the only option available in elderly unfit patients. Carbenoxolone must be used with caution in these patients. The major problem with medical treatment is the lesser likelihood of complete control of reflux. Perhaps newer drugs such as the proton pump inhibitor omeprazole may in combination with Gaviscon enhance medical control of reflux. Cisapride may also be of value in improving acid clearance from the lower oesophagus. The almost complete abolition of reflux which can be achieved by successful anti-reflux surgery (Figure 4.5) ensures better control of symptoms, reduces oesophagitis and allows ulcers to heal. Strictures may need to be dilated although Seaman and Wyllie [56] reported resolution of a stricture after hiatal hernia repair. With control of reflux the proximal progression of aberrant epithelium is arrested and regression of columnar

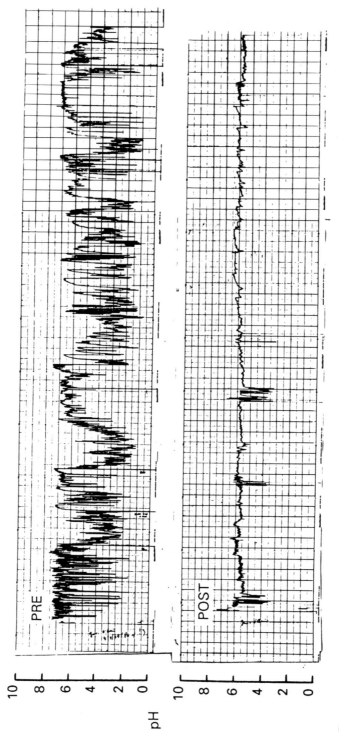

Figure 4.5 The dramatic change in pH profile after anti-reflux surgery

epithelium may occur. Brand *et al.* [95] reported regression of columnar epithelium in four out of ten patients undergoing anti-reflux surgery. They also noted that although most patients in the group obtained relief of symptoms three patients in whom columnar epithelium persisted had more postoperative reflux than those in whom regression of Barrett's epithelium took place. The authors' criteria for regression were based on assessment of the level of the squamocolumnar junction pre- and postoperatively. Alterations in the anatomy brought about by the surgery may make such measurements difficult. Skinner *et al.* [67] observed a different kind of regression in which islands of squamous epithelium spread over the residual columnar epithelium. They also noted regression of columnar epithelium until the ectopic mucosa was completely replaced by the distally progressing new squamous epithelium. Reappearance of normal mucosa in patches offers more convincing evidence of regression. One report exists of regression to squamous epithelium on medical treatment [96]. The regimen included bethanechol, cimetidine, Gaviscon and antacids. The author also noted resolution of dysplastic change. Other authors [65,97,98] have failed to observe regression after anti-reflux surgery but no objective evidence of control of reflux by postoperative pH studies was available in most of these patients.

The most frequently chosen anti-reflux procedure is the Nissen fundoplication. Successful regression of columnar epithelium has also been recorded after the Hill posterior gastropexy. Some reflux usually occurs after the Belsey Mark IV operation and although it is effective in relieving symptoms of gastro-oesophageal reflux it may not be an appropriate procedure for Barrett's oesophagus. Few comparative studies have been carried out on the effectiveness of the available anti-reflux procedures.

DeMeester *et al.* [99] compared the results of Nissen fundoplication, Hill posterior gastropexy and the Belsey Mark IV procedure and concluded that the Nissen fundoplication was superior to the others. Stuart *et al.* [100] found the Nissen fundoplication superior to the Angelchik prosthesis. At present the Nissen fundoplication would appear to be the procedure of choice (Table 4.2).

To what extent successful anti-reflux surgery can reduce the risk of adenocarcinoma is unknown. When reflux continues after surgery the risk undoubtedly remains. In one of Brand's cases where postoperative reflux was confirmed by pH monitoring an adenocarcinoma developed 4 years later.

Table 4.2 An outline treatment plan for patients with Barrett's oesophagus

	Elderly or unfit patients	*Young fit patients*
Barrett's oesophagus with or without symptoms	1. Postural measures, weight loss 2. H$_2$-receptor antagonists 3. Alginate	Anti-reflux surgery
Barrett's oesophagus with stricture	Dilatation and 1–3 above	Dilatation plus anti-reflux surgery
Barrett's oesophagus with ulcer	1–3 above	Anti-reflux surgery
Intractable Barrett's ulcer	Resection if possible	Resection
Low grade dysplasia	Anti-reflux surgery if possible plus 6-monthly endoscopic surveillance with biopsy and cytology	Anti-reflux surgery plus 6-monthly endoscopic surveillance with biopsy and cytology
High grade dysplasia	Anti-reflux surgery and endoscopic surveillance	Resection

1

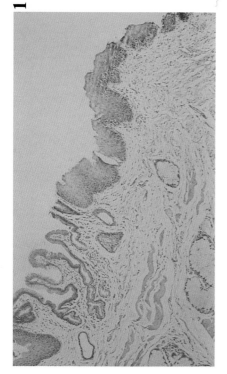

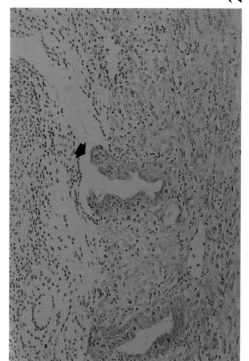

2b

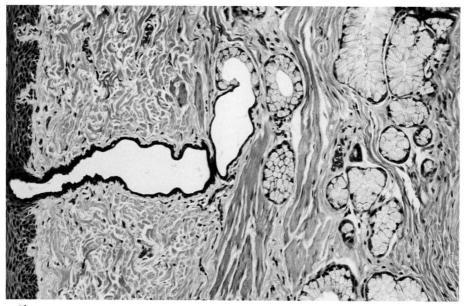

2a

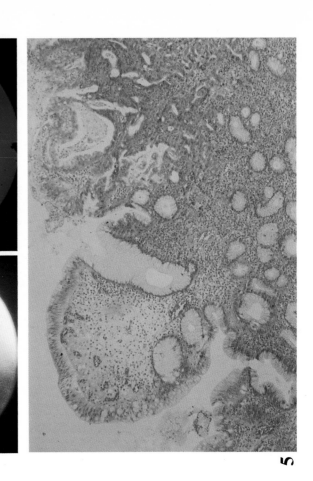

4

3

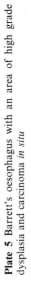

5

Plate 1 Reflux-induced columnar epithelial regeneration above a squamous barrier in a canine model

Plate 2a Oesophageal gland duct lined in its distal part by squamous epithelium.
Plate 2b Erosion of surface layers by reflux may expose deeper part of duct lined by cuboidal epithelium allowing regeneration with columnar epithelium to occur

Plate 3 Barrett's ulcer

Plate 4 Endoscopic view of Barrett's oesophagus showing the deep red appearance of the columnar epithelium in contrast to the paler appearance of the squamous epithelium

Plate 5 Barrett's oesophagus with an area of high grade dysplasia and carcinoma *in situ*

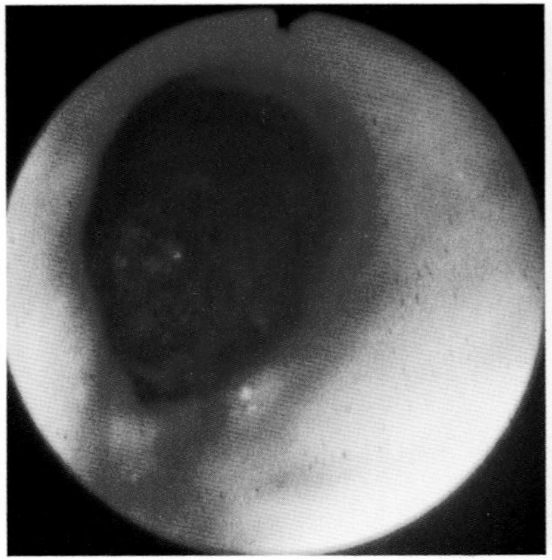

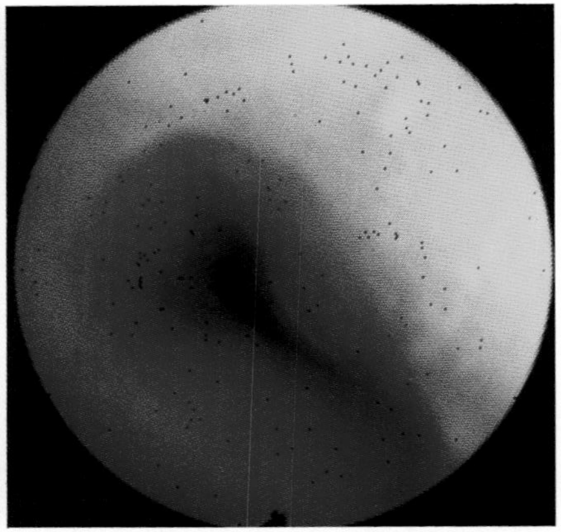

Surveillance

Patients with asymptomatic Barrett's oesophagus, particularly if elderly, may not require treatment. Elderly or unfit patients with symptoms may be treated medically but those fit enough to undergo surgery should have an anti-reflux procedure carried out. The authors' own preference is the Nissen fundoplication. The outcome of surgery should be assessed by 24-hour pH monitoring. Subsequently patients should be checked endoscopically and histologically by multiple biopsy at yearly intervals to see how much, if any, regression takes place or alternatively to note the development of dysplasia if it occurs. For patients in whom dysplastic change has occurred 6-monthly endoscopy with wash and brush cytology and biopsy is advisable. Areas of dysplasia may be identified with toluidine blue. The test lacks specificity, however, because erosions and ulcers may also give a positive result. Serious consideration should be given to resection in cases with progressive dysplasia.

Controversy surrounds the question of establishing endoscopic surveillance programmes for patients with Barrett's oesophagus. Endoscopic surveillance has the potential advantage of identifying a carcinoma at an asymptomatic or even pre-invasive stage when treatment is more likely to be successful. The American Cancer Society [101] in its recommendations on procedures for the early detection of cancer has put forward the following proposals: there should be good evidence that the procedure is effective in reducing morbidity or mortality; the medical benefits should outweigh the risks; the costs should be reasonable when related to the benefits; the procedures should be practical and feasible. It is difficult to provide evidence that endoscopic surveillance is effective in reducing the morbidity and mortality of oesophageal cancer in patients with Barrett's oesophagus. In three studies [74,75,102], the risk has been established as being 30–40 times greater than that of the general population of the USA. Based on the incidence of adenocarcinoma reported in these studies Spechler [103] has calculated that the overall incidence is 500 : 100 000 (i.e. 500 adenocarcinomas per 100 000 patients with Barrett's oesophagus). He estimated that in order to demonstrate a reduction in mortality from endoscopic surveillance at least 2000 patients would need to be followed up for 10 years.

Fulfilment of the second requirement presents no difficulty as any reduction in mortality would outweigh the risks of endoscopy which are negligible. A response to the third proposal is difficult because it involves the philosophical consideration of cost *vs* patient benefit. The costs of endoscopic surveillance are significant and Achker and Carey [104] have calculated the costs of a screening programme at $31 000 per cancer detected; but a reduction in mortality from cancer could be held to be of incalculable value to patients. Compliance with the last condition is easy as regular endoscopy is both practical and feasible. Atkinson [105] has examined the possibility of screening only very high-risk patients with Barrett's oesophagus. He points out that, while smoking and alcohol are known risk factors in squamous carcinoma of the oesophagus, their role in promoting adenocarcinoma in Barrett's oesophagus is less certain. The length of the columnar lining was not less than 10 cm in the four patients with adenocarcinoma in the series of van der Veen *et al.* [102] and extended Barrett's mucosa may warrant closer monitoring [106]. Specialized intestinal epithelium and sulphomucin secretion are both too common in Barrett's oesophagus to be useful in identifying special risk patients.

The severity of the reflux has not received attention as a special risk factor, but it may be of interest to note that in the one patient in the authors' series who developed an adenocarcinoma during surveillance a pH < 4 was recorded during 75% of the monitored 24 hours.

Atkinson has also pointed out that in elderly unfit patients endoscopic monitoring would be a useless exercise since even if an early carcinoma was detected curative treatment could not be offered. Such patients may succumb to other conditions before an early oesophageal carcinoma becomes symptomatic. In the studies of van der Veen *et al.* [102] and Cameron *et al.* [74] no difference in survival was seen between patients with Barrett's oesophagus and a control population.

While the controversy cannot be resolved on the evidence available at present, some guidelines might be considered. There is probably little benefit in providing surveillance for elderly patients with short segments of columnar epithelium. On the other hand most centres have a relatively small number of patients with Barrett's oesophagus and the costs of a screening programme are not prohibitive. Endoscopy is safe and easily available. It seems reasonable to screen younger patients, those with extensive metaplastic epithelium and especially those with dysplasia. A procedure which could lead to early diagnosis and curative treatment of a potentially fatal disease must be worth while. Reid *et al.* [69] have highlighted a number of points which they consider important for successful endoscopic biopsy surveillance. Specimens should be taken at 2 cm intervals throughout the columnar epithelium, large biopsy forceps should be used and all visible lesions, no matter how slight, should be biopsied. Labelling of specimens should be performed according to level so that re-biopsy can be carried out where diagnosis is equivocal. Mounting specimens on a support medium of monofilament plastic mesh is helpful. The addition of Alcian blue to the staining process makes the diagnosis of dysplasia and carcinoma easier.

Treatment of Barrett's ulcer

The two major manifestations of Barrett's ulcer are bleeding and an associated stricture. Although healing has been reported in response to medical treatment and anti-reflux surgery, the life-threatening nature of the haemorrhage and the possibility of perforation into the mediastinum with fatal consequences makes resection mandatory where healing is not prompt. Fatal haemorrhage has occurred in at least three instances before surgery could be performed [107–109]. Emergency resection for haemorrhage was reported by Ranson *et al.* [106]. Successful resection after perforation into the pericardium was reported by Cyrlak *et al.* [109]. Three of Postlethwait's [110] four patients had to have resection for haemorrhage despite intensive medical treatment. Most authors have commented on the poor response to conservative measures and advocate resection.

Treatment of Barrett's stricture

Strictures associated with Barrett's oesophagus may resolve with successful anti-reflux surgery as reported by Seaman and Wylie [56]. The authors' own experience is that they require regular dilatation even after Nissen fundoplication. Some strictures consist of dense transmural scarring and are undilatable or recur very quickly after dilatation. In these circumstances resection is necessary. Limited resection with intrathoracic anastomosis may not be adequate and further reflux may occur. Three-stage oesophagectomy with oesophagogastric anastomosis in the neck or replacement of the thoracic oesophagus by isoperistaltic left colon would seem to offer more advantages.

Treatment of adenocarcinoma associated with Barrett's oesophagus

When a carcinoma is identified the treatment of choice is resection. The resection margins should include all the ectopic mucosa and the aim should be to provide 10 cm margins on either side of the tumour. Three-stage oesophagectomy is probably the most appropriate procedure. The tumours are usually advanced and prognosis is poor. Mean survival is around 12 months. Survival does not appear to be influenced by tumour type. In advanced cases palliative intubation or laser treatment may be adopted. Adenocarcinomas respond moderately to radiotherapy and palliative treatment with 40–45 Gy may afford considerable relief of dysphagia.

References

1. Barrett, N. R. Chronic peptic ulcer of the oesophagus and oesophagitis. *Br. J. Surg.* 1950; **38**: 175–182

2. Allison, P. R. and Johnstone, A. S. The oesophagus lined by gastric mucous membrane. *Thorax* 1953; **8**: 87–101

3. Barrett, N. R. The lower oesophagus lined by columnar epithelium. *Surgery* 1957; **41**: 881–894

4. Savary, M. and Mounier, P. Diagnosis, pathophysiology and adenocarcinogenesis of Barrett's oesophagus. In DeMeester, T. R. and Skinner, D. B., Eds. *Esophageal Disorders: Pathophysiology and therapy.* New York: Raven Press. 1985: 101–108

5. Schridde, H. Uber Magenschleimhaut-Inseln vom Bau der Cardialdrusenzone und Fundusdrusenregion und anderen osophageglen Cardialdrusen gleichenden Drusen im obersten Oesophagusabschnitt. *Virchows Arch. Pathol. Anat. Physiol. Klin. Med.* 1904; **175**: 1–16

6. Johns, B. A. E. Developmental changes in the oesophageal epithelium in man. *J. Anat.* 1952; **86**: 431–442

7. Frindlay, L. and Kelley, A. B. Congenital shortening of the oesophagus and the thoracic stomach resulting therefrom. *Proc. R. Soc. Med.* 1931; **24**: 1561–1578

8. Everhart, C. W. Jr, Holtzapple, P. G. and Humphries, T. J. Barrett's oesophagus: inherited epithelium or inhibited reflux. *J. Clin. Gastroenterol.* 1983; **5**: 357–358

9. Gerfand, M. D. Barrett's oesophagus in sexagenarian identical twins. *J. Clin Gastroenterol.* 1983: **5** 251–253

10. Hague, A. K. and Merkel, M. Total columnar lined oesophagus. *Arch. Pathol. Lab. Med.* 1981; **105**: 546–548

11. Dahms, B. B. and Rothstein, F. C. Barrett's oesophagus in children: a consequence of chronic gastro-oesophageal reflux. *Gastroenterology* 1984; **86**: 318–323

12. Hamilton, S. R. Pathogenesis of columnar cell-lined (Barrett) esophagus. In: Spechler, S. J. and Goyal, R. K., Eds. *Barrett's Oesophagus: Pathophysiology, Diagnosis and Management.* New York: Elsevier Science. 1985: 29–37

13. Iascone, C., DeMeester, T. R., Little, A. G. and Skinner, D. B. Barrett's oesophagus: Functional assessment, proposed pathogenesis and surgical therapy. *Arch. Surg.* 1983; **118**: 543–549

14. Flook, D. and Stoddard, C. J. Gastro-oesophageal reflux (GOR) in patients with oesophagitis or a columnar lined (Barrett's) oesophagus (Abstract). *Gut* 1983; 24:A1007

15. Gillen, P., Keeling, P., Byrne, P. J. and Hennessy, T. P. J. Barrett's oesophagus: pH profile. *Br. J. Surg.* 1987; **74**: 774–776

16. Katzka, D. A., Reynolds, J. C., Saul, S. H. *et al.* Barrett's metaplasia and adenocarcinoma of the esophagus in scleroderma. *Am. J. Med.* 1987; **82**: 46–52

17. Andreollo, N. A. and Earlam, R. J. Heller's myotomy for achalasia: is an anti-reflux procedure necessary? *Br. J. Surg.* 1987; **74**: 765–769

18. Kortin, P., Warren, R. E., Gardner, J., Ginsberg, R. J. and Diamant, N. E. Barrett's esophagus in a patient with surgically treated achalasia. *J. Clin. Gastroenterol.* 1981; **3**: 357–360

19. Feczko, P. J., Ma, C. K., Halpert, R. D. and Batra, S. K. Barrett's metaplasia and dysplasia in postmyotomy achalasia patients. *Am. J. Gastroenterol.* 1983; **78**: 265–268

20. Mossberg, S. M. The columnar lined oesophagus (Barrett's syndrome) an acquired condition. *Gastroenterology* 1965; **50**: 671–676

21. Goldman, M. C. and Bechman, R. C. Barrett's syndrome: case report with discussion about concepts of pathogenesis. *Gastroenterology* 1960; **39**: 104–110

22. Hamilton, S. R. and Yardley, J. H. Regeneration of cardiac type mucosa and acquisition of Barrett mucosa after esophagogastrostomy. *Gastroenterology* 1977; **72**: 669–675

23. Hayward, J. The treatment of fibrous stricture of the oesophagus associated with hiatal hernia. *Thorax* 1961; **16**: 45–55

24. Creamer, B., Shorter, R. G. and Bamforth, J. The turnover and shedding of epithelial cells. Part 1 The turnover in the gastro-intestinal tract. *Gut* 1961; **2**: 110–118

25. Borrie, J. and Goldwater, L. Columnar cell lined oesophagus: assessment of aetiology and treatment. A 22 year experience. *J. Thorac. Cardiovasc. Surg.* 1976; **71**: 825–834

26. Johnson, D. A., Winters, C., Spurling, T. J., Chobanian, S. J. Jr and Cattal, E. L. Jr. Esophageal acid sensitivity in Barrett's esophagus. *J. Clin. Gastroenterol.* 1987; **9**: 23–27

27. Bremner, C. G. In: Silber E., Ed. *Carcinoma of the Oesophagus.* Capetown: Balkema, 1978: 132–138

28. Gillen, P., Keeling, P., Byrne, P. J., Healy, M., O'Moore, R. R. and Hennessy, T. P. J. Implications of duodenogastric reflux in the pathogenesis of Barrett's oesophagus. *Br. J. Surg.* 1988; **75**: 540–543

29. Paull, G. and Yardley, J. H. Gastric and esophageal *Campylobacter pylori* in patients with Barrett's esophagus. *Gastroenterology* 1988; **95**: 216–218

30. Van de Kerckhof, J. and Gahagan, T. Regeneration of the mucosal lining of the oesophagus. *Med. Bull. Henry Ford Hospital* 1963; **11**: 129–134

31. Hennessy, T. P. J., Edlich, R. F., Buchin, R. J., Tsung, M. S., Prevost, M. and Wangensteen, O. H. Influence of gastro-esophageal incompetence on regeneration of esophageal mucosa. *Arch. Surg.* 1968; **97**: 105–107

32. Bremner, C. G., Lynch, V. P. and Ellis, E. H. Jr. Barrett's esophagus: congenital or acquired? An experimental study of esophageal mucosal regeneration in the dog. *Surgery* 1970; **69**: 209–216

33. Allison, P. R. and Johnstone, A. S. The oesophagus lined by gastric mucous membrane. *Thorax* 1953; **8**: 87–101

34. Trier, J. S. Morphology of the epithelium of the distal oesophagus in patients with mid-oesophageal stricture. *Gastroenterology* 1970; **58**: 441–461

35. Meyer, W., Vollmer, F. and Barr, W. Barrett oesophagus following total gastrectomy. *Endoscopy* 1979; **11**: 121–126

36. Gillen, P., Keeling, P., Byrne, P. J., West, A. B. and Hennessy, T. P. J. Experimental columnar metaplasia in the canine oesophagus. *Br. J. Surg.* 1988; **75**: 113–115

37. Thompson, J. J., Zinsser, K. R. and Enterline, H. T. Barrett's metaplasia and adenocarcinoma of the esophagus and gastro-esophageal junction. *Human Pathol.* 1983; **14**: 42–61

38. Rothery, G. A., Patterson, J. E., Stoddard, C. J. and Daw, D. W. Histological and histochemical changes in the columnar lined (Barrett's) oesophagus. *Gut* 1986; **27**: 1062–1068

39. Paull, A., Trier, J. S., Dalton, M. D., Camp, R. C., Loeb, P. and Goyal, R. K. The histologic spectrum of Barrett's esophagus. *N. Engl. J. Med.* 1976; **295**: 477–480

40. Trier, J. S. Morphology of the epithelium of the distal esophagus in patients with mild esophageal peptic stricture. *Gastroenterology* 1970; **58**: 444–460

41. Pederson, S. A., Hage, E., Nielsen, P. A. and Sorenson, H. R. Barrett's syndrome: morphological and physiological characteristics. *Scand. J. Thorac. Cardiovasc. Surg.* 1971; **5**: 191–205

42. Mangla, J. C., Schenk, E. A., Desbraillets, L., Guarasci, G., Kubasih, N. P. and Turner, M. D. Pepsin secretion pepsinogen and gastrin in Barrett's esophagus. *Gastroenterology* 1976; **70**: 669–676

43. Dayal, Y. and Wolfe, H. G. Gastrin producing cells in ectopic gastric mucosa of developmental and metaplastic origins. *Gastroenterology* 1978; **75**: 655–660

44. Dalton, M. D., McGuigan, J. E., Camp, R. C. and Goyal, R. K. Gastrin content of columnar mucosa lining the lower (Barrett's) oesophagus. *Am. J. Dig. Dis.* 1977; **22**: 97

45. Berensen, M. M., Herbst, J. J. and Freston, J. W. Esophageal columnar epithelial β-galactosidase and β-glucuronidase. *Gastroenterology* 1975; **68**: 1417–1419

46. Jass, J. R. Role of intestinal metaplasia in the histogenesis of gastric carcinoma. *J. Clin. Pathol.* 1980; **33**: 801–810

47. Lei, D. N. and Yu, J. Y. Types of mucosal metaplasia in relation to the histogenesis of gastric carcinoma. *Arch. Pathol. Lab. Med.* 1984; **108**: 220–224

48. Jass, J. R. Mucin histochemistry of the columnar epithelium of the oesophagus: a retrospective study. *J. Clin. Pathol.* 1981; **34**: 866–870

49. Savary, M. and Miller, G. In: Savary, M. and Miller, G., Eds. *The Esophagus: Handbook and Atlas of Endoscopy.* Solothurn, Switzerland: A. G. Gassman. 1978: 160–167

50. Trier, J. S., Curtis, R. L. and Sherlock, P. In: Jerzy Glass G., Ed. *Progress in Gastroenterology.* New York: Grune & Stratton. 1983: 231–237

51. Burbidge, E. J. and Radigan, J. Characteristics of columnar cell lined (Barrett's) esophagus. *Gastrointest. Endosc.* 1979; **25**: 133–136

52. Robbins, A. H., Vincent, M. E., Saini, M. and Schimmel, E. M. Revised radiologic concepts of the Barrett esophagus. *Gastrointest. Radiol.* 1978; **3**: 377–381

53. Levine, M. S., Knessel, H. Y., Caroline, D. F., Laufer, I., Herlinger, H. and Thompson, J. J. Barrett esophagus: Reticular pattern of the mucosa. *Radiology* 1983; **146**: 663–667

54. Barrett, N. R. In: James, A., Ed. *Modern Trends in Gastroenterology.* London: Butterworths. 1958

55. Pierce, J. W. and Creamer, B. The diagnosis of the columnar lined oesophagus. *Clin. Radiol.* 1963; **14**: 64–69

56. Seaman, W. B. and Wylie, R. H. Observations on the nature of the stricture in Barrett's esophagus (Allison and Johnstone's anomaly). *Radiology* 1966; **87**: 30–32

57. Westdorp, I. C. E., Bartelsman, J., Schipper, M. E. I. and Tytgat, G. N. Effect of long-term treatment with cimetidine and antacids in Barrett's oesophagus. *Gut* 1981; **22**: 724–727

58. Heitmann, P., Csendes, A. and Struzer, T. Esophageal strictures and lower esophagus lined with columnar epithelium. *Am. J. Dig. Dis.* 1971; **16**: 307–320

59. Patel, G. K., Clift, S. A. and Read, R. C. Mechanism of gastroesophageal reflux (GER) in patients with Barrett's esophagus (Abstract). *Gastroenterology* 1982; **82**: 1146

60. DeMeester, T. R., Lafontaine, E., Joelsson, B. E. *et al.* The relationship of a hiatal hernia to the function of the body of the esophagus and the gastroesophageal junction. *J. Thorac. Cardiovasc. Surg.* 1981; **82**: 547–558

61. Vidins, E. L., Fox, J. A. and Bech, I. T. Transmural potential difference (PD) in the body of the esophagus in patients with esophagitis. Barrett's epithelium and carcinoma of the esophagus. *Am. J. Dig. Dis.* 1971; **16**: 991–999

62. Orlando, R. C., Powell, D. W., Bryson, J. C. *et al.* Esophageal potential difference measurements in esophageal disease. *Gastroenterology* 1982; **83**: 1026–1032

63. Orlando, R. C., Powell, D. W., and Carney, C. N. Pathophysiology of acute acid injury in rabbit esophageal epithelium. *J. Clin. Invest.* 1981; **68**: 268–293

64. Berquist, T. H., Nolan, N. G., Carlson, H. C. and Stephens, D. H. Diagnosis of Barrett's esophagus by pertechnetate scintigraphy. *Mayo Clin. Proc.* 1973; **48**: 276–279

65. Bremner, C. G. Barrett's oesophagus In: Watson, A. and Celestin, L. R., Eds. *Disorders of the Oesophagus: Advances and controversies.* London: Pitman. 1984: 94–104

66. Chobanian, S. J., Cattau, E. L. Jr, Winters, C. Jr *et al.* In vitro staining with toluidine blue as an adjunct to the endoscopic detection of Barrett's esophagus. *Gastrointest. Endosc.* 1987; **33**: 99–101

67. Skinner, D. B., Walther, B. C., Riddell, R. H., Schmidt, H., Iascone, C. and DeMeester, T. R. Barrett's esophagus. Comparison of benign and malignant esophagus: comparison of benign and malignant cases. *Ann. Surg.* 1983; **198**: 546–554

68. Bozymski, E. M. Barrett's oesophagus: endoscopic characteristics. In: Spechler, S. J. and Goyal, R. K., Eds. *Barrett's Esophagus: Pathophysiology, diagnosis and management.* New York: Elsevier Science. 1985: 113–120

69. Reid, B. J., Weinstein, W. M., Lewin, K. J. *et al.* Endoscopic biopsy can detect high-grade dysplasia or early adenocarcinoma in Barrett's esophagus without grossly recognizable neoplastic lesions. *Gastroenterology* 1988; **94**: 81–90

70. Herbst, J. J., Berenson, M. M., McCloskey, D. W. and Wiser, W. C. Cell proliferation in esophageal columnar epithelium (Barrett's esophagus). *Gastroenterology* 1978; **75**: 683–687

71. Pellish, L. J., Hermos, J. A. and Eastwood, G. L. Cell proliferation in three types of Barrett's epithelium. *Gut* 1980; **21**: 26–31

72. Tamura, H. and Schulman, S. Barrett-type esophagus associated with squamous epithelium. *Chest* 1971; **59**: 330–333

73. Eller, J. L., Ziter, T. F. and Brott, W. Inflammatory polyp: A complication in esophagus lined by columnar epithelium. *Radiology* 1971; **98**: 145–146

74. Cameron, A. J., Ott, B. J. and Payne, W. S. The incidence of adenocarcinoma in columnar-lined (Barrett's) oesophagus. *N. Engl. J. Med.* 1985; **313**: 857–859

75. Spechler, S. J., Robbins, A. H., Rubins, H. B. *et al.* Adenocarcinoma and Barrett's esophagus: an overrated risk? *Gastroenterology* 1984; **87**: 927–933

76. Kalich, R. J., Clancy, P. E., Orringer, M. B. and Appelman, H. D. Clinical, epidemiologic and morphologic comparison between adenocarcinomas arising in Barrett's esophageal mucosa and in the gastric cardia. *Gastroenterology* 1984; **86**: 461–467

77. Griffin, M. and Sweeney, E. C. The relationship of endoscopic cells dysphagia and carcinoembryonic antigen in Barrett's mucosa to adenocarcinoma of the oesophagus. *Histopathology* 1987; **11**: 53–62

78. Smith, R. R. L., Boitnott, J. K., Hamilton, S. R. and Rogers, E. L. The spectrum of carcinoma arising in Barrett's esophagus. *Am. J. Surg. Pathol.* 1984; **8**: 563–573

79. Haggitt, R. C., Tryzeluar, J., Ellis, F. H. and Coliler, H. Adenocarcinoma complicating columnar epithelium-lined (Barrett's) esophagus. *Am. J. Clin. Pathol.* 1978; **70**: 1–5

80. Skinner, D. B., Walther, B. C., Riddell, R. H., Schmidt, H., Iascone, C. and DeMeester, T. R. Barrett's oesophagus: comparison of benign and malignant cells. *Ann. Surg.* 1983; **198**: 554–565

81. Reid, B. J., Haggitt, R. C., Rubin, C. E. and Rabinovitch, P. S. Barrett's. Correlation between flow cytometry and histology in detection of patients at risk for adenocarcinoma. *Gastroenterology* 1987; **93**: 1–11

82. McKinley, M. J., Budman, D. R., Gruenberg, D., Bronzo, R. L., Weissman, G. S. and Kahn, E. DNA content in Barrett's esophagus and esophageal malignancy. *Am. J. Gastroenterol.* 1987; **82**: 1012–1015

83. Peuchmaur, M., Potet, F. and Goldfain, D. Mucin histochemistry of the columnar epithelium of the oesophagus (Barrett's oesophagus): a prospective biopsy study. *J. Clin. Pathol.* 1984; **37**: 607–610

84. Haggitt, R. C., Reid, B. J., Rabinovitch, P. S. and Rubin, C. E. Barrett's esophagus: correlation between mucin histochemistry, flow cytometry and histological diagnosis for predicting increased cancer risk. *Am. J. Pathol.* 1988; **131**: 53–61

85. Garewal, H. S., Gerner, E. W., Sampliner, R. E. and Roe, D. Ornithine decarboxylase and polyamine levels in columnar upper gastrointestinal mucosa in patients with Barrett's esophagus. *Cancer Res.* 1988; **48**: 3288–3291

86. Garewal, H. S., Sampliner, R., Gerner, E. W., Steinbronn, K., Alberts, D. S. and Kendall, D. S. Ornithine decarboxylase activity in Barrett's esophagus: a potential marker for dysplasia. *Gastroenterology* 1988; **94**: 819–821

87. Metcalf, B. W., Bey, P., Danzin, C., Jung, M. J., Cassura, P. and Vevert, J. P. Catalytic irreversible inhibition of mammalian ornithine decarboxylase by substrate and product analogs. *J. Am. Chem. Soc.* 1978; **100**: 2551–2553

88. Sontag, S. F., Chejfec, G., Stanley, M. *et al.* Barrett's esophagus and colonic tumours. *Lancet* 1985; **i**: 946–948

89. Tripp, M. R., Sampliner, R. E., Kogan, F. J. and Morgan, T. R. Colorectal neoplasms and Barrett's esophagus. *Am. J. Gastroenterol.* 1986; **81**: 1063–1064

90. Ramage, J. K. Barrett's oesophagus. *Lancet* 1987; **ii**: 851

91. Cooper, B. T. and Barbezat, G. O. Barrett's oesophagus: a clinical study of 52 patients. *Q. J. Med.* 1987; **62**: 97–108

92. Thompson, W. G. and Barr, R. Pharmacotherapy of an ulcer in Barrett's esophagus: carbenoxolone and cimetidine. *Gastroenterology* 1977; **73**: 808–810

93. Kothari, T., Mangla, J. C. and Kalra, T. M. S. Barrett's ulcer and treatment with cimetidine. *Arch. Intern. Med.* 1980; **140**: 475–477

93a. Lee, F. I. and Isaccs, P. E. T. Peptic ulcer of the oesophagus (Barrett's ulcer) healing in response to standard dose ranitidine, high dose ranitidine and omeprazole. *Am. J. Gastroenterol.* 1987; **82**: 926

93b. Hameetman, W. and Tytgat, G. N. Healing of chronic Barrett's ulcer with omeprazole. *Am. J. Gastroenterol.* 1986; **81**: 764–766

94. Everhart, C. W. and Humphries, T. J. Medical treatment of Barrett's esophagus with bethanechol: report of three cases with prolonged follow-up. *Gastroenterology* 1978; **74**: 1033

95. Brand, D. L., Ylvisaker, J. T., Gelfand, M. and Pope, C. E. Regression of columnar esophageal (Barrett's) epithelium after anti-reflux surgery. *N. Engl. J. Med.* 1980; **302**: 844–848

96. Patel, G. K., Clift, S. A., Schaefer, R. A., Read, R. C. and Texter, E. C. Resolution of severe dysplastic (Ca. in situ) changes with regression of columnar epithelium in Barrett's esophagus on medical treatment (Abstract). *Gastroenterology* 1982; **82**: 1147

97. Dooner, J. and Cleator, I. G. Selective management of benign esophageal strictures. *Am. J. Gastroenterol.* 1982; **77**: 172–177

98. Endo, M. and Kobayashi Kozu T. A case of Barrett's epithelialisation followed up for 5 years. *Endoscopy* 1974; **6**: 48–51

99. DeMeester, T. R., Johnson, L. F. and Kent, A. H. Evaluation of current operations for prevention of gastroesophageal reflux. *Ann. Surg.* 1974; **180**: 511–525

100. Stuart, R. C., Dawson, K., Keeling, P., Byrne, P. J. and Hennessy, T. P. J. A prospective randomized trial of Angelchik prosthesis versus Nissen fundoplication. *Br. J. Surg.* 1989; **76**: 86–89

101. American Cancer Society. Guidelines for the cancer-related check-up: recommendations and rationale. *Cancer* 1980; **80**: 194–240

102. Van der Veen, A. H., Dees, J., Blankenstrijn, J. D. and van Blankenstein, M. Adenocarcinoma in Barrett's oesophagus: an overrated risk. *Gut* 1989; **30**: 14–18

103. Spechler, S. J. Endoscopic surveillance for patients with Barrett esophagus: does the cancer risk justify the practice? *Ann. Intern. Med.* 1987; **106**: 902–904

104. Achker, E. and Carey, W. The cost of surveillance for adenocarcinoma complicating Barrett's esophagus. *Am. J. Gastroenterol.* 1988; **83**: 291–294

105. Atkinson, M. Barrett's oesophagus – to screen or not to screen? *Gut* 1989; **30**: 2–5

106. Ranson, J. M., Patel, G. K., Clift, S. A., Womble, N. E. and Read, R. C. Extended and limited types of Barrett's esophagus in the adult. *Ann. Thorac. Surg.* 1982; **33**: 895–907

107. Sokol, E. M., Schechterman, L. and Frucht, H. L. Fatal perforating ulcer of the esophagus lined by columnar epithelium. *NY State J. Med.* 1968; **68**: 2193

108. Wright, J. T. Allison and Johnstone's anomaly. *Am. J. Roentgenol.* 1965; **94**: 308–320

109. Cyrlak, D., Cohen, A. J. and Dunn, E. R. Esophago pericardial fistula: causes and radiographic features. *Am. J. Radiol.* 1983; **141**: 141–177

110. Postlethwait, R. W., (Ed.) Other congenital anomalies. In: *Surgery of the Esophagus.* Norwalk: Appleton-Century-Crofts. 1986: 39–82

Chapter 5

Motility disorders in gastro-oesophageal reflux disease

J. S. de Caestecker and R. C. Heading

Introduction

Gastro-oesophageal reflux (GOR) results from a motor disorder of the oesophagus and the gastro-oesophageal junction. The evidence for this contention is summarized in Chapter 1. The incidence of and extent to which motor abnormality of the lower oesophageal sphincter (LOS), oesophageal body and upper oesophageal sphincter are primary or secondary to GOR will form the subject of part of this chapter. Oesophageal clearance of acid depends on oesophageal peristalsis and swallowed saliva, so it should be anticipated that patients with oesophagitis would have abnormal primary peristalsis. The contribution of abnormalities of oesophageal motility to symptoms arising from refluxed acid is controversial and will be examined in the next section.

Motility disorders and acid-induced oesophageal pain

Early investigation of oesophageal motility suggested that the symptoms of heart-burn were associated with peristaltic waves or a rise in the mean intraoesophageal pressure [1]. The observation that heartburn could be produced by oesophageal balloon distension was felt to be in keeping with a motility-induced mechanism [2,3]. Heartburn could also be produced by intraoesophageal injection of acid, alkali, cold water, gastric contents or barium into the lower oesophagus [2,4]. The speed of injection and volume of fluid injected appear to have a direct bearing on the production and intensity of heartburn [4]. Furthermore, fluoroscopic examination with barium after heartburn had been produced by one of these fluids showed the presence of either spasm or reverse peristalsis [2,4] and indeed the severity of the symptoms appeared to vary with the subsidence or reappearance of the peristaltic wave [4]. Bernstein and Baker, who introduced the diagnostic oesophageal acid perfusion test into clinical practice, aroused controversy by finding that oesophageal motility did not change during symptomatic acid perfusion in five subjects [5]. Siegel and Hendrix [6] performed oesophageal acid perfusion in 25 patients with GOR symptoms and 25 controls. During the acid perfusion, they monitored oesophageal motility, and found motor abnormalities in all patients in whom acid perfusion reproduced symptoms, but only in four controls. In two of the controls, the abnormal motility was present also during the saline perfusion and, in all four, occurred as sporadic motor abnormalities in contrast to the sustained motor activity which was seen during the symptomatic periods in the heartburn group. In a number of the symptomatic patients, the motility changes preceded the development of heartburn, but grew more marked as symptoms developed. Three patterns of abnormal motility were described, many symptomatic patients showing all three. These were:

1. Increased peristaltic amplitude and duration.
2. Spontaneous non-propagating contractions.
3. A gradual rise in intraluminal pressure which was interpreted as an indication of increased oesophageal tone.

The last abnormality may simply be an effect of the fluid accumulating in the oesophagus, because the patients were studied in the supine position. Tuttle and colleagues observed a similar gradual rise in intraluminal pressure with both saline and acid perfusion [7]. Although the majority of their patients had no motility changes during acid-induced heartburn, they noted that some patients developed heartburn without a simultaneous fall in pH during belching. They observed a transient elevation in intraluminal pressure following the belch and reasoned that heartburn resulted in these cases from oesophageal distension. In another study, they described 4 patients (out of 124 studied) with sustained elevation of intraoesophageal pressure above fundic pressure in addition to demonstrable GOR and suggested that this was a manifestation of diffuse oesophageal spasm [8]. Creamer and colleagues found a similar pattern in a series of patients with diffuse oesophageal spasm [9], and it has since been pointed out that diffuse oesophageal spasm may occur with GOR [10].

The acidified barium swallow has been advocated as a test for GOR, a positive test requiring delayed clearance and motility abnormalities observed. fluoroscopically following acid, but not neutral barium [11]. Among subjects with GOR symptoms, 60% had an abnormal test, but 30% of controls also had an abnormal test [11]. Although these results show the test to lack specificity and symptoms were not recorded in this study, they provide some support for the contention that acid provokes motility disturbances.

Atkinson and Bennett studied 40 patients with reflux oesophagitis and 14 controls [12]. Non-peristaltic contractions occurred in 10 patients during saline perfusion, and in 28 patients and 5 controls during acid perfusion. In the majority, these were intermittent and in only 4 did the onset of heartburn coincide with a striking alteration in the motility pattern. In 3 other patients, although non-peristaltic contractions appeared before the onset of pain, the occurrence of spasms of pain coincided with the contractions. Infusion of 0.1 M sodium bicarbonate rapidly relieved symptoms in the majority of patients without altering motility, while an intravenous anticholinergic drug did not abolish symptoms in any of the 21 patients to whom it was administered. This was despite abolition of all motor activity in 15 of the 21, although 4 patients reported lessening of symptoms after the drug. They concluded that acid could induce pain and motility changes, and that they were usually (but not always) independent of one another.

All these studies were performed with water-filled, but non-perfused, intraluminal manometry catheters, which are known to underestimate intraoesophageal pressure. There have been a number of recent studies using perfused catheter systems. Two studies found that there were no significant differences in simultaneous and repetitive contractions during acid perfusion between controls and GOR patients, and that the production of heartburn was not associated with any disturbance of motility [13,14].

However, these and two other studies found a significant increase in duration of peristalsis and a decrease in propagation velocity [13–16]. Whilst this might be simply an effect of liquid bolus volume [17], the effect was only seen with acid [13,16], and in patients who became symptomatic during the test [13,15]. This implies that acid perfusion results in an alteration of primary peristalsis, although this may not be related to symptoms.

These findings are pertinent to patients presenting with chest pain atypical of reflux. In one study, the increases in peristaltic amplitude and duration were significantly greater in patients experiencing chest pain during acid perfusion than in those who did not [18]. Some of these patients did not have independent evidence (by prolonged intraoesophageal pH monitoring) of abnormal GOR, implying that, whilst they were not refluxers, they had an abnormally acid-sensitive oesophagus. This confirms the findings of another group, who coined the term 'irritable oesophagus' for such patients [19].

Thus, most evidence seems to suggest that the symptom of heartburn occurs independently of any change in oesophageal motility. This implies a direct action of acid on oesophageal pain receptors. In a minority of patients, motility disorders coincide with the development of symptoms, suggesting a subsidiary role of abnormal motility in the production of heartburn. Acid perfusion does induce changes in the primary peristaltic wave, and this may be more marked in patients with chest pain atypical for GOR, in whom other investigations often fail to demonstrate pathological GOR. This emphasizes that the acid perfusion test measures oesophageal sensitivity to acid and is not in itself a test for GOR [20].

Gastro-oesophageal reflux and the lower oesophageal sphincter

Gastro-oesophageal reflux was commonly believed to be a consequence of a poorly functioning LOS. As discussed in Chapter 1, it is now recognized that a low basal LOS pressure is not necessary for pathological GOR to occur, and indeed an atonic LOS is rarely encountered. However, with increasing severity of oesophagitis, it is known that the resting LOS pressure measured by sampling methods decreases progressively [21,22]. Dent and colleagues found an inverse relationship between basal LOS pressure and the severity of reflux disease, also observing that the proportion of reflux events occurring across an atonic sphincter (as compared to other mechanisms) increased with the severity of oesophagitis [23]. This raises the question of whether low basal LOS pressure is a primary event or secondary to oesophagitis. A number of experimental animal studies in which oesophagitis was induced by acid perfusion have demonstrated that LOS pressure decreased [24,25] and rose again to control values with healing of the oesophagitis [24]. Studies in a cat model have indicated that the ultrastructure of the LOS from the inflamed oesophagus appeared normal and that the response of the LOS to bethanechol, a direct cholinergic stimulant, remained normal despite lowered basal LOS pressures [26]. However, response to edrophonium and pentagastrin, which both have an indirect cholinergic stimulating effect, was subnormal, suggesting that basal hypotension was the result of damage to cholinergic nerves [26]. Further studies have indicated that treatment with indomethacin prevented LOS hypotension and the attenuated response to edrophonium associated with experimental oesophagitis [27].

Furthermore, indomethacin treatment of animals with established oesophagitis prompted a more rapid return of LOS pressure to normal. These observations suggest that the functional impairment of LOS pressure has a neural basis and may be related to prostaglandins released by the acutely inflamed oesophageal tissues. Biancani and colleagues were unable to demonstrate any protective effect on LOS pressure in cats pre-treated with indomethacin or prostaglandins [28]. They found changes in the in vitro mechanical properties of strips of LOS muscle from cats with oesophagitis: principally a reduction in basal tone in all animals and a reduction in the maximal contraction induced by potassium chloride only in animals with the most severe histological grades of oesophagitis. These changes were specific to the LOS and could not be demonstrated from strips of muscle taken from the adjacent oesophagus. They also reported early changes of damage to LOS smooth muscle by electron microscopy and proposed that the organelle damage might alter calcium handling by the LOS smooth muscle and thus account for the observed dysfunction.

It is always difficult to know how far to extrapolate animal studies to the situation in human disease. The fact that even patients with low basal LOS pressures are able to generate normal pressures at some periods during prolonged measurements [23] would suggest that the LOS smooth muscle is still able to respond to stimulation, favouring functional impairment as in experimental animal studies [26–28].

If the cat experimental model is to parallel the human disease, improvement in LOS basal pressure would be expected with medical healing of oesophagitis. Katz and colleagues did not find any improvement in LOS pressure after healing of oesophagitis in 13 patients with GOR disease [29]. Baldi and co-workers found, following medical healing of oesophagitis, that LOS basal pressure did not fall postprandially, as was the case prior to treatment [30]. The pressure was comparable before and after healing (as measured by a Dent sleeve) at other times. Despite these findings, this group reported that the amount of acid GOR was unchanged following a healing course of medical treatment. Two trials using cimetidine failed to show an improvement in LOS pressure after treatment, although only about two-thirds of patients in each study had healed oesophagitis [31,32].

Motor function of the oesophageal body in gastro-oesophageal reflux disease

The prevalence and nature of dysmotility

Olsen and Schlegel reported a study of oesophageal motility in 50 patients with oesophagitis. Only 28% had normal peristaltic activity, the remainder having evidence of motor incoordination (32%), low amplitude peristalsis (37%) or complete motor failure (8%). As the degree of oesophagitis became more severe, so the proportion of patients with low amplitude peristalsis or total motor failure increased [21]. Kahrilas and colleagues supported these findings in a study of 177 patients with GOR disease and asymptomatic volunteers. They observed that peristaltic dysfunction was more prevalent with increasing severity of oesophagitis, occurring in 25% of patients with mild oesophagitis and 48% of those with severe oesophagitis [22]. The peristaltic dysfunction they reported included failed peristalsis after more than 50% of wet swallows (either no peristaltic wave or an incompletely propagating peristaltic wave after swallows) and diminished peristaltic amplitude in the distal oesophagus. Both abnormalities were more commonly found with more severe grades of oesophagitis. However, considerable overlap occurred with healthy controls, in that many

GOR patients had normal peristalsis. Gill and co-workers also found peristaltic amplitudes in 32 patients with GOR disease (half had oesophagitis) to be significantly lower at all levels in the oesophagus than a cohort of 18 controls [33]. Peristaltic failure (either a local (76%) or general failure (8%) of oesophageal contraction or synchronous waves (16%) after a swallow) was significantly more common in patients with GOR disease with or without oesophagitis than in patients without abnormal GOR [34]. In 26 children with GOR, peristaltic amplitude was significantly lower in patients with severe oesophagitis compared with those with minimal or absent oesophagitis and with controls. Non-specific motor abnormalities were also more common in the former group of patients [35]. In another study, aperistalsis and non-specific motor disorders were found in 64% of patients in benign GOR-related strictures compared to 32% of patients with GOR but no stricture [36]. However, a quarter of the patients with stricture had scleroderma or Raynaud's phenomenon, and these accounted for all the patients with aperistalsis.

Thus, motility disorders occur in a substantial minority of patients with GOR disease, the most common features being low amplitude peristalsis and failure of peristaltic propagation. The prevalence of abnormal motility seems to increase with the severity of oesophagitis.

Abnormal motility: primary or secondary to reflux?

In a baboon model, acute oesophagitis induced by acid perfusion resulted in a significant reduction of peristaltic amplitude compared to control animals [25]. Healing of oesophagitis after anti-reflux surgery is associated with a significant improvement in peristaltic amplitude [33,37], although, with the exception of a report of two individual patients [38] and a group of children with oesophagitis [35], medical healing of oesophagitis has not been followed by a change in oesophageal motility [29,30]. In the patients studied after anti-reflux surgery, peristaltic duration also increased significantly [33,37]. In view of the finding that lower oesophageal sphincter relaxation was incomplete in a majority of patients after fundoplication [33], it is possible that the improvement in oesophageal peristaltic amplitude and duration reflected a response to a degree of obstruction at the level of the lower sphincter.

Thus, although there is some evidence that abnormalities of peristalsis are secondary to acid GOR and recover when reflux is eliminated, the evidence is not conclusive. The existence of a primary abnormality of oesophageal motility is, by contrast, supported by the results of Russell and colleagues, who found that prolonged transit of a radionuclide-labelled fluid bolus, observed in 52% of GOR patients preoperatively, persisted after a surgical anti-reflux procedure [39].

The importance of abnormal motility in the pathophysiology of gastro-oesophageal reflux disease

There are two areas in which disorders of oesophageal motility may have a bearing on GOR disease. First, failed or non-conducted primary peristalsis may be the initiating event for many reflux episodes in normal human volunteers and patients with GOR. Mittal and McCallum have found mylohyoid electromyographic complexes, small oesophageal contractions and proximal non-conducting oesophageal contractions occurring at the outset of a large number of transient lower oesophageal relaxations accompanied by GOR [40,41], Longhi and Jordan, who observed this phenomenon some 20 years ago, referred aptly to the 'unguarded moment of sphincter relaxation' [42].

The second important area is that of oesophageal clearance. Acid clearance from the oesophagus depends chiefly on primary peristalsis which not only clears the oesophagus of the bulk of the volume of refluxed acid but delivers saliva to the distal oesophagus. As discussed in Chapter 1, saliva is crucial to neutralization of residual intraoesophageal acid. Stanciu and Bennett found that, in patients with GOR disease and abnormal motility (either low amplitude peristalsis or more than 25% of swallows followed by non-peristaltic waves), 90% had an abnormal acid clearance test. However, many patients with delayed acid clearing had apparently normal motility detected by standard manometric studies [43]. This discordance has been noted in studies using radionuclide oesophageal transit measurements. Russell and colleagues found an incidence of manometric abnormality in 18% from among 29 GOR patients compared to 52% with abnormalities of liquid bolus oesophageal transit [39]. Delayed liquid transit in GOR subjects without motility disorders on standard oesophageal manometry has been documented in other studies [44,45]. Similar results have been found using a chewed solid bolus in subjects seated upright [46–48], a test which appears to be more physiological than liquid oesophageal transit time assessed in supine patients. There is some evidence that the incidence of delayed solid transit is unrelated to the presence of oesophagitis [47,48] and that delayed liquid or solid bolus transit persists after surgical correction of abnormal GOR [39,48]; both of these findings imply that delayed clearance is a primary event and not secondary to GOR itself or to oesophagitis.

Thus, while abnormalities demonstrable by manometry contribute to the pathophysiology of GOR disease, the abnormalities of oesophageal clearance are not wholly explained. The evidence suggests that abnormal oesophageal liquid and solid bolus clearance persist after surgical correction of abnormal GOR, in contrast to the improvement in oesophageal peristalsis documented after surgery [33].

Most importantly, non-specific abnormalities of oesophageal motility, even if associated with dysphagia, are not a contraindication to surgical treatment for GOR. Bancewicz and colleagues found that dysphagia in these patients almost invariably resolved several months following successful anti-reflux surgery, and this was despite rarely observing a change in oesophageal manometry from abnormal to normal postoperatively [49].

Gastro-oesophageal reflux and the upper oesophageal sphincter

The functions of the upper oesophageal sphincter (UOS) have been suggested as prevention of oesophageal distension during respiration and protection against oesophagopharyngeal regurgitation and subsequent tracheobronchial aspiration [50].

With regard to the latter, it might be expected that increased UOS tone would occur in patients with abnormal GOR as a protective mechanism. There is good evidence that UOS responds to oesophageal distension by balloon [51,52] or liquid [52,53] by increasing its pressure. The magnitude of the response is related to bolus volume, the speed of oesophageal distension and the distance of the stimulus below the UOS [51–53], One group has found the response to acid to be greater than that during saline infusion of the oesophagus [53], although this has not been confirmed [52,54]. The clinical evidence that increased UOS pressure occurs in GOR patients is less convincing. One study found the resting UOS pressure to be higher in GOR patients with or without cricopharyngeal dysphagia compared to controls [55].

However, this study suffers from serious limitations, in that no account was taken of the marked radial asymmetry of the UOS, and non-perfused, water-filled catheters were used, which underestimate luminal pressure. Five subsequent studies using methods which took account of these factors failed to find any significant differences between patients with GOR disease and controls [54,56–59].

Additionally, no increase in UOS pressure was found with increasing severity of oesophagitis [54], nor was a hypotonic LOS related to any consistent changes in UOS pressure [57]. Kahrilas and colleagues, in a study using a modified sleeve device to study UOS function in normal volunteers, found no changes in UOS pressure postprandially or during spontaneous episodes of GOR [60]. This does not, of course, exclude the possibility of the effect of an episode of GOR on UOS pressure in reflux patients, in whom the volume of refluxate may be greater.

Nevertheless, the UOS may fail in patients with GOR who also have symptoms of oesophagopharyngeal regurgitation. In such patients, Gerhardt and co-workers have demonstrated diminished peristaltic amplitude in the oesophageal body, upper oesophageal sphincter hypotension and a diminished upper oesophageal sphincter response to acid or saline oesophageal infusion [59]. Conversely, some GOR subjects have cricopharyngeal dysphagia which may persist following surgical correction of abnormal GOR [58]. Henderson and Marryat reported successful treatment of this condition by cricopharyngeal myotomy, and found that a careful history was the most sensitive indicator of this problem [58]. Few of their patients had radiological abnormalities, while just over one half of those studied with manometry exhibited evidence of intermittent cricopharyngeal incoordination [58]. Finally, although one group has reported that globus hystericus is a complication of GOR [61], this has not been substantiated in a large study using prolonged intraoesophageal pH monitoring to detect abnormal GOR [62].

In conclusion, there is good evidence that the UOS can respond to intraoesophageal distension, particularly by an acid bolus, but little evidence for any change in basal UOS pressure in the majority of GOR patients. Nevertheless, a minority with symptoms of oesophagopharyngeal regurgitation or cricopharyngeal dysphagia does appear to have functional abnormalities of the UOS.

References

1. Payne, W. W. and Poulton, E. P. Visceral pain in the upper alimentary tract. *Q. J. Med.* 1923; **17**: 53–80
2. Jones, C. M. and Richardson, W. Observations on the nature of heartburn (Abstract). *J. Clin. Invest.* 1926; **2**: 610
3. Polland, W. S. and Bloomfield, A. L. Experimental referred pain from the gastrointestinal tract. Part 1: the oesophagus. *J. Clin. Invest.* 1931; **10**: 435–452
4. Jones, C. M. Digestive Tract Pain: Diagnosis and Treatment. New York: Macmillan. 1938.
5. Bernstein, L. M. and Baker, L. A. A clinical test for esophagitis. *Gastroenterology* 1958; **34**: 760–781
6. Siegel, C. I. and Hendrix, T. R. Esophageal motor abnormalities induced by acid perfusion in patients with heartburn. *J. Clin. Invest.* 1963; **42**: 686–695
7. Tuttle, S. G., Rufin, F. and Bettarello, A. The physiology of heartburn. *Ann. Intern. Med.* 1961; **55**: 292–300
8. Tuttle, S. G., Bettarello, A. and Grossman, M. I. Esophageal acid perfusion test and a gastroesophageal reflux test in patients with esophagitis. *Gastroenterology* 1960; **38**: 861–872
9. Creamer, B., Donoghue, F. E. and Code, C. F. Patterns of esophageal motility in diffuse spasm. *Gastroenterology* 1958; **34**: 782–796

10. Bennett, J. R. and Hendrix, T. R. Diffuse esophageal spasm: a disorder with more than one cause. *Gastroenterology* 1970; **59**: 273–279

11. Benz, L. J., Hootkin, L. A., Margulies, S., Donner, M. W., Cauthorne, R. T. and Hendrix, T. R. A comparison of clinical measurements of gastroesophageal reflux. *Gastroenterology* 1972; **62**: 1–5

12. Atkinson, M. and Bennett, J. R. Relationship between motor changes and pain during esophageal acid perfusion. *Am. J. Dig. Dis* 1968; **13**: 346–350

13. Richter, J. E., Johns, D. N., Wu, W. C. and Castell, D. O. Are esophageal motility abnormalities produced during the intraesophageal acid perfusion test? *J. Am. Med. Assoc.* 1985; **253**: 1914–1917

14. Burns, T. W. and Venturatos, S. G. Esophageal motor function and response to acid perfusion in patients with symptomatic reflux esophagitis. *Dig. Dis. Sci.* 1985; **30**: 529–535

15. Kjellen, G. and Tibbling, L. Oesophageal motility during acid provoked heartburn and chest pain. *Scand. J. Gastroenterol.* 1985; **20**: 937–940

16. Traube, M. and McCallum, R. W. Effect of acid infusion on esophageal motility in the normal esophagus (Abstract). *Gastroenterology* 1986; **90**: 1670

17. Hollis, J. B. and Castell, D. O. Effect of dry swallows and wet swallows of different volumes on esophageal peristalsis. *J. Appl. Physiol.* 1975; **38**: 1161–1164

18. de Caestecker, J. S., Pryde, A. and Heading, R. C. Comparison of intravenous edrophonium and oesophageal acid perfusion during oesophageal manometry in patients with non-cardiac chest pain. *Gut* 1988; **29**: 1029–1034

19. Vantrappen, G., Janssens, J. and Ghillebert, G. The irritable oesophagus – a frequent cause of angina-like pain. *Lancet* 1987; **i**: 1232–1234

20. Richter, J. E. Acid perfusion (Bernstein) test. In: Castell, D. O., Wu, N. C. and Ott, D. J., Eds. *Gastroesophageal Reflux Disease: Pathogenesis, diagnosis, therapy.* New York: Futura Co. 1985: 139–148

21. Olsen, A. M. and Schlegel, J. F. Motility disturbances caused by oesophagitis. *J. Thorac. Cardiovasc. Surg.* 1965; **50**: 607–612

22. Kahrilas, P. J., Dodds, W. J., Hogan, W. J., Kern, D. M., Arndorfer, R. C. and Reece, A. Esophageal peristaltic dysfunction in peptic esophagitis. *Gastroenterology* 1986; **91**: 897–904

23. Dent, J., Holloway, R. H., Toouli, J. and Dodds, W. J. Mechanisms of lower oesophageal sphincter incompetence in patients with symptomatic gastro-oesophageal reflux. *Gut* 1988; **29**: 1020–1028

24. Eastwood, G. L., Castell, D. O. and Higgs, R. H. Experimental esophagitis in cats impairs lower oesophageal sphincter pressure. *Gastroenterology* 1975; **69**: 146–153

25. Sinar, D. R., Fletcher, J. R., Cordova, C. C., Eastwood, G. L. and Castell, D. O. Acute acid induced esophagitis impairs esophageal peristalsis in baboons (Abstract). *Gastroenterology* 1981; **80**: 1286

26. Higgs, R. H., Castell, D. O. and Eastwood, G. L. Studies in the mechanism of esophagitis induced lower esophageal sphincter hypotension in casts. *Gastroenterology* 1976; **71**: 51–57

27. Eastwood, G. L., Beck, B. D., Castell, D. O., Brown, F. C. and Fletcher, J. R. Beneficial effect of indomethacin on acid-induced esophagitis in cats. *Dig. Dis. Sci.* 1981; **26**: 601–608

28. Biancani, P., Barwick, K., Selling, J. and McCallum, R. Effects of acute experimental esophagitis on mechanical properties of the lower esophageal sphincter. *Gastroenterology* 1984; **87**: 8–16

29. Katz, P. O., Knuff, T. E., Benjamin, S. B. and Castell, D. O. Abnormal esophageal pressures in reflux esophagitis: cause or effect? *Am. J. Gastroenterol.* 1986; **81**: 744

30. Baldi, F., Ferrarini, F., Longanesi, A. *et al.* Oesophageal function before, during and after healing of erosive oesophagitis. *Gut* 1988; **29**: 157–160

31. Behar, J., Brand, D. L., Brown, F. L. *et al.* Cimetidine in the treatment of symptomatic gastroesophageal reflux: a double blind controlled trial. *Gastroenterology* 1978; **74**: 441–448

32. Wesdorp, E., Bartelsman, J., Pape, K., Dekker, W. and Tytgat, G. N. Oral cimetidine in reflux esophagitis: a double blind controlled trial. *Gastroenterology* 1978; **74**: 821–824

33. Gill, R. C., Bones, K. L., Murphy, P. D. and Kingman, Y. J. Esophageal motor abnormalities in gastroeosophageal reflux and the effects of fundoplication. *Gastroenterology* 1986; **91**: 364–369

34. Heddle, R., Dent, J., Toouli, J. and Lewis, I. Esophageal peristaltic dysfunction in peptic esophagitis (Abstract). *Gastroenterology* 1984; **86**: 1109

35. Cucchiara, S., Staiano, A., DiLorenzo, C. *et al.* Esophageal motor abnormalities in children with gastrooesophageal reflux and peptic esophagitis. *J. Pediatr.* 1986; **108**: 1109

36. Ahtaridis, G., Snape, W. J. and Cohen, S. Clinical and manometric findings in benign peptic strictures of the esophagus. *Dig. Dis. Sci.* 1979; **24**: 858–861

37. Gonis, G., Anggiansah, A., Rokkas, T., McCullagh, M. and Diven, W. J. Does oesophageal motor activity improve after surgical treatment of gastro-oesophageal reflux (GOR)? (Abstract) *Gut* 1988; **29**: A1448

38. Marshall, J. B. and Gerhardt, D. C. Improvement in esophageal motor dysfunction with treatment of reflux esophagitis: a report of 2 cases. *Am. J. Gastroenterol.* 1982; **77**: 351–354

39. Russell, C. O. H., Pope, C. E., Gannan, R. M., Allen, F. D., Velasco, N. and Hill, L. D. Does surgery correct esophageal motor dysfunction in gastroesophageal reflux? *Ann. Surg.* 1981; **194**: 290–295

40. Mittal, R. K. and McCallum, R. W. Characteristics of transient lower esophageal sphincter relaxation in humans. *Am. J. Physiol.* 1987; **252**: G636–G641

41. Mittal, R. K. and McCallum, F. W. Characteristics and frequency of transient relaxations of the lower esophageal sphincter in patients with reflux esophagitis. *Gastroenterology* 1988; **95**: 593–599

42. Longhi, E. H. and Jordan, P. H. Pressure relationships responsible for reflux in patients with hiatal hernia. *Surg. Gynecol. Obstet.* 1969; **129**: 734–748

43. Stanciu, C. and Bennett, J. R. Oesophageal acid clearing: one factor in the production of reflux oesophagitis. *Gut* 1974; **15**: 852–857

44. Tolin, R. D., Malmud, R. S., Reilley, J. and Fisher R. S. Esophageal scintigraphy to quantitate esophageal transit (quantitation of esophageal transit). *Gastroenterology* 1979; **76**: 1402–1408

45. de Caestecker, J. S., Blackwell, J. N., Adam, R. D., Hannan, W. J., Brown, J. and Heading, R. C. Clinical value of radionuclide oesophageal transit measurement. *Gut* 1986; **27**: 659–666

46. Cranford, C. A., Sutton, D., Sadek, S. A., Kennedy, N. and Cuschieri, A. New physiological method of evaluating oesophageal transit. *Br. J. Surg.* 1987; **74**: 411–415

47. Eriksen, C. A., Sadek, S. A., Cranford, C., Sutton, D., Kennedy, D. and Cuschieri, A. Reflux oesophagitis and oesophageal transit: evidence for a primary oesophageal motor disorder. *Gut* 1988; **29**: 448–452

48. Maddern, G. J. and Jamieson, G. G. Oesophageal emptying in patients with gastro-oesophageal reflux. *Br. J. Surg.* 1986; **73**: 615–617

49. Bancewicz, J., Osugi, H. and Marples, M. Clinical applications of abnormal oesophageal motility. *Br. J. Surg.* 1987; **74**: 416–419

50. Winship, D. H. Upper esophageal sphincter: does it care about reflux? *Gastroenterology* 1983; **85**: 470–472

51. Creamer, B. and Schlegel, J. Motor responses of the esophagus to distension. *J. Appl. Physiol.* 1957; **10**: 498–504

52. Andreollo, N. A., Thompson, D. G., Kendall, G. P. N. and Earlam, R. J. Functional relationship between cricopharyngeal sphincter and oesophageal body in response to graded intraluminal distension. *Gut* 1988; **29**: 161–166

53. Gerhardt, D. C., Shuck, T. J., Bordeaux, R. A. and Winship, D. H. Human upper esophageal sphincter: response to volume, osmotic and acid stimuli. *Gastroenterology* 1978; **75**: 268–274

54. Stanciu, C. and Bennett, J. R. Upper oesophageal sphincter yield pressure in normal subjects and in patients with gastro-oesophageal reflux. *Thorax* 1974; **29**: 459–462

55. Hunt, P. S., Connell, A. M. and Sunley, T. B. The cricopharyngeal sphincter in gastric reflux. *Gut* 1970; **11**: 303–306

56. Winnans, C. S. The pharyngoesophageal closure mechanism: a manometric study. *Gastroenterology* 1972; **63**: 768–777

57. Berte, L. E. and Wimans, C. S. Lower esophageal sphincter function does not determine resting upper esophageal sphincter pressure. *Dig. Dis.* 1977; **22**: 877–880

58. Henderson, R. D. and Marryat, G. Cricopharyngeal myotomy as a method of treating cricopharyngeal dysphagia secondary to gastroesophageal reflux. *J. Thorac. Cardiovasc. Surg.* 1977; **74**: 721–725

59. Gerhardt, D. E., Castell, D. O., Winship, D. H. and Shuck, T. J. Esophageal dysfunction in esophagopharyngeal regurgitation. *Gastroenterology* 1980; **78**: 893–897

60. Kahrilas, P. J., Dodds, W. J., Dent, J., Haeberle, B., Hogan, W. J. and Arndorfer, R. C. Effect of sleep, spontaneous gastroesophageal reflux and a meal on upper esophageal sphincter pressure in

normal human volunteers. *Gastroenterology* 1987; **92**: 466–471

61. Delahunty, J. E. and Ardan, G. M. Globus hystericus – a manifestation of reflux esophagitis? *J. Laryngol. Otol.* 1970; **84**: 1049–1054

62. Wilson, J. A., Heading, R. C., Maran, A. G. D., Pryde, A., Piris, J. and Allan, P. L. Globus sensation is not due to gastro-oesophageal reflux. *Clin. Otolaryngol.* 1987; **12**: 271–275

Chapter 6

Medical therapy for gastro-oesophageal reflux

John R. Bennett

Background

Symptomatic gastro-oesophageal reflux is so common that it would be a major problem in medicine were it not the case that the symptoms are often mild, and readily treated by simple medication. Recent UK figures [1] suggest that over 60% of the population have, or have had, dyspepsia and 69% of this dyspepsia includes heartburn. Of those with dyspepsia currently, 73% treat themselves, only 27% seeking medical advice. Nevertheless, this indicates a substantial number of patients with a condition likely to be chronic or recurrent; only a small proportion go on to receive surgery, so medical treatment will continue for many years. In order to give the patient the best result, and to use the resources most effectively, a clear understanding of the principles of medical therapy is desirable.

Aims of medical therapy

Gastro-oesophageal reflux varies in severity from a mild and infrequent inconvenience to a severe condition with life-threatening complications. The therapeutic approach needs modifying according to the circumstances, and the physician should be aware of what is achievable.

Occasional mild symptoms
Many people experience occasional heartburn and rely on self-medication, never seeking medical advice. If they do eventually visit a physician he should ascertain whether the patient came simply because he thought 'it was time' to do so, or whether there has some been change in the pattern or severity of the symptoms, If the former, it may be sufficient to confirm that continuing self-medication is acceptable; if the latter, investigation is needed to explain the deterioration before deciding on a therapeutic regimen.

'Average' regular symptoms
Here the aim is to reduce to tolerable levels, and perhaps entirely abolish, the symptoms. To do so treatment needs tailoring to the individual's specific symptoms: predominantly day-time pain may require intensive antisecretory and antacid medication; night pain may respond to nocturnal dosing and/or postural measures; regurgitation may be more responsive to weight reduction, postural measures and motility enhancing drugs; respiratory symptoms need appropriate non-competitive combinations of anti-reflux and bronchodilator drugs.

Endoscopic oesophagitis
It is still unclear how far the physician should be influenced in his therapy by the degree of endoscopically visible oesophagitis. As in duodenal ulceration, the patient's concern is to be rid of his symptoms; does it matter if a symptom-free patient nevertheless has oesophagitis? Theoretically, the abolition of oesophagitis might be important to reduce further complications, but evidence is lacking (from the literature or from personal experience) that such progression is likely or common. The point is unresolved, but the author's personal practice is to be more vigorous in initial medication if oesophagitis is marked, to be satisfied with adequate symptomatic improvement even if oesophagitis persists, although to be more disposed to continue 'maintenance therapy'. Some studies of long-term outcome indicate that prognosis and the need for maintenance therapy are predictable from the extent of oesophagitis [2].

Severe symptoms
If the symptoms are severe, significantly interfering with the patient's life and pleasure, treatment may have to be intensive and prolonged, using several therapeutic agents, and it is likely that some continued maintenance therapy will be required. If adequate remission cannot be achieved or sustained, surgery must be considered.

Complications
Ulcer   An ulcer may be 'junctional' (at the oesophagogastric junction), a gastric ulcer in the hiatus hernia or an ulcer in a columnar-lined oesophagus. In practice, the treatment is the same, and most ulcers heal well with medical therapy including antisecretory drugs.

Barrett's oesophagus   This is discussed in detail in Chapter 4, but so far no medical therapy has convincingly been shown to lead to regression of the metaplastic epithelium. Treatment is therefore based on patient symptoms, which are frequently mild.

Stricture   When the patient has reflux symptoms as well as stricture-induced dysphagia, treatment is necessary to control those symptoms. In the many patients who have dysphagia but no other reflux symptoms the need for drugs is uncertain. So far studies have not produced evidence that medical therapy alters the rate of narrowing of such strictures, although it seems reasonable to recommend standard anti-reflux measures, particularly if the stricture tends to narrow down quickly, or if there is marked oesophagitis. Indeed, in some patients with a stricture the dysphagia may be disproportionate to the degree of narrowing, due mainly to oesophagitis and, perhaps, peristaltic failure. In these circumstances, intensive medication may achieve more than repeated bougie dilatations.

The aetiological basis of therapy

The causative factors which lead to the development of gastro-oesophageal reflux disease can be discussed under five headings: the gastro-oesophageal barrier, gastric factors, oesophageal clearing, the refluxed juice and mucosal defences. For each of these the possible therapeutic options can be determined.

Gastro-oesophageal barrier

The anatomical structures which assist in forming the gastro-oesophageal barrier cannot be influenced by medical measures, unless they are helpfully changed by reduction of obesity. Weight reduction is undoubtedly extremely beneficial in reflux, but the mechanism by which improvement occurs is unknown. There have been few studies, but one report showed no correlation between body weight and resting gastro-oesophageal sphincter tone [3].

Resting tone of the gastro-oesophageal sphincter can be altered by drugs; the tone is raised by *metoclopramide* [4–7] and perhaps by *domperidone* [8,9] although others failed to demonstrate a rise [10,11] acting as dopamine antagonists, by *cisapride*, which facilitates acetylcholine release from myenteric nerves [12,13] and by the cholinergic drug *bethanechol* [14]. Bethanechol, metoclopramide and domperidone all raise the sphincter pressure by an amount proportional to its resting tone [15], limiting their usefulness in patients with weak sphincters and their effect is much less obvious when administered orally [9]. Cisapride's effect is not so related to basal tone [16] but its effects differ according to the phases of the interdigestive complex [13]. Cisapride orally reduces acid reflux [17].

An aromatic oil, *guaiacol* taken orally, increased gastro-oesophageal sphincter pressure [18] but its use has not been tested in a clinical trial. Although bethanechol has the additional useful effect of increasing salivation, it also stimulates gastric secretion.

Certain factors reduce sphincter tone, so if avoided reflux may be diminished. Fat ingestion [19], coffee [20,21], chocolate [23], peppermint [23] and alcohol [24,25] have all been shown to lower resting sphincter pressure. Alcohol also stimulates gastric secretion and delays gastric emptying. Cigarette smoking also has the effect of lowering sphincter pressure and increasing reflux [15,26].

Several drugs, administered for other indications, have adverse effects which may promote gastro-oesophageal reflux.

Although theophylline-like drugs under experimental conditions lower sphincter tone [27,28], they may not have noticeable adverse effects in clinical use [29,30]. Nevertheless, prudence suggests that they should be used cautiously in patients with both reflux and obstructive airway disease [31]. Nitroglycerin and isosorbide dinitrate are well known to lower oesophageal sphincter tone [32]. Progestational agents used in oral contraceptives may also exacerbate reflux [33].

Anticholinergics [34], calcium-channel blocking drugs [35] and β-adrenergic agonists [8,36] lower sphincter tone and may delay gastric emptying [37,38].

Oesophagitis itself reduces sphincter pressure in experimental animals [39] and effective medical treatment of oesophagitis improves resting sphincter tone [40].

Physical exertion increases intra-abdominal pressure and, although the sphincter responds to this by increasing its own tone, this reflex is less marked in patients with reflux disease. A rise in intragastric pressure may be a trigger for inappropriate sphincter relaxation [41].

The gastro-oesophageal barrier may be improved, or supplemented, by alginate compounds. After contact with gastric acid they form a viscous 'raft' on the gastric contents. This raft has been shown by scintiscanning and intraoesophageal pH monitoring [42,43] to reduce gastro-oesophageal reflux.

Experiments with injections of sclerosants under the mucosa of the gastro-oesophageal junction have shown a rise in barrier pressure, and a consequent reduction in reflux [44] but the improvement diminishes over the course of 12 months. The technique has not reached the stage of practical application.

Transient 'inappropriate' relaxation of the sphincter may be an important mechanism of reflux [45]. As their cause is still uncertain, no therapeutically beneficial way of reducing them is known.

Gastric factors

Gastric emptying

Uncertainty exists about the importance of changes in gastric emptying in gastro-oesophageal reflux. Of eleven studies of this factor, six showed delayed emptying in up to 40% of reflux patients compared with normal subjects; it is likely that in some reflux patients delayed gastric emptying is a relevant contribution. Gastric emptying can be accelerated by metoclopramide [46], domperidone [47,48] and cisapride [17,49,50], although the contribution of this effect to improving gastro-oesophageal reflux has not been convincingly demonstrated.

Duodenogastric reflux

Reports of abnormal degrees of duodenogastric reflux in patients with gastro-oesophageal reflux [51] suggested that this might be a causative factor, and it could be the case even though bile salts are present in tiny amounts in the oesophagus of reflux patients with an intact stomach [52,53]. In practice, the prokinetic drugs which accelerate gastric emptying (see above) are thought also to diminish duodenogastric reflux.

Gastric contents volume

It is logical to suppose that reflux may be increased if the volume of gastric contents is high although good evidence of this is lacking, except for studies showing that extremes of distension lead to gastro-oesophageal sphincter relaxation [41,54]. The volume of contents can obviously be minimized by eating only small meals, by reducing gastric secretion with an antisecretory drug, and by accelerating emptying. Clearly meals shortly before reflux-inducing activities or posture (physical work, bending or going to bed) should be avoided.

Oesophageal clearing

Peristalsis

The oesophagus returns refluxed gastric contents to the stomach by gravity combined with peristaltic contraction, which may be *primary*, induced by a swallow or *secondary*, as a response to oesophageal distension especially by acid [55].

The frequency of primary peristaltic waves can be increased by encouraging swallowing – such as sucking a tablet or lozenge. The force of peristaltic contractions can be increased by metoclopramide [15], bethanechol [56] and cisapride [12,49]. Oesophageal clearance appears to be uninfluenced by changes in peristaltic force [45] although cisapride was shown to increase oesophageal emptying [57]. Oesophagitis is associated with peristaltic failure [57a].

Saliva

Residual oesophageal acid, not emptied by peristalsis, is neutralized by swallowed bicarbonate-containing saliva [45]. Therapeutically salivary flow may be stimulated by the cholinergic bethanechol but more effectively and conveniently by sucking a lozenge [45].

Gravity
When the patient is recumbent, gravity does not aid oesophageal emptying (clearing). Bed-head elevation by 20 cm, or raising the shoulders by a foam wedge under the mattress [58], accelerates oesophageal emptying and reduces oesophageal acid exposure [59]. It improves oesophagitis and reflux symptoms used alone, and improves the effectiveness of antisecretory drugs in reducing symptoms and endoscopic oesophagitis [60].

Nature of refluxed material

Acid
Gastric hydrochloric acid is still considered the predominant material in the refluxate which causes symptoms and oesophagitis.

Antacids neutralize small amounts of acid in the oesophagus and often give prompt relief of heartburn. In large amounts they can reduce intragastric acidity [61], making the refluxate less acid [62], but this is seldom used in practice today.

The addition of silicones (polymethylsiloxane) has been considered by some to improve antacid effectiveness [63] but their use does diminish the effectiveness of alginate raft production.

Antisecretory drugs produce noticeable reductions in volume and acidity of gastric juice, depending on the drug and its dose. For effective healing of oesophagitis it seems necessary to use doses either higher or more frequent than those employed in treating duodenal ulcers. Their convenience and safety have made this range of drugs the stand-by treatment of moderate to severe reflux and oesophagitis.

Pepsin
No specific antipepsin drugs are available, although antisecretory drugs reduce pepsin secretion by amounts proportional to their acid-reducing power. Sucralfate inhibits peptic activity by adsorbing pepsin [64].

Bile
It has been suggested that bile may be an important element in causing oesophagitis. After gastric surgery this may be so, but most of the evidence about bile damage comes from animal experiments using high concentrations of bile [65,66]. Two studies of bile concentrations in the oesophageal juice of reflux patients show there to be little or no bile acids [52,53]. In any case, no practical medical treatment to remove or inhibit bile exists. Cholestyramine is a theoretical possibility [67], but cannot be kept in contact with the oesophagus for long enough to be effective, and so proved disappointing in a clinical trial [68]. Sucralfate may have some effect in adsorbing bile.

Mucosal defences

The oesophageal mucosa has a natural resistance to damage by refluxed gastric juice or swallowed irritants. Experiments have shown that resistance can be diminished by bile salts [68a] and cigarette smoke [68b].

It is also known that certain drugs can damage the mucosa, either through their own irritant effect or by diminishing resistance to the entry of H^+ ions. A list of drugs known to do this is given in Table 6.1.

Non-steroidal anti-inflammatory drugs may be a particular problem. Although

Table 6.1 Drugs which induce oesophagitis

Emepronium
Potassium chloride
Tetracycline and other antibiotics
Theophylline
Ascorbic acid
Naftidrofuryl
Carbachol
Fluorouracil
Iron compounds
Non-steroidal anti-inflammatory drugs

their role in the aetiology of uncomplicated reflux oesophagitis is presumed rather than proved, there does seem to be a definite association between their use and the occurrence of oesophageal stricture [69,70]. All such drugs should be avoided by patients with gastro-oesophageal reflux.

Two drugs are thought to have possible beneficial effects on the oesophageal mucosa – carbenoxolone and sucralfate.

Carbenoxolone, given in combination with alginate as the preparation Pyrogastrone, increases mucosal repair mechanisms [71]. The only randomized trial of its use showed improved healing of oesophageal ulcers and oesophagitis compared with alginate alone [72] but it has not gained widespread use, perhaps because of anxieties about the aldosterone-like side effects. Sucralfate, used as a slurry, can be shown to attach itself to inflamed oesophageal mucosa [73]. It enhances resistance of the mucosa to acid diffusion [74] and clinical studies have given encouraging results (see below).

Therapeutic trials in gastro-oesophageal reflux

Formal therapeutic trials in gastro-oesophageal reflux disease present many problems.

The first is of diagnosis and definition. There is no single criterion upon which the diagnosis can be firmly based (unlike, for example, the presence or absence of a peptic ulcer) (see Chapter 3).

Symptoms are unreliable; endoscopic appearances are subject to observer error and are absent in perhaps 30% of patients considered on other grounds to have reflux; all methods for demonstrating reflux are fallible. So whatever diagnostic criterion is used, some patients will be wrongly included, and the trial group will not contain the full spectrum of reflux disease. Thus, if endoscopic oesophagitis is a qualification for entry, the 30% or so of reflux patients who do not exhibit mucosal changes will be excluded.

The second, and related, problem is to judge the end-point of success or failure. Symptom scores and 'escape' antacid consumption give an indication of patient satisfaction but are subject to all the vagaries of human behaviour; changes in endoscopic oesophagitis are dependent on observer accuracy; alterations in degree of reflux (e.g. by pH monitoring) do not necessarily reflect benefit or failure of treatment of the whole reflux syndrome.

Duration of therapy is a third difficulty. Reflux disease tends to improve slowly, so trials need to be considerably longer than those for peptic ulcer healing. Many published trials have been for only 4–6 weeks, probably too short for full benefit to accrue.

Single-agent therapy can be tested relatively well despite these problems, but in practical clinical medicine several therapeutic approaches are deployed simultaneously. So, in a trial, is it ethical to give the patient no advice about diet, weight, posture, smoking etc. and, if some patients do alter these, is the trial valid? Assessing more than a single entity in one trial raises great difficulties, requiring large numbers of individuals particularly if an untreated placebo group is to be included. Cross-over studies can be misleading because of a marked potential carry-over effect of initial improvement.

Against this background, any assessment of the results of therapeutic trials must be cautious. Every trial differs from its predecessors, and several trials of the same agent may be markedly different in design. The review of some trials which follows should be read with these provisos in mind.

Antacids

Despite the frequency with which antacids are used in reflux disease (or, perhaps, because of it) there have been few formal trials of their efficacy. Behar *et al.* [75] showed symptomatic benefit in mild oesophagitis; Graham and Paterson [76] showed no significant difference in symptoms between antacid (560 mmol/day) and placebo over 5 weeks although in a cross-over study by Grove *et al.* [77] antacid (850 mmol/day) was superior to placebo for symptom relief.

Antacids with silicone

Dimethylpolysiloxane preparations reduce surface tension and act as defoaming agents. The theory that this is of benefit has been put to the test only once: Ogilvie and Atkinson [63] compared antacid and dimethicone with antacid alone and found similar rates of improvement of symptoms and oesophagitis for both; there was a marginally greater improvement of oesophagitis in the dimethicone group.

Antacids with alginate

Alginic acid forms a floating raft of high pH alginate foam on the gastric contents. When combined with antacid it reduces gastro-oesophageal reflux, as shown by oesophageal pH monitoring [42], or by scintiscanning [78]. Several groups found a reduction in reflux symptoms when compared with placebo or antacid [42,79–81], although others [82,83] found no difference from antacids. No randomized trial has shown improvement in oesophagitis due to alginate preparation alone.

Acid secretory antagonists

These drugs diminish the volume, acid concentration and pepsin content of gastric juice to varying degrees.

Cimetidine, the first commercially available histamine H_2-receptor antagonist, showed its superiority to placebo in diminishing reflux symptoms in several studies at a dose of 1.2–1.6 g/day [84,85] although many of them had only small numbers of patients [86–88]. Endoscopic changes sometimes improved [87,89,90] but more often did not. An intraluminal pH study showed only a modest reduction in acid reflux

[91]. Cimetidine was superior to bethanechol [92], Pyrogastrone [93] and antacid–alginate.

Although one study [94] suggested that cimetidine 800 mg at night was as effective as 400 mg four times daily, the continued occurrence of reflux episodes throughout the day suggests that more frequent dosing may be more reliable.

One report suggests that cimetidine may be more effective when administered in suspension than as a tablet [95].

Ranitidine 300 mg a day was also superior to a placebo [96–98], to metoclopramide [99] and to antacid [77], but not to domperidone [100] or to cimetidine [101–103], although Brunner had some success in treating cimetidine failures with ranitidine [104]. Endoscopic healing has been more often reported than with cimetidine [96,97,105,106] including a large study (vs placebo) by Sontag et al. [98]. The milder degrees of oesophagitis healed faster than more extensive erosions [2] but more prolonged treatment may heal more severe lesions [97]. Smoking did not adversely affect the improvement [107]. A single 300 mg bed-time dose was as effective as 150 mg twice daily [108].

In a study in which a higher dose (300 mg twice daily) produced endoscopic healing in only half the cases after 6 weeks, improvement seemed related to the amount by which measurable acid reflux had been suppressed [109]. A night-time dose of 300 mg seems equivalent to 150 mg twice daily [109a]. However, in patients who did poorly on 150 mg twice daily an increase in dose to 600–1500 mg daily produced impressive healing of oesophagitis and reduction in symptoms.

Famotidine is also effective and as its dose increases from 40 mg at night to 40 mg twice daily, oesophageal acid exposure diminishes [110].

Nizatidine 300 mg twice daily gave better symptom relief but similar endoscopic healing to 300 mg at night (unpublished data).

In summary, histamine H_2-receptor antagonists have been a considerable advance in the management of reflux disease, but on their own will only control and heal the disease in 60–70% of patients. Their great advantage is their convenience and safety.

Pirenzepine

Pirenzepine is a tricyclic compound which inhibits gastric secretion [111] by antimuscarinic effects. Its antisecretory activity is less powerful than histamine H_2-receptor antagonists, and there is the theoretical possibility that it might reduce gastro-oesophageal sphincter tone as it does when given parenterally [112,113]. However, no measurable effect on the sphincter has been detected after oral dosing [114–117].

In therapeutic trials the drug improved symptoms, reduced endoscopic oesophagitis [118,119] and reduced acid exposure measured by pH monitoring [120].

Omeprazole

This proton pump inhibitor is the most powerful gastric secretory blocking drug currently available [121] but has no perceptible effect on oesophageal motility. It reduces oesophagitis quickly, as shown in a 4-week open study [122], and is more effective than ranitidine in symptom relief and oesophagitis healing [123–127a]. A dose of 40 mg a day heals slightly faster than 20 mg daily [128]. Patients who had not improved on cimetidine at a high dose of 3.2 g daily usually improved when changed to omeprazole [129] and in one study all 'ranitidine failures' healed with omeprazole [124]. Intraluminal pH measurements indicate a greater reduction in acid exposure by omeprazole 20 mg daily, than ranitidine 150 mg twice daily [129a]. Used alone, omeprazole will increase healing rates of oesophagitis to 90%.

Motility enhancing drugs

This group of drugs (sometimes known as prokinetic agents) comprises bethanechol, metoclopramide, domperidone and cisapride. Other drugs with similar effects exist but are either not commercially available or have not been widely used.

Bethanechol

This is a muscarinic agent which raises gastro-oesophageal pressure [130]. It also accelerates oesophageal clearance of an acid load, an effect once thought to be due to peristaltic stimulation but shown by Helm and colleagues [45] to be mediated mainly by salivary stimulation. It reduces acid exposure in the recumbent posture [131]. Thanik et al. [92] demonstrated a similar effectiveness to cimetidine, but a good trial by Saco et al. [132] demonstrated no greater benefit from antacid with bethanechol 25 mg four times daily than from antacid alone.

Some patients on the drug experience abdominal cramps or urinary frequency.

Metoclopramide

This benzamide derivative probably acts by dopamine antagonism together with possible acetylcholine release, and antagonism of 5-hydroxytryptamine (5HT or serotonin) receptors. It reduces reflux [133], improves symptoms better than placebo [134,135] and in one trial did so as effectively as cimetidine [136], but ranitidine was better at healing oesophagitis [99].

Tiredness affects about a third of patients taking 30–40 mg daily, and severe extrapyramidal side effects occasionally occur.

Domperidone

Domperidone relieved symptoms better than placebo [11,137], as well as ranitidine [100], but oesophagitis was not often healed, while other studies failed to show benefit [10].

Hyperprolactinaemia can occur with long-term use, causing galactorrhoea or amenorrhoea.

Cisapride

This may be the most effective prokinetic agent at present. Trials in reflux disease have shown its superiority to placebo [138,139] and to metoclopramide [140] in symptom and oesophagitis improvement, and a similar effectiveness to ranitidine [141] and cimetidine [142]. It improved the effectiveness of cimetidine when used in combination [143]. Diarrhoea and abdominal cramps occur in up to 5% of patients on the drug.

Mucosal protective agents

The available drugs which seem to act by this mechanism are carbenoxolone, sucralfate and tripotassium dicitratobismuthate (TDB). The chief problem of such agents is the relatively short contact time of any swallowed drug with the oesophageal mucosa compared with the longer period the drug will be in the stomach or duodenum.

Carbenoxolone

This agent has several effects on columnar epithelium which accelerate healing of gastric and duodenal ulcers, but the effects on squamous epithelium might not be the same. Nevertheless, the only double-sided study showed a carbenoxolone–alginate preparation to be more effective than antacid in healing oesophageal ulcers [72], and a retrospective open study of 104 patients suggested good symptomatic endoscopic responses; some patients had been treated for over a year continuously without major ill effects [144]. At a dose of 100 mg daily it produced speedier symptom improvement than antacid–alginate, but no better endoscopic healing [145]. In a comparison with cimetidine there was similar symptomatic and endoscopic benefit [93].

Sucralfate

This aluminium salt of sucrose sulphate becomes viscous and adhesive when mixed with gastric acid. It binds to protein causing resistance to proteolysis, and also adsorbs pepsin and inhibits its activity.

Studies in vitro show that it increases the resistance of oesophageal mucosa to acid, pepsin and bile [74] and it increases resistance to artificially induced oesophagitis in animals [146]. Perhaps surprisingly one study suggested that it diminished acid reflux after 12 weeks' treatment [147].

Therapeutic trials have given equivocal results; against placebo one large trial demonstrated no benefit [148], but others demonstrated better symptom relief, especially in mild minimal-change oesophagitis [149–151]. It was as effective as an antacid–alginate in reducing symptoms and a little better at healing oesophagitis [152,153]. Yet it has been shown to give marginally poorer or similar benefit to cimetidine [154] and ranitidine [155]. Ros *et al.* [156] were successful in using sucralfate in some patients with oesophagitis resistant to H$_2$-receptor antagonists.

In these studies the sucralfate was given as a suspension. There is uncertainty whether it is as effective in tablet form, and as to the best intervals and timing in relation to meals at which it should be administered.

Tripotassium dicitratobismuthate (TDB)

This agent is effective in healing gastric and duodenal ulcers, possibly because of its effectiveness at suppressing *Campylobacter pylori*. It has been used in reflux disease and anecdotes suggest benefit, but formal trials are lacking.

Physical methods

Weight reduction, avoidance of bending, diets low in fat, chocolate and coffee, cessation of smoking and avoidance of alcohol are usually advised on the basis of short-term studies showing that the various agents increase reflux, or an observation that they regularly precipitate symptoms. The effectiveness of avoidance measures has not been put to formal trial.

Elevation of the bed-head, shown by intraluminal pH measurements, to reduce reflux, has been tested in an interesting four-way comparison of placebo, ranitidine and bed-head elevation. Ranitidine and bed elevation each gave benefit (symptoms and endoscopic healing) but their combined effect was greatest [60].

Combined therapy

As indicated in the introduction, studies of drug combination in reflux disease are not easy (despite the fact that combined therapy is often deployed in clinical practice) and few have been done.

The good study of ranitidine combined with bed-elevation has been mentioned above [60].

The only other studies of combined therapy have been with cimetidine and alginate, and cimetidine with metoclopramide or cisapride.

The first large study of metoclopramide 30 mg daily with cimetidine 1600 mg showed no benefit, and a high incidence of adverse effects [157]. However, Lieberman and Keeffe [158] added metoclopramide to cimetidine in patients doing poorly on cimetidine alone and showed benefit.

Cisapride 40 mg daily improved the results of cimetidine 1 g daily, both for symptoms and oesophagitis healing [143] but 20 mg combined with 300 mg ranitidine was no better than ranitidine alone [159].

Cimetidine 1600 mg daily increased the clinical benefit of antacid–alginate [160] and reduced acid reflux (Cuschieri, A., 1987, unpublished results).

Long-term therapy

Gastro-oesophageal reflux disease is well known to be a chronic and relapsing condition, so it is surprising that there are few data about long-term outcome, and not many studies of medication for periods longer than 8–12 weeks. Yet it is of prime importance to know what the likely long-term course is to be for a patient, and to have clearer ideas of the best approach to maintenance therapy.

Not all patients relapse quickly after a course of therapy and, for many, simple medication (perhaps on-demand antacids alone) suffices. As many patients do not seek medical advice but rely on self-medication the whole picture is difficult to see.

Of those who are treated medically by physicians, perhaps half relapse soon after a course of treatment, and a few relapse subsequently, but up to 40% remain in remission [161], although 24 patients in Norway followed for 36 weeks after a 12-week course of cimetidine all maintained their improvement whether they were on placebo or cimetidine 400 mg daily [162]. However, Koelz et al. [2] found relapse in over a third of their healed patients within 6 months, whether they were given placebo or ranitidine 150 mg daily. Higher doses of ranitidine continuously does seem to prevent relapse, however [96,163].

Practical approach to therapy

Once the diagnosis of gastro-oesophageal reflux disease has been established, a clear explanation should be given to the patient of the cause and mechanism of his problem, so that he can understand his role in management. Many patients have been told, or suspect, that they have a 'hiatus hernia', a diagnosis which may cause them unnecessary concern, with its implications of hernia complications and the likelihood of needing surgery.

It is essential at an early stage to stress the general measures which are so important. These must include weight reduction for the obese, cessation of smoking, reduction of (or temporary abstinence from) alcohol, avoidance of fat and chocolate, and only modest amounts of coffee. Caution should be taken in drinking citrus juices and eating spices.

For some patients these measures (particularly weight reduction) may be all that is required, but they should be prescribed a supply of palatable antacid tablets to suck as frequently as they wish, particularly after meals and if heartburn occurs. This can be supplemented by an antacid–alginate preparation, after meals and particularly at bedtime.

If symptoms are troublesome or oesophagitis is evident at endoscopy, greater medication is necessary. Most convenient and safe is to add a histamine H_2-receptor antagonist. Initially this can be given as a standard 'ulcer-healing' course (single bedtime dose) but if response is inadequate more frequent and higher doses (e.g. cimetidine 400 mg four times or ranitidine 300 mg twice daily) will give a better result.

The patient's progress should be reviewed after 4–6 weeks on this regimen. If response has been good it should be continued undiminished for a total of 12 weeks. If response has been unsatisfactory, something more is needed.

There can be no doubt that a course of omeprazole will produce a marked improvement in most patients and, if the response is inadequate, the diagnosis should be reviewed. Eight weeks of omeprazole seems entirely safe. In our present state of knowledge it remains uncertain whether longer courses are justified, except in problem patients.

If nocturnal pain or regurgitation is a particular problem bed-head elevation should be arranged, and this can be a helpful measure even if the symptoms are mainly diurnal. Addition of another drug should be considered. Both mucosal protective agents and prokinetics can be used in combination with the preceding drugs, and there are no guides as to the likely success of one or the other. If nausea, fullness, satiety or belching are prominent a prokinetic drug is logical. If odyno-phagia and heartburn are the main symptoms, sucralfate might be preferred. If there is real difficulty in symptom control, both can be deployed.

Whatever combination is used, if benefit is derived it should be continued for a minimum of 12 weeks, the aim being to allow 'healing' – diminution of oesophagitis and reduction of mucosal sensitivity, and perhaps improvement in gastro-oeso-phageal sphincter tone [40]. At this point a tentative reduction in drug therapy may begin, emphasizing the importance of continuing dietary and weight control.

Some patients will find that they can gradually reduce their medication to nothing; others will discover that a certain level of maintenance is required – trial and error will determine the optimum but it may be a nocturnal dose of alginate or H_2-receptor antagonist, supplemented by antacids whenever needed, although some will require intensive medication.

References

1. Jones, R. and Lydeard, S. Prevalence of dyspepsia in the community. *Br. Med. J.* 1989; **298**: 30–32
2. Koelz, H. R., Birchler, R., Bretholz, A. *et al.* Healing and relapse of reflux esophagitis during treatment with ranitidine. *Gastroenterology* 1986; **91**: 1198–1205
3. Backman, L., Granstom, L., Lindahl, J. and Melcher, A. Manometric studies of lower esophageal sphincter in extreme obesity. *Acta Chir. Scand.* 1983; **149**: 193–197
4. Stanciu, C. and Bennett, J. R. Smoking and gastro-oesophageal reflux. *Br. Med. J.* 1972; **3**: 793–795
5. Schulze-Delrieu, K. Metoclopramide. *Gastroenterology* 1979; **77**: 768–779
6. Wallin, L., Boesby, S. and Madsen, T. Effect of oral metoclopramide on oesophageal peristalsis and gastro-oesophageal pressure. *Scand. J. Gastroenterol.* 1979; **14**: 923–927
7. Durazo, F., Gramisu, M. and Valenzuela, J. E. Effect of metoclopramide on the mechanism of gastroesophageal reflux. *Gastroenterology* 1987; **92**: 1378
8. Weihrauch, T. R., Forster, C. R. F. and Kriegelstein, J. Evaluation of the effect of domperidone on human esophagus and gastroduodenal motility by intraluminal manometry. *Postgrad. Med. J.* 1979; **55**: 7–11
9. Wallin, L., Madsen, T. and Boesby, S. Effect of domperidone on gastro-oesophageal function in normal human subjects. *Scand. J. Gastroenterol.* 1985; **20**: 150–154

10. Blackwell, J. N., Heading, R. C. and Fettes, M. R. Effects of domperidone on lower esophageal sphincter pressure and gastro-esophageal reflux in patients with peptic esophagitis. In: *Progress with Domperidone, Royal Society of Medicine International Congress and Symposium*, Vol. 36. 1981: 57–67

11. Valenzuela, J. E. Effects of domperidone on the symptoms of reflux oesophagitis. In *Progress with Domperidone, Royal Society of Medicine International Congress and Symposium*, Series No. 36. 1981: 51–57

12. Janssens, J., Ceccatelli, P. and Vantrappen, G. Cisapride restores the decreased lower esophageal sphincter pressure in reflux patients. *Dig. Dis. Sci.* 1986; **31**: 285

13. Smout, A. J. P. M., Bogaard, J. W., Grade, A. C., Tenthie, O. J., Akkermans, L. M. and Wittebol, P. Effects of cisapride, a new gastrointestinal prokinetic substance, on interdigestive and post-prandial motor activity of the distal oesophagus. *Gut* 1986; **26**: 246–251

14. Farrell, R. L., Roling, G. T. and Castell, D. O. Cholinergic therapy of chronic heartburn. *Ann. Intern. Med.* 1974; **80**: 573–576

15. Stanciu, C. and Bennett, J. R. Metoclopramide in gastro-oesophageal reflux. *Gut* 1973; **14**: 275–279

16. Ceccatelli, P., Janssens, J., Vantrappen, G. and Cucciara, S. Cisapride restores the decreased lower oesophageal sphincter pressure in reflux patients. *Gut* 1988; **29**: 631–635

17. Collins, B. J., Spence, R. A. J., Ferguson, R., Laird, J. and Love, A. H. G. Cisapride: influence on oesophageal and gastric emptying and gastro-oesophageal reflux in patients with reflux oesophagitis. *Hepato-gastroenterology* 1987; **34**: 113–116

18. Heatley, R. V., Evans, B. K., Rhodes, J. *et al.* Guaiacol – a new compound in the treatment of gastro-oesophageal reflux. *Gut* 1982; **23**: 1044–1047

19. Nebel, O. T. and Castell, D. O. Inhibition of the lower oesophageal sphincter by fat – a mechanism for fatty food intolerance. *Gut* 1973; **14**: 270–274

20. Cohen, S. Pathogenesis of coffee-induced gastro-intestinal symptoms. *N. Engl. J. Med.* 1980; **303**: 122–124

21. Salmon, P. R., Fedail, S. S., Wurzner, H. P., Harvey, R. F. and Read, A. E. Effect of coffee on human lower esophageal function. *Digestion* 1981; **21**: 69–73

22. Wright, L. E. and Castell, D. O. The adverse effect of chocolate on lower esophageal sphincter pressure. *Am. J. Dig. Dis.* 1975; **20**: 703–707

23. Sigmund, C. J. and McNally, E. F. The action of a carminative on the lower esophageal sphincter. *Gastroenterology* 1969; **56**: 13–18

24. Hogan, W. J., Viegas de Andrade, S. R. and Winship, D. H. Ethanol-induced esophageal motor dysfunction. *J. Appl. Physiol.* 1972; **32**: 755–760

25. Kaufman, S. E. and Kaye, M. D. Induction of gastro-oesophageal reflux by alcohol. *Gut* 1978; **19**: 336–338

26. Dennish, S. W. and Castell, D. O. Inhibitory effect of smoking on the lower esophageal sphincter. *N. Engl. J. Med.* 1971; **284**: 1136–1137

27. Stein, M. R., Towner, T. G., Weber, R. W. *et al.* The effect of theophylline on the lower esophageal sphincter pressure. *Ann. Allergy* 1980; **45**: 238–241

28. Johannesson, N., Andersson, K. E., Joelsson, B. *et al.* Relaxation of lower esophageal sphincter and stimulation of gastric secretion and diuresis by anti-asthmatic xanthines. *Am. Rev. Respir. Dis.* 1985; **131**: 26–31

29. Hubert, D., Gaudric, M., Marsac, I. *et al.* Theophylline does not increase gastroesophageal reflux in asthmatic patients. *Am. Rev. Respir. Dis.* 1986; **133**: 320A

30. Lynrenas, E., Abrahamsson, H. and Dovetail, G. Effect of β_2-adrenergic stimulation on human esophageal peristalsis. *Gastroenterology* 1986; **90**: 1528A

31. Goldman, J. and Bennett, J. R. Gastro-oesophageal reflux and respiratory disorders in adults. *Lancet* 1988; **ii**: 493–494

32. Kikkendall, J. W. and Mellon, M. H. Effect of sublingual nitroglycerine and long-lasting nitrate preparation on esophageal motility. *Gastroenterology* 1980; **79**: 703–706

33. Van Thiel, D. H., Gavaler, J. S. and Stremple, J. F. Lower esophageal sphincter pressure in women using sequential oral contraceptives. *Gastroenterology* 1976; **71**: 232–235

34. Fournet, J., Bost, R., Hostein, J. *et al.* Effets de la propantheline sur l'activite motrice de l'oesophage chez l'homme normale. *Gastroenterol. Clin. Biol.* 1983; **7**: 457–464

35. Castell, D. O. Calcium-channel blocking agents for gastro-intestinal disorders. *Am. J. Cardiol.* 1985; **55**: 210B–213B

36. Misiewicz, J. J., Waller, S. L. and Anthony, P. P. Achalasia of the cardia: pharmacology and histopathology of isolated cardiac-sphincter muscle from patients with and without achalasia. *Q. J. Med.* 1969; **38**: 17–30

37. Rees, M. R., Clark, R. A., Holdsworth, C. D. *et al.* The effect of β-adrenoreceptor agonists and antagonists on gastric emptying in man. *Br. J. Pharmacol.* 1980; **10**: 551–554

38. Santander, R., Mena, I. and Valenzuela, J. E. Effect of nifedipine on gastric emptying and gastro-intestinal motility in man. *Gastroenterology* 1986; **90**: 1614A

39. Biancini, P., Barwick, K., Selling, J. and McCallum, R. Effects of acute experimental esophagitis on mechanical properties of the lower esophageal sphincter. *Gastroenterology* 1984; **87**: 8–10

40. Baldi, F., Ferrarini, F., Longanesi, A. M. *et al.* Oesophageal function before, during and after healing of erosive oesophagitis. *Gut* 1988; **29**: 157–160

41. Holloway, R. H., Hongo, M., Berger, K. *et al.* Gastric distension: a mechanism for postprandial gastro-esophageal reflux. *Gastroenterology* 1985; **89**: 779–784

42. Stanciu, C. and Bennett, J. R. Alginate–antacid in the reduction of gastro-oesophageal reflux. *Lancet* 1974; **i**: 109–111

43. Bortolotti, M., Bersoni, G., Calleti, T., Longanesi, A., Fischi, S. and Labo, E. Evaluation of the effectiveness of a treatment for gastroesophageal reflux with a new portable pH-monitoring apparatus. *Abstracts of the International Society for Diseases of the Esophagus* 1983: M-16

44. O'Connor, K. W. and Lehman, G. A. Endoscopic placement of collagen at the lower esophageal sphincter to inhibit gastroesophageal reflux: a pilot study of 10 medically intractable patients. *Gastrointest. Endosc.* 1988; **34**: 106–112

45. Helm, J. F., Dodds, W. J., Riedel, D. R. *et al.* Determinants of esophageal clearance in normal subjects. *Gastroenterology* 1983; **85**: 607–612

46. McCallum, R. W., Kline, M. M., Curry, N. *et al.* Effects of metoclopramide and bethanechol on delayed gastric emptying present in gastroesophageal reflux patients. *Gastroenterology* 1983; **68**: 1114–1118

47. Corinaldesi, R., Stanghellini, V., Zarabini, G. E. *et al.* The effect of domperidone on the gastric emptying of solid and liquid phases of a mixed meal in patients with dyspepsia. *Curr. Therapeut. Res.* 1983; **34**: 982–986

48. Del Genio, A., Di Martino, N., Piccolo, S., Maffetone, V., Landolfi, V. and Salvatore, M. The effect of domperidone on gastric emptying in reflux esophagitis: a radio-isotope study. *J. Nucl. Med. Allied Sci.* 1984; **28**: 251–256

49. Corazziari, E., Scopinaro, F., Bonteripo, I. *et al.* Effect of R 51619 on distal oesophageal motor activity and gastric emptying. *Ital. J. Gastroenterol.* 1983; **15**: 185–186

50. Schuurkes, J. A. F., Akkermans, L. M. A. and Van Nevten, J. M. Stimulating effects of cisapride on antroduodenal motility in the conscious dog. In: Roman, C., Ed. *Gastrointestinal Motility.* Lancaster: MTP Press. 1984: 95–102

51. Crumplin, M. K. H., Stol, D. W., Murphy, G. M. and Collis, J. L. The pattern of bile salt reflux and acid secretion in sliding hiatus hernia. *Br. J. Surg.* 1974; **61**: 611–616

52. Smith, M. R., Buckton, G. K. and Bennett, J. R. Bile acid levels in stomach and oesophagus in patients with acid gastro-oesophageal reflux. *Gut* 1984; **25**: A556

53. Mittal, R. K., Reuben, A., Whitney, J. O. and McCallum, R. W. Do bile acids reflux into the esophagus? *Gastroenterology* 1987; **92**: 371–375

54. Muller-Lissner, S. A. and Blum, A. Fundic pressure rise lowers sphincter pressure in man. *Hepatogastroenterology* 1982; **29**: 151–152

55. Madsen, T., Wallin, L., Boesby, S. and Hojkjaer Larsen, V. Spontaneous peristaltic activity in the oesophagus after imitated acid gastro-oesophageal reflux. *Scand. J. Gastroenterol.* 1982; **17**: 811–815

56. Phaosawasdi, K., Malmud, L. S., Tolin, R. D. *et al.* Cholinergic effects on esophageal transit and clearance. *Gastroenterology* 1981; **81**: 915–920

57. Horowitz, M., Maddox, A., Harding, P. E. *et al.* Effect of cisapride on gastric and esophageal emptying in insulin-dependent diabetes mellitus. *Gastroenterology* 1987; **92**: 1899–1907

57a Kahrilas, P. J., Dodds, W. J., Hogan, W. J. *et al.* Esophageal peristaltic function in peptic esophagitis. *Gastroenterology* 1986; **91**: 897–904

58. Hamilton, J. W., Boisen, R. J., Yamamoto, D. T., Wagner, J. L. and Reichelderfer, M. Sleeping on a wedge diminishes exposure of the esophagus to acid. *Dig. Dis. Sci.* 1988; **33**: 518–522

59. Stanciu, C. and Bennett, J. R. Effects of posture on gastro-oesophageal reflux. *Digestion* 1977; **15**: 104–109

60. Harvey, R. F., Gordon, P. C., Hadley, N. *et al.* Effects of sleeping with the bed-head raised and of ranitidine in patients with severe peptic oesophagitis. *Lancet* 1987; **ii**: 1200–1203

61. Isenberg, J. L. Therapy of peptic ulcer. *J. Am. Med. Assoc.* 1975; **233**: 540–542

62. Deschalliers, J. P., Galmiche, J. P., Touchais, J. Y., Denis, P. and Colin, R. Ranitidine, cimetidine, antacids and gastro-oesophageal reflux: results of a 20 hour oesophageal pH study. *J. Clin. Pharmacol. Res.* 1984; **4**: 217–222

63. Ogilvie, A. L. and Atkinson, M. Does dimethicone increase the efficacy of antacids in the treatment of reflux oesophagitis? *J. R. Soc. Med.* 1986; **79**: 584–587

64. Brogden, R. N., Heel, R. C., Speight, T. M. *et al.* Sucralfate: a review of its pharmacodynamic properties and therapeutic use in peptic ulcer disease. *Drugs* 1984; **27**: 194–209

65. Gillison, E. W., Venancio, A. M., Nyhus, L. M., Kusakari, K. and Bombeck, C. T. The significance of bile in reflux oesophagitis. *Surg. Gynecol. Obstet.* 1972; **134**: 419–424

66. Gillison, E. W., Kusakari, K., Bombeck, C. T. and Nyhus, L. M. The importance of bile in reflux esophagitis and the success of its prevention by surgical means. *Br. J. Surg.* 1972; **59**: 794–798

67. Rees, W. and Rhodes, J. Bile reflux in gastro-oesophageal disease. *Clin. Gastroenterol.* 1977; **61**: 179–200

68. Meshkinpour, H., Elashoff, J. and Stewart, H. Effect of cholestyramine on the symptoms of reflux gastritis. *Gastroenterology* 1977; **73**: 441–443

68a. Safie-Shirazi, S., DenBester, L. and Zike, W. L. Effect of bile salts on the ionic permeability of the esophageal mucosa and their role in the production of esophagitis. *Gastroenterology* 1975; **68**: 728–733

68b. Orlando, R. C., Bryson, J. C. and Powek, D. W. Effect of cigarette smoke on esophageal epithelium of the rabbit. *Gastroenterology* 1986; **91**: 1536–1542

69. Heller, S. R., Fellows, I. W., Ogilvie, A. L. and Atkinson, M. Non-steroidal anti-inflammatory drugs and benign oesophageal stricture. *Br. Med. J.* 1982; **285**: 167–168

70. Wilkins, W. E., Ridley, M. S. and Pozniak, A. L. Benign stricture of the oesophagus: role of non-steroidal anti-inflammatory drugs. *Gut* 1984; **25**: 478–480

71. Park, D. V. The pharmacology and biochemistry of carbenoxolone. In: Beck, I. T., Ed. *Proceedings of the Symposium on Carbenoxolone.* Amsterdam: Excerpta Medica. 1976: 19–32

72. Reed, P. I. and Davies, W. A. Controlled trial of a new dosage form of carbenoxolone (Pyrogastrone) in the treatment of reflux esophagitis. *Am. J. Dig. Dis.* 1978; **23**: 161–165

73. Nagashima, R. (1981) Development and characteristic of sucralfate. *J. Clin. Gastroenterol.* 1981; **3**: 103–110

74. Orlando, R. C. and Powell, D. W. Effect of sucralfate on esophageal epithelial resistance to acid in the rabbit. *Gastroenterology* 1984; **86**: 1201

75. Behar, J., Sheahan, D. G., Biancini, P., Spiro, H. M. and Storer, E. H. Medical and surgical management of reflux esophagitis. *N. Engl. J. Med.* 1975; **293**: 263–268

76. Graham, D. Y. and Patterson, D. J. Double-blind comparison of liquid antacid and placebo in the treatment of symptomatic reflux esophagitis. *Dig. Dis. Sci.* 1983; **28**: 559–563

77. Grove, O., Bekker, C. and Jeppe Hansen, N. G. Ranitidine and high-dose antacid in reflux oesophagitis. *Scand. J. Gastroenterol.* 1985; **20**: 457–461

78. Malmud, L. S., Charkes, N. D., Littlefield, J. *et al.* The mode of action of alginic acid in the reduction of gastroesophageal reflux. *J. Nucl. Med.* 1979; **20**: 1023–1028

79. Beeley, N. and Warner, J. O. Medical treatment of symptomatic hiatus hernia with low-density compounds. *Curr. Med. Res. Opin.* 1972; **1**: 63–69

80. Barnardo, D. E., Lancaster-Smith, M., Strickland, I. D. and Wright, J. T. A double-blind controlled trial of Gaviscon in patients with symptomatic gastro-oesophageal reflux. *Curr. Med. Res. Opin.* 1975; **3**: 338–391

81. Chevrel, B. A comparative crossover study in the treatment of heart-burn and epigastric pain: liquid Gaviscon and magnesium–aluminium antacid gel. *J. Int. Med. Res.* 1980; **8**: 300–302

82. Graham, D. Y., Lanza, F. and Dorsch, E. R. Symptomatic reflux oesophagitis: a double-blind controlled comparison of antacids and alginate. *Curr. Therapeut. Res.* 1977; **22**: 653–658

83.   McHardy, G. A multicentre, randomised trial of Gaviscon in reflux. *S. Med. J.* 1978; **71**: 16–21
84.   Behar, J., Brand, D. L., Brown, F. C. *et al.* Cimetidine in the treatment of symptomatic gastro-esophageal reflux. *Gastroenterology* 1978; **74**: 441–448
85.   Fiasse, R., Hanin, C., Lepot, A. *et al.* Controlled trial of cimetidine in reflux oesophagitis. *Dig. Dis. Sci.* 1980; **25**: 750–755
86.   Powell-Jackson, P., Barkley, H. and Northfield, T. C. Effect of cimetidine in symptomatic gastroesophageal reflux. *Lancet* 1978; **ii**: 1068–1069
87.   Wesdorp, E., Bartelsman, J., Pape, K., Dekker, W. and Tytgat, G. N. Oral cimetidine in reflux esophagitis: a double blind controlled trial. *Gastroenterology* 1978; **74**: 821–824
88.   Greaney, M. G. and Irvin, T. T. Cimetidine for the treatment of symptomatic gastro-oesophageal reflux. *B. J. Clin. Pract.* 1981; **35**: 21–24
89.   Ferguson, R., Dronfield, M. W. and Atkinson, M. Cimetidine in the treatment of reflux oesophagitis with peptic stricture. *Br. Med. J.* 1979; **2**: 472–474
90.   Druguet, M. and Lambert, R. Oral cimetidine in reflux oesophagitis: a double blind controlled trial. In: Dress, A., Barbier, F., Harvengt, C. and Tytgat, G. N. *Proceedings of the Second National Symposium.* Amsterdam: Excerpta Medica. 1980: 30–36
91.   Bennett, J. R., Buckton, G. K. and Martin, H. D. Cimetidine in gastro-oesophageal reflux. *Digestion* 1983; **26**: 166–172
92.   Thanik, K., Chey, W. Y., Shak, A., Hamilton, D. and Nadelson, N. Bethanechol or cimetidine in the treatment of symptomatic reflux esophagitis. *Arch. Intern. Med.* 1982; **142**: 1479–1481
93.   Krasner, N., Walker, R. J., Morris, A. I. and Haas, H. D. Comparison of pyrogastrone, cimetidine and placebo in peptic oesophagitis and ulceration. *Scand. J. Gastroenterol.* 1982; **17** (suppl. 78): 136
94.   Dawson, J., Barnard, J. and Delatre, M. Cimetidine 800 mg at bedtime in reflux oesophagitis: multicentre trial. In: Siewert, J. R. and Holscher, A. H., Eds. *Proceedings of the International Esophageal Week.* Munich: Demeter Verlag. 1986: 189
95.   Thor, K. Treatment of reflux esophagitis with cimetidine in a liquid suspension. *Gastroenterology* 1986; **90**: 1966A
96.   Sherbaniuk, R., Wensel, A., Bailey, R., Trautmann, A. *et al.* Ranitidine in the short-term management of symptomatic gastro-oesophageal reflux. *J. Clin. Gastroenterol.* 1984; **6**: 9–15
97.   Wesdorp, E., Dekker, W. and Klinkenberg-Knol, E. C. Treatment of reflux oesophagitis with ranitidine. *Gut* 1983; **24**: 921–924
98.   Sontag, S., Robinson, M., McCallum, R. W., Barwick, K. W. and Nardi, R. Ranitidine therapy for gastroesophageal reflux disease. Results of a large double-blind trial. *Arch. Intern. Med.* 1987; **147**: 1485–1491
99.   Guslandi, A., Testoni, P. A. Passaretti, S. *et al.* Ranitidine vs. metoclopramide in the medical treatment of reflux oesophagitis. *Hepatogastroenterology* 1983; **30**: 96
100. Masci, E., Testoni, P. A., Passaretti, S., Gazzone, G. and Tittobello, A. Efficacia della ranitidina del domperidone maleato e della associazione dei due farmacia nel trattmento dell'esofagite da reflusso. Sezione Lombardo della SIED. *Drugs Exp. Clin. Res.* 1985; **11**: 687–692
101. Fielding, J. F. and Doyle, G. D. Comparison between ranitidine and cimetidine in the treatment of reflux oesophagitis. *Irish Med. J.* 1984; **77**: 356–357
102. Noya, G. Dettori, G., Muscas, A., Spirito, R., Niolo, P. and Marongiu, G. Cimetidine versus ranitidine in the treatment of peptic oesophagitis. *Minerva Med.* 1983; **74**: 787–788
103. Kimmig, J. M. Cimetidine and ranitidine in the treatment of reflux esophagitis. *Z. Gastroenterol.* 1984; **22**: 373–378
104. Brunner, G., Losgen, H. and Harke, U. Ranitidine in the treatment of cimetidine-resistant ulceration of the upper gastro-intestinal tract. *Therapiewercke* 1982; **32**: 4154
105. Elizalde, R. O., Manauta, J. P., Sanjurjo, J. Z. *et al.* Ranitidine treatment of reflux esophagitis and duodenal and gastric ulcer. *Invest. Med. Int.* 1983; **10**: 3–6
106. Hine, K. R., Holmes, K. T., Melikian, V., Lucey, M. and Fairclough, P. D. Ranitidine in reflux oesophagitis. *Digestion* 1984; **29**: 119–123
107. Berenson, M. M., Sontag, S., Robinson, M. G. and McCallum, R. M. Effect of smoking in a controlled study of ranitidine treatment in gastro-esophageal reflux disease. *J. Clin. Gastroenterol.* 1987; **9**: 499–503
108. Halvorsen, L., Lee, F. I., Wesdorp, I. C. E., Johnson, N. J., Mills, J. G. and Wood, J. R. Acute

treatment of reflux oesophagitis: a multi-centre study to compare 150 mg ranitidine twice daily with 300 mg at bedtime. *Aliment. Pharmacol. Therapeut.* 1989; **3**: 171–181

109. Robertson, D. A. F., Aldersley, M. A., Shepherd, H., Lloyd, R. S. and Smith, C. L. H_2 antagonists in the treatment of reflux oesophagitis: can physiological studies predict the response? *Gut* 1987; **28**: 946–949

109a. Bovero, E., Chali, L. *et al.* Short-term treatment of reflux oesophagitis with ranitidine 300 mg nocte. *Hepatogastroenterology* 1987; **34**: 155–159.

110. Orr, W. C., Robinson, M. G., Humphries, T. J. *et al.* Dose response effects of famotidine on gastroesophageal reflux. *Gastroenterology* 1987; **92**: 1562.

111. Carmine, A. A. and Brogden, R. N. Pirenzipine: a review of its pharmacodynamic and pharmaco-kinetic properties and therapeutic efficacy in peptic ulcer disease and other allied diseases. *Drugs* 1985; **30**: 85–126

112. Stacher, G., Bauer, P. and Schmierer, G. The effect of intramuscular pirenzipine on esophageal contractile activity and lower esophageal sphincter pressure under fasting conditions and after a standard meal. *Int. J. Clin. Pharmacol. Biopharm.* 1979; **17**: 442–448

113. Pandolfo, N., Borgonovo, G., Torre, G. L. *et al.* Response to pirenzipine of the human lower esophageal sphincter. *Curr. Therapeut. Res.* 1981; **30**: 38–43

114. Denis, P., Galmiche, J. P., Gibon, J. P. *et al.* Effet due pirenzipin sur la motricite oesophagienne chez l'adulte sain. *Gastroenterol. Clin. Biol.* 1982; **6**: 27–32

115. Dent, J., Downton, J., Heddle, R. *et al.* Effects of omeprazole on peptic oesophagitis and oesophageal motility and pH. *Scand. J. Gastroenterol.* 1986; **21** (suppl. 118): 181

116. Texter, E. C., Patel, G. K., Navab, F. *et al.* Effect of oral pirenzipine, a muscarinic antagonist, and oral atropine, on lower esophageal sphincter pressure, esophageal manometry and scintiscans and gut peptides. *Clin. Res.* 1983; **31**: 766A

117. Castell, D. O., Blackwell, J. N. and Dalton, C. B. Pirenzipine: a unique anti-cholinergic on the esophagus. In: Bettarello, A., Ed. *New Aspects in Research and Therapy.* Amsterdam: Excerpta Medica. 1985: 142–149

118. Evreux, M. and Bouvet, B. Pirenzipine and peptic pathology of the esophagus. In: Cheli, E. and Molinari, F., Eds. *Pirezipine: Knowledge and new trends.* New York: Raven Press. 1986: 15–16

119. Niemela, S., Jaaskelainen, T., Lehtola, J. *et al.* Pirenzipine in the treatment of reflux esophagitis. *Scand. J. Gastroenterol.* 1986; **21**: 1193–1199

120. Garcia-Albarran, A., Ruiz de Leon, A. and Diaz-Rubro, M. Gastro-esophageal reflux. Study of the treatment with pirenzipine. *Dig. Dis. Sci.* 1986; **31**: 467S

121. Walt, R. P., Gomes, M. de F. A., Wood, E. C., Logan, L. H. and Pounder, R. E. Effects of daily oral omeprazole on 24-hour intragastric acidity. *Br. Med. J.* 1983; **287**: 12–14

122. Downton, J., Dent, J., Heddle, R. *et al.* Elevation of gastric pH heals peptic oesophagitis – a role for omeprazole. *J. Gastroenterol. Hepatol.* 1987; **2**: 317–324

123. Damman, H. G., Blum, A. L., Lux, G. *et al.* Omeprazole is superior to ranitidine in the treatment of reflux esophagitis. *Gastroenterology* 1986; **90**: 85A

124. Klinkenberg-Knol, E. C., Festen, H. P. M., Jansen, J. M. B., Meuwissen, S. G. M. and Lamers, C. B. H. W. Double blind multicentre comparison of omeprazole and ranitidine in the treatment of reflux oesophagitis. *Lancet* 1987; **i**: 349–350

125. Vantrappen, G., Rutgeerts, L., Schurmans, P. and Coenegrachts, J-L. Omeprazole (40 mg) is superior to ranitidine in short-term treatment of ulcerative reflux esophagitis. *Dig. Dis. Sci.* 1988; **33**: 523–529

126. Havelund, T., Laursen, L. S., Skoubo-Kristensen, E., Andersen, B. N., Pedersen, S. A. and Jensen, K. B. Omeprazole and ranitidine in the treatment of reflux oesophagitis: double-blind comparative trial. *Br. Med. J.* 1988; **296**: 89–92

127. Sandmark, S., Carlsson, R., Fausa, O. and Lundell, L. Omeprazole or ranitidine in the treatment of reflux esophagitis. *Scand. J. Gastroenterol.* 1988; **23**: 625–632

127a. Sandmark, S., Carlsson, R., Fausa, O. and Lundell, L. Omeprazole or ranitidine in the treatment of reflux oesophagitis. *Scand. J. Gastroenterol.* 1988; **23**: 625–632

128. Hetzel, D. J., Dent, J., Reed, W. D. *et al.* Healing and relapse of severe peptic oesophagitis after treatment with omeprazole. *Gastroenterology* 1988; **95**: 903–912

129. Bardhan, K. D., Morris, P., Thompson, M. *et al.* Value of omeprazole in the management of erosive oesophagitis refractory to high dose cimetidine. *Gastroenterology* 1987; **92**: 1306

129a. Ruth, M., Enbom, M., Lundell, L., Lönroth, H., Sandberg, N. and Sandmark, S. The effect of omeprazole or ranitidine treatment on 24-hour esophageal acidity in patients with reflux esophagitis, *Gastroenterol. Int.* 1988; **1**: 723

130. Bettarello, A., Tuttle, G. G. and Rossman, M. I. Effect of autonomic drugs on gastroesophageal reflux. *Gastroenterology* 1960; **39**: 340–346

131. Johnson, L. F. and DeMeester, T. R. Evaluation of elevation of the head of the bed, bethanechol, and antacid foam tablets on gastroesophageal reflux. *Dig. Dis. Sci.* 1981; **36**: 673–680

132. Saco, L. S., Orlando, R. C. and Levinson, S. L. Double-blind controlled trial of bethanechol and antacid versus placebo and antacid in the treatment of erosive esophagitis. *Gastroenterology* 1982; **82**: 1369

133. Behar, J. and Biancini, P. Effect of oral metoclopramide on gastro-esophageal reflux in the post-cibal state. *Gastroenterology* 1976; **70**: 331–335

134. McCallum, R. W., Ippoliti, A. F., Cooney, C. and Sturdevant, R. A. L. A controlled trial of metoclopramide in symptomatic gastroesophageal reflux. *N. Engl. J. Med.* 1977; **296**: 345–357

135. McCallum, R. W., Fink, S. M., Winnar, G. R., Auella, J. and Callaghan, C. Metoclopramide in gastroesophageal reflux: rationale for its use and results of a double-blind trial. *Am. J. Gastroenterol.* 1984; **79**: 165–172

136. Bright-Asare, P., Behar, J. and Brand, D. L. Cimetidine, metoclopramide or placebo in the treatment of symptomatic gastro-esophageal reflux. *Gastroenterology* 1980; **82**: 1025

137. Goethals, C. Domperidone in the treatment of post-prandial symptoms suggestive of gastroesophageal reflux. *Curr. Therapeut. Res.* 1979; **26**: 874–880

138. Baldi, F., Bianchi Porro, G., Iascone, C. *et al.* Placebo-controlled study of the effect of cisapride on lesions and symptoms of reflux oesophagitis. In: *Progress in the Treatment of Gastrointestinal Motility.* Frankfurt: Alte oper. 1986; 32–33

139. Lepoutre, L., Van der Linden, I., Bolleri, S. *et al.* Controlled trial of cisapride in the treatment of Grade II and III oesophagitis. In: *Progress in the Treatment of Gastrointestinal Motility.* Frankfurt: Alte oper. 1986:

140. Rode, H., Stunden, R. J., Millar, A. J. W. and Cywes, S. Esophageal pH assessment of gastro-oesophageal reflux in 18 patients and the effect of two prokinetic agents: cisapride and metoclopramide. *J. Pediatr. Surg.* 1987; **22**: 931–934

141. Janisch, H. D. and the CISRAN Study Group. Double blind multicenter trial to compare the efficacy of cisapride and ranitidine in the acute treatment of gastro-esophageal reflux disease. *Gastroenterology* 1986; **90**: 1475A

142. Evreux, M., Filoche, B., Fournet, J. *et al.* Endoscopic and clinical evaluation of cisapride and cimetidine in reflux esophagitis. *Gastroenterology* 1988; **94**: A120

143. Galmiche, J. P., Vitaux, J., Brandstatter, G. *et al.* Benefit of adding cisapride to cimetidine in the treatment of severe reflux esophagitis. *Gastroenterology* 1987; **92**: 1400

144. Markham, C. and Reed, P. I. Pyrogastrone treatment of peptic oesophagitis: analysis of 104 patients treated during a three and a half year period. *Scand. J. Gastroenterol.* 1980; **15**: 73–82

145. Young, G. P., Nagy, G. S., Myren, J. *et al.* Treatment of reflux oesophagitis with a carbenoxolone/antacid/alginate preparation. *Scand. J. Gastroenterol.* 1986; **21**: 1098–1100

146. Schweitzer, E. J., Bass, B., Johnson, L. F. and Harmon, J. W. Sucralfate prevents experimental peptic esophagitis in rabbits. *Gastroenterology* 1985; **88**: 611–619

147. Elsborg, L., Beck, B. and Stubgaard, M. Effect of sucralfate on gastro-esophageal reflux in esophagitis. *Hepatogastroenterology* 1985; **32**: 181–184

148. Williams, R. M., Orlando, R. C., Bozymski, E. M. *et al.* Multicentre trial of sucralfate suspension for the treatment of reflux esophagitis. *Am. J. Med.* 1987; **83**: 61–66

149. Weiss, W., Brunner, H., Byttner, G. R. *et al.* Oesophagite peptique. Traitment par le sucralfate. *Med. Chir. Dig.* 1984; **17**: 17

150. Kairaluoma, M. I., Hentilae, R., Alavaikku, P. *et al.* Sucralfate versus placebo in treatment of non-ulcer dyspesia. *Am. J. Med.* 1987; **83**: 51–55

151.   Carling, L., Cronstedt, J., Kagevi, I. *et al.* Sucralfate vs placebo in reflux esophagitis. *Gastroentero-logy* 1987; **92**: 1338A

152.   Laitinen, S., Stahlberg, M., Kairaluoma, M. I. *et al.* Sucralfate and alginate/antacid in reflux esophagitis. *Scand. J. Gastroenterol.* 1985; **20**: 229–232

153.   Evreux, M. Sucralfate versus alginate/antacid in the treatment of peptic esophagitis. *Am. J. Med.* 1987; **83**: 48–50

154.   Tytgat, G. N. J. Clinical efficacy of sucralfate in reflux esophagitis. *Am. J. Med.* 1987; **83**: 38–41

155.   Simon, R. and Mueller, P. Comparison of the effect of sucralfate and ranitidine in reflux esophagitis. *Am. J. Med.* 1987; **83**: 43–47

156.   Ros, E., Pugol, A., Bordas, J. and Grande, L. Sucralfate in refractory esophagitis. *Dig. Dis. Sci.* 1986; **31** (suppl.): 497

157.   Temple, J. G., Bradby, G. V. H., O'Connor, F. *et al.* Cimetidine and metoclopramide in oesophageal reflux disease. *Br. Med. J.* 1983; **1**: 1863–1864

158.   Lieberman, D. A. and Keeffe, E. B. Treatment of severe reflux esophagitis with cimetidine and metoclopramide. *Ann. Intern. Med.* 1986; **104**: 21–26

159.   Wienbeck, M., Biefeld, P., Enck, P. *et al.* Does a motor-stimulating agent improve the therapeutic effect of H_2-blockers in reflux esophagitis? *Gastroenterology* 1986; **90**: 1691

160.   Bennett, J. R., Buckton, G. K., Martin, H. D. and Smith, M. R. Effect of adding cimetidine to alginate-antacid in treating gastro-oesophageal reflux. In: Siewart, J. R. and Holscher, A. H., Eds. *Diseases of the Esophagus.* Berlin: Springer Verlag. 1988: 1111–1115

161.   Lieberman, D. A. Medical therapy for chronic reflux esophagitis. *Arch. Intern. Med.* 1987; **147**: 1717–1720

162.   Kaul, B., Petersen, H., Erichsen, H. Y. *et al.* Gastroesophageal reflux disease: acute and mainten-ance treatment with cimetidine. *Scand. J. Gastroenterol.* 1986; **21**: 139–145

163.   McCallum, R. W., Sontag, S. J. and Vlahcevic, Z. R. Ranitidine versus placebo in long-term treatment of gastroesophageal reflux. *Am. J. Gastroenterol.* 1985; **80**: 864

Chapter 7

Surgical treatment of reflux disease

A. Cuschieri

Introduction

The generally held view among surgeons that the commonly used anti-reflux operations are successful in some 80% of patients is based on incompletely audited experience and remains unsubstantiated. Moreover, gastroenterologists remain sceptical about the long-term efficacy of anti-reflux surgery. A more objective evaluation of the current position is that surgical treatment of oesophageal reflux disease remains problematical. Since the introduction of the anatomical repair of the gastro-oesophageal junction by Allison [1,2], who originated the concept of reflux-induced damage to the oesophageal mucosa, there has been a proliferation of anti-reflux procedures. This in itself is a sure indication that the ideal operation for this common condition has not been established. All these procedures have their limitations and recurrent reflux after surgical treatment of this disorder is much higher than appreciated [3]. The reasons for the present unsatisfactory state relating to the surgical management of reflux disease are:

1. The paucity of prospective long-term studies to evalute relative efficacy and long-term benefit of the various procedures.
2. The vast majority of retrospective reports on which current practice is based have been poorly audited and have incomplete or short follow-up periods.
3. Reflux disease presents a varying problem in the individual patient in terms of the requirements for a successful outcome after surgical treatment and therefore no one operation may be universally applicable to all patients suffering from the disease. Thus patient selection for the appropriate procedure depending on build, technical feasibility and assessment of the pathological anatomy is an important aspect which has not been adequately addressed.
4. Some anti-reflux operations achieve effective control of reflux at the expense of altered physiology of the upper gastrointestinal tract leading to persistent untoward symptoms not related to reflux which detract from an otherwise successful clinical result.

Indications for anti-reflux surgery

The currently accepted indications for surgical treatment are shown in Table 7.1. Several qualifications to these indications for surgery need to be addressed. In the

Table 7.1 Indications for surgical treatment for gastro-oesophageal reflux disease

1. Failure of medical therapy
   Persistent symptoms despite medication
   Intractable oesophagitis
   Non-compliance with treatment
2. Development of complications
   Stricture, Barrett's metaplasia
3. Reflux and motility disorders and oesophageal chest pain
   Reflux-induced motility disorders
   Motility disorders causing reflux
   Reflux following myotomy
4. Reflux in infants and children
5. Reflux after upper abdominal surgery
   Neutral/alkaline
   Acid

first instance practice varies from centre to centre and some gastroenterologists are reluctant to refer patients for surgery despite failure of medical therapy to control symptoms. The fitness of the patient for surgery and the presence of co-morbid cardiorespiratory disease are important considerations in the selection of patients for surgical treatment.

Failure of medical therapy

This is the most common indication with persistence of symptoms and oesophagitis despite medical therapy. The problem concerns the definition of failure of medical treatment and terms such as 'intractable oesophagitis'. The duration of medical therapy after which treatment is said to have failed is not generally agreed. Most antacids including H_2-receptor antagonists and alginates control reflux symptoms. There is evidence that combined alginate–H_2-receptor blocker therapy is more effective in controlling symptoms and promoting healing of the oesophagitis than either agent alone [4]. These agents do not cure the reflux diathesis and for this reason symptoms recur on cessation of therapy. In practice therefore patients are referred for surgery either because symptoms persist despite medication, or recur soon after withdrawal, or because the patient is non-compliant with his medication.

In the short term, omeprazole has proved more effective in healing oesophagitis and in controlling chronic bleeding from this disorder [5]. There are justifiable fears regarding the long-term consequences of this Na^+/K^+ ATPase inhibitor emanating from the total achlorhydria it induces. However, this consideration need not concern the aged patient whose oesophagitis cannot be controlled by less powerful antacid therapy.

Development of complications of reflux disease

These usually arise on a background of long-standing history of reflux symptoms but may on occasion constitute the presenting complaint, as exemplified by the onset of dysphagia due to an oesophageal peptic stricture in the elderly. Although generally regarded as indications for surgical treatment, the management of patients with oesophageal strictures and Barrett's oesophagus is by no means standardized and to a large extent is influenced by the age and general condition of the patient.

Reflux associated with oesophageal motility disorders

The established association between reflux and disorders of oesophageal motility remains poorly understood and requires further study. In the first instance gastro-oesophageal reflux may initiate non-specific motility disorders of the oesophagus and induce non-cardiac chest pain with clinical features which are virtually indistinguishable from those due to coronary artery disease. Secondly, certain motility disorders which lead to hypo- or aperistalsis of the oesophageal musculature, e.g. scleroderma, are often accompanied by acid reflux which tends to be particularly severe because of the grossly defective oesophageal clearance of the refluxate. Thirdly reflux may be precipitated by various myotomy procedures performed for certain specific motility disorders of the oesophagus.

Reflux in infancy and childhood

Reflux disease in infancy and childhood requires early recognition and active intervention because of the immediate risks which include serious respiratory complications, and the possibility of the infant apnoea syndrome which is thought to account for some cot deaths and failure to thrive. Untreated or inadequately controlled reflux in children leads to oesophageal shortening which in the past was confused with 'congenital short oesophagus'. Most are agreed, however, that conservative treatment should be persisted with whenever possible until the age of 2 years because of the tendency to spontaneous resolution and the undoubted inferior results in infants.

Reflux developing after previous abdominal surgery

Reflux, both acid and neutral, may develop after upper abdominal operations particularly gastric surgery, e.g. gastrectomy (partial and total), vagotomy (truncal with drainage and highly selective) and cholecystectomy. Refluxate containing activated pancreatic enzymes, bile salts and lysolecithin is stated to be particularly injurious to the oesophageal mucosa [6,7] and may lead to intractable stricture formation of the oesophagus over a relatively short period of time, although the exact pathogenesis of this neutral–alkaline reflux remains unclear. It cannot be detected by pH monitoring because of its neutral pH and is diagnosed by endoscopy and biopsy. The combination of gastric surgery and cholecystectomy is particularly prone to result in symptomatic neutral reflux. The management of these patients is difficult. There is no effective medical therapy. Mucosal protective agents, such as sucralfate and bile salt binding agents may give some relief but these agents are ineffective in the long term.

Surgery for uncomplicated reflux

Choice of operation

The choice of operation for reflux is determined by certain considerations, as follows.

Patient's build
Any subdiaphragmatic procedure is difficult to perform adequately and with safety if the patient has a deep-set subdiaphragmatic compartment with a narrow subcostal

angle, or is obese. A transthoracic operation, e.g. Belsey, is safer and more likely to yield a satisfactory outcome in these patients.

Previous abdominal surgery

This affects the technical feasibility of the procedure which can be performed. A previous extensive partial gastrectomy often precludes a safe total fundoplication because of insufficient stomach to ensure a loose wrap without any tension.

Presence of oesophageal shortening

When significant, this requires a gastroplasty to achieve oesophageal lengthening in addition to an anti-reflux operation. Although intrathoracic fundoplication is practised by some, this procedure is not generally recommended because of its propensity to serious complications.

Impaired oesophageal motility

Impaired oesophageal motility may be primary or secondary to gastro-oesophageal reflux. In either case, it is one of the most important factors in determining the severity of reflux disease and the need for surgical intervention. When motility is grossly disturbed, e.g. aperistalsis, the nature of the anti-reflux operation requires careful consideration. Thus a complete fundal wrap is likely to obstruct the gastro-oesophageal junction in this situation.

Delayed gastric emptying

Although not a significant feature of adult gastro-oesophageal reflux disease, delayed gastric emptying is encountered in some infants with reflux particularly in the presence of neurological deficits and in adult patients after gastric and previous failed anti-reflux surgery. When delayed gastric emptying is demonstrated by the appropriate isotope studies, a drainage operation, usually a pyloroplasty, is added to the anti-reflux operation.

Fundoplication

The most commonly used operation is fundoplication performed through the abdominal route. The major disadvantage of this operation is the creation of a supercompetent sphincter which is unphysiological and the high incidence of persistent untoward symptoms. Modifications have been introduced over the years designed to overcome this intrinsic problem. These include loose, complete and partial wraps.

Complete wraps (360°)

The complete wrap was first described by Nissen [8]. The component steps of this operation are mobilization of the gastro-oesophageal junction with ligature and division of the upper two to three short gastric vessels, crural repair with interrupted non-absorbable sutures, and a complete 3–5 cm fundal wrap with the sutures taking bites of the anterior wall of the abdominal oesophagus (Figure 7.1). There is no question about the efficacy of this operation in abolishing reflux. Herein lies its disadvantage. It creates a supercompetent one-way valve abolishing 'physiological reflux'. Apart from technical complications, the operation is attended by unpleasant sequelae which detract from an otherwise successful outcome. Generally referred to as the gas-bloat syndrome, these include early satiety, inability to vomit and belch,

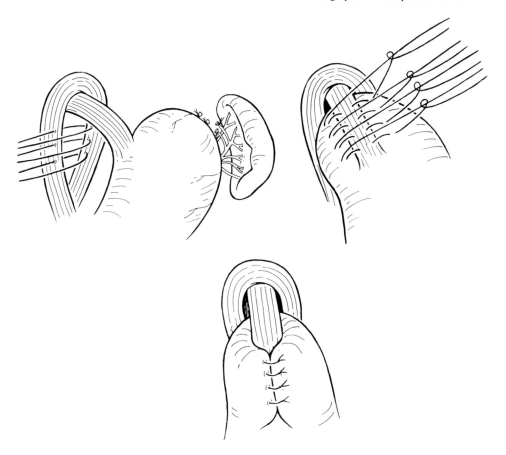

Figure 7.1 The classic Nissen total fundoplication. The wrap sutures take bites on the anterior wall of the oesophagus

abdominal distension, alterations in the swallowing pattern and upper abdominal pain [9–12]. It is difficult to ascertain the exact cause of these symptoms. They have been attributed, without any material evidence, to the wrap being too tight. The aetiological role of diminished gastric volume and gastroparesis with delayed gastric emptying or loss of adaptive relaxation, following inadvertent vagotomy, in the production of these non-reflux related symptoms has not been evaluated.

The Rosetti–Hell modification was devised in an attempt to reduce the super-competence and risk of vagal damage of the classic Nissen fundoplication [13]. The hiatal dissection is limited to division of the phreno-oesophageal membrane to enable finger mobilization without the necessity of division of the short gastric vessels. The crural defect is repaired and the anterior wall of the stomach is pushed behind the oesophagus to emerge on its right margin. It is then sutured back to the anterior wall of the stomach by three to four non-absorbable sutures (Figure 7.2). This modifi-cation, which was designed to take advantage of the responsiveness of the fundic muscle to neuromuscular stimuli, appears to result in a lesser incidence of dysphagia and gas-bloat symptoms than the classic Nissen fundoplication although there have not been any prospective comparative studies.

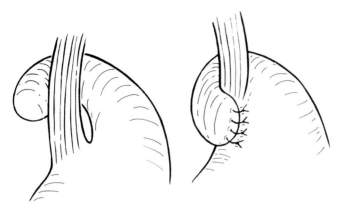

Figure 7.2 The Rosetti–Hell modification of the classic Nissen procedure. The hiatal dissection is limited. The fundus is pushed behind the oesophagus to emerge on its right margin. It is then stitched back to the anterior wall of the stomach near the lesser curve

Complications of complete wraps

These are technical resulting from faulty technique (tight wrap, wrap disruption, slipped wrap and para-oesophageal hernia), recurrent reflux, ulcerative sequelae (gastric ulcer in the wrap, gastrobronchial fistula, gastrointestinal bleeding) and the development of persistent and disabling non-reflux symptoms, loosely categorized as the gas-bloat syndrome, precipitated by food intake and which often lead to weight loss from a diminished dietary intake. In addition, abdominal fundoplication is accompanied by a high incidence of iatrogenic trauma necessitating splenectomy in 10%. In the author's view this inordinately high reported incidence of operative splenic injury is the result of indiscriminate adoption of the abdominal route, in patients in whom upper abdominal surgery is difficult because of a deep-set subdiaphragmatic compartment compounded by a narrow subcostal angle, or because of obesity.

A realistic failure rate of Nissen and other complete wraps based on all of these complications is of the order of 40%. The majority of published retrospective reports claiming 80% success rates are based on defining a successful result as the absence of reflux symptoms and ignore the non-reflux related consequences.

In an attempt to overcome some of the problems including early dysphagia, the tendency has been to fashion increasingly loose and short complete wraps. Thus the current recommendation is the creation of a 1.0 cm wrap with a size F60 bougie [14].

Incomplete wraps (270–180°)

These leave varying segments of the anterior wall of the oesophagus unbuttressed (240–270° wraps) to reduce supercompetence and allow eructation [15,16]. The disadvantage of these operations lies in the two rows of sutures placed longitudinally along the anterior wall of the oesophagus which pull in opposite directions favouring disruption, especially in the presence of significant peri-oesophagitis where there is a tendency for sutures to cut out (Figure 7.3).

The most physiological variation is the posterior 180–240° crurally fixed wrap first described by Toupet [17] and subsequently modified by Boutelier and Jonsell [18].

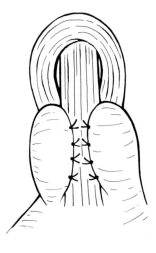

Figure 7.3 Incomplete wraps leave varying segments of the anterior wall of the oesophagus unbuttressed. The disadvantage of these operations lies in the two parallel rows of sutures on the anterior wall of the oesophagus which pull in opposite directions favouring disruption

(a)   (b)

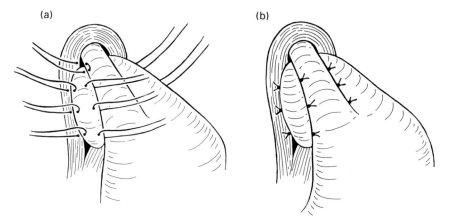

Figure 7.4 Toupet crurally fixed fundoplication favoured by the author

The peritoneum and phreno-oesophageal ligament are divided, the crura of the diaphragm are dissected and the cardia and the oesophagus fully mobilized. The right vagus is freed from the oesophagus, following which the fundus and upper portion of the posterior wall of the stomach are sutured to the right crus behind the oesophagus. A second row of sutures approximates the right border of the oesophagus to the fundus. Similar fixation is carried out on the left side. This step is facilitated by the insertion of the left crural sutures prior to fixation of the right side (Figure 7.4). The fixation of the partial wrap to the crura of the diaphragm is important because, not only does it prevent herniation through the hiatus but, more importantly, it abolishes any drag on the oesophageal sutures. The author increasingly favours this operation as his procedure of choice in patients with uncomplicated reflux because of the virtual absence of non-reflux associated sequelae. This procedure most closely approximates to the Belsey Mark IV operation and fulfils the important criteria for the ideal anti-reflux operation.

Another technique, first described by Dor *et al.* in 1962 [19] and reported favourably by others [20], is the anterior 180° wrap. The mobilized fundus is brought in front of the oesophagus and maintained in this position by the placement of two lines of sutures between the oesophagus and the stomach, with the highest sutures anchored to the right crus of the diaphragm.

Combined anti-reflux gastroplasties

These include the Collis–Belsey and the Collis–Nissen procedures which are indicated in the presence of significant oesophageal shortening. The uncut Collis–Nissen procedure [21,22] performed by stapling the stomach over a length of 5–7 cm without division (Figure 7.5) has had favourable reports in the short term [23,24]. Whilst it might offer some advantages over the classic cut Collis–Nissen procedure in patients who have not been operated on, it is probably unwarranted in patients undergoing re-intervention after previous operations for reflux (see below).

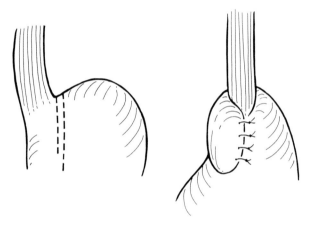

Figure 7.5 The uncut stapled Collis–Nissen procedure. This procedure is unwise in re-do procedures but is perfectly safe in first interventions in patients with short oesophagus

Angelchik prosthesis

First introduced by Angelchik and Cohen [25], this anti-reflux prosthesis controls gastro-oesophageal reflux effectively but does so at the expense of a significant late morbidity: gas-bloat syndrome, dysphagia in 30–50%, prosthesis migration, erosion into the gastrointestinal tract, slippage or rotation with obstruction of the gastro-oesophageal junction [26–28]. The risk of erosion is increased when the prosthesis is placed adjacent to a suture line and after previous unsuccessful anti-reflux surgery. Although one clinical trial comparing the use of the prosthesis with fundoplication [29] reported equally good results with the two procedures, the follow-up period of this trial was very short (1–2 years). A subsequent clinical trial from another institution involving a total of 61 patients randomized to either the Angelchik prosthesis ($n = 30$) or fundoplication ($n = 31$) with a longer follow-up (mean of 38 months, range 18–56 months) reported a much less favourable outcome in the prosthesis group [30]. In this study clinical assessment confirmed a better outcome in the fundoplication group with 94% being graded as Visick I as opposed to 77% in the prosthesis group. Moreover, long-term endoscopic follow-up revealed grade III oesophagitis in seven patients in the Angelchik group with none in patients treated by fundoplication. In this study, three prostheses (10%) required removal, two for persistent dysphagia and one because of sepsis. Removal of the prosthesis because of late complications has been reported to be necessary in 10–25%. At present the Angelchik prosthesis cannot be recommended for routine use in anti-reflux surgery and is contraindicated after previous subdiaphragmatic surgery.

Hill's posterior gastropexy

This operation first reported by Hill in 1967 [31] is less commonly used than fundoplication despite being more physiological. In experienced hands, the success rate of this procedure is high and it is relatively free of untoward sequelae [32,33]. Its disadvantages include technical difficulty, the need for intraoperative manometry during the construction of the medially placed wrap and the risk of damage to the coeliac axis and the pancreas.

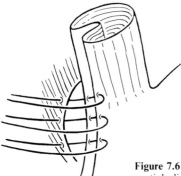

Figure 7.6 Hill's posterior gastropexy. This creates a medially situated partial plication which is fixed to the arcuate ligament. The operation requires intraoperative manometry

The principle of the Hill repair is simultaneous plication of the lower oesophagus and maintenance of an intra-abdominal length of oesophagus by fixation of the repair to the median arcuate ligament. After mobilization of the abdominal oesophaagus and the proximal portion of the lesser curve of the stomach, interrupted sutures are passed through (in order) the anterior leaf of the lesser omentum at the lesser curve, the gastric seromuscular layer of the lesser curve and the posterior leaf of the lesser omentum. Then they catch the median arcuate ligament to which they are tied. The number of sutures required and the degree of infolding of the medial wall of the oesophagus is determined by intraoperative manometry, the objective being to create a high pressure zone of 45–55 mmHg. In essence this procedure creates a medially placed partial longitudinal fixed buttress of infolded lower oesophagus. This results in a long intra-abdominal segment gently curving to the right (Figure 7.6).

Belsey Mark IV

The favoured thoracic operation is the Belsey Mark IV [34], although this approach is less commonly employed by general surgeons. The Belsey procedure is a good operation with a long-term proven efficacy but is technically exacting. Its main disadvantage is persistent thoracotomy pain which can be prevented by a high thoracotomy, limited rib resection and loose periosteal sutures.

Following mobilization, the hernial sac is excised, the stomach mobilized further by division of the upper short gastric vessels, the right crus repaired posteriorly and the fundus of the stomach wrapped twice around the anterior three-quarters of the lower 3–5 cm of the oesophagus by means of two rows of sutures, the second overlapping the first. In addition, the second layer of sutures is carried through the hiatus to the diaphragm and, when tied, results in reduction of the gastro-oesophageal junction below the diaphragm and firm fixation of the repair to this structure (Figure 7.7).

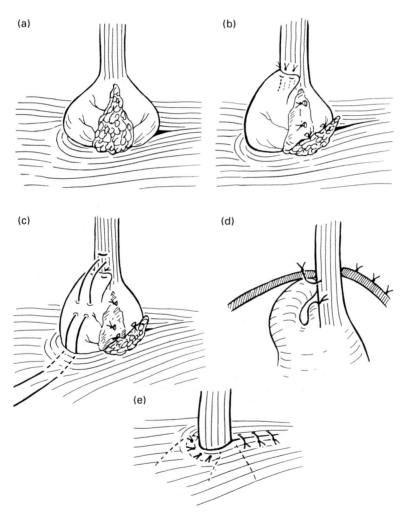

Figure 7.7 Belsey Mark IV operation. In the author's view this is the best thoracic operation and is indicated in patients in whom abdominal approach is difficult because of obesity or narrow subcostal angle. It consists of a double incomplete anterior wrap (a,b,c). The second larger wrap is fixed to the undersurface of the diaphragm and is buttressed by the posterior crural repair (d,e)

Other anti-reflux operations

In addition to the anatomical repair of Allison, there are several other anti-reflux procedures which have been described over the years. Some of these, such as the anterior gastropexy of Boerema [35], are of historical interest only. Others, such as fixation of the gastro-oesophageal junction by a sling of the ligamentum teres [36], have never been adequately evaluated. Vagotomy, antrectomy and Roux-en-Y diversion is a procedure which is useful in selected cases of complicated reflux [37].

Surgery for complicated reflux

The important major complications of reflux disease are persistent oesophagitis, aspiration pneumonia, stricture formation, bleeding and Barrett's columnar cell metaplasia. Practice is again not standardized particularly with regard to the management of patients with reflux strictures. There is general agreement that dilatation alone constitutes inadequate therapy since the recurrence rate is high and averages 40% [38], whereas dilatation combined with anti-reflux medical treatment is effective in 70%. Whilst the wisdom of this management could not be disputed in the elderly and the infirm, should this approach be applied to all in the first instance? There have been few controlled clinical trials to outline the optimum subsequent management of these patients following relief of dysphagia and conflicting anecdotal statements based largely on uncontrolled and retrospective data remain. There are restrospective reports which indicate a successful long-term outcome with a decreased tendency to re-stricture by medical anti-reflux regimens [39,40]. Other retrospective reports indicate that the results of dilatation followed by surgical treatment are better than can be achieved by medical anti-reflux measures [41,42].

There is little doubt that major gastro-oesophageal reflux of acid continues and may indeed be enhanced subsequent to dilatation of reflux stricture [43]. In this study both the cumulative oesophageal exposure to acid and reflux event analysis showed that acid reflux was more pronounced and was associated with slower oesophageal clearance in patients with strictures when compared to patients without. Some 20–30% of patients in 11 reported series of dilatation followed by medical treatment required frequent dilatation and were considered fit enough for anti-reflux surgery. In one of the few controlled clinical trials comparing dilatation and medical therapy *vs* dilatation and anti-reflux surgery, 56% of the medically treated group needed more than one dilatation as opposed to 25% in the surgical group [44].

Thus it would seem prudent to suggest that these patients ought to be treated medically in the first instance and surgical treatment performed if the stricture recurs and the patient is fit for operation.

Oesophageal shortening is a major problem and, if substantial, precludes a simple anti-reflux operation of any type. It results from long-standing severe oesophagitis with contracture and fibrosis of the oesophageal musculature, the peristaltic motility of which may be impaired. It is often accompanied by peptic stricture formation. The best results are obtained by the combined Collis–Nissen procedure (cut or uncut) which is superior to the Collis–Belsey counterpart in these patients.

Supradiaphragmatic wraps
These have been performed for the surgical correction of reflux in patients with an acquired oesophageal shortening. The procedure is usually carried out through a left

thoracotomy. Following dilatation of any strictures, the hiatus is dilated and the mobilized stomach is wrapped round the distal oesophagus without taking suture bites in the oesophagus and over a size 42 bougie. The upper border of the wrap is anchored to the oesophagus by interrupted non-absorbable sutures and the main portion of the wrap sutured to the dilated hiatus to prevent herniation of the abdominal contents into the chest. This operation, though favoured by some [45], has been reported to have a high morbidity with the development of gastric ulcers in the wrap, para-oesophageal colon hernia and outlet obstruction of the wrap following its herniation through the hiatus [46].

Treatment of Barrett's oesophagus is considered in Chapter 4. A proximal gastric vagotomy should be added to the anti-reflux procedure in these patients [47].

Re-operation for failed anti-reflux surgery

The common causes for failure of an anti-reflux operation are technical errors due to inexperience, defects in the design of the procedure itself, oesophageal shortening from chronic oesophagitis and age of the patient. Infants and the elderly have high recurrence rates because of poor tensile strength of their tissues. All operations seem to have the same failure rate which increases with the duration of follow-up [48].

The interval from the most recent failed anti-reflux procedure to revisional surgery is variable but half of the symptomatic recurrences occur during the first 5 years. Aside from age, risk factors for recurrence include obesity, chronic obstructive airway disease and previous gastric surgery [49].

The symptoms of patients coming to revisional surgery are usually those of recurrent reflux: heartburn, regurgitation and dysphagia. Others present with weight loss, evidence of aspiration, oesophageal spasm or obstruction, or gastrointestinal bleeding or the gas-bloat syndrome.

The management of these patients is difficult, and requires careful assessment and case selection based on thorough investigation. In addition to the usual tests for reflux disease, these patients require assessment of oesophageal motility and transit and, in some instances, gastric emptying studies. An additional gastric drainage operation, usually a pyloroplasty, is required in 10–20 of these patients.

The surgical treatment depends on the nature of the previous surgery, the number of operative interventions and the degree of oesophageal shortening. Irrespective of the operation used the objectives include restoration of the gastro-oesophageal junction some 3–5 cm below the diaphragm, repair without tension, correction of any pathology attributed to the previous interventions and crural approximation using adequate bites of crural musculature and tendinous diaphragm. A transthoracic or thoracoabdominal approach is advisable for all patients and is mandatory after multiple previous anti-reflux operations [50,51].

Re-do procedures

These are indicated for first re-operations either because of recurrent reflux or because of complications or persistent non-reflux symptoms. The approach may be abdominal or thoracic depending on preference and familiarity. Their success depends on the absence of oesophageal shortening. They are particularly applicable to failed 'anatomical repairs', the slipped, disrupted or obstructed Nissen repair and the complicated Angelchik repair. Whichever anti-reflux procedure is decided upon (fundoplication, Hill's posterior gastropexy, Belsey Mark IV), it must be performed after adequate mobilization of the abdominal oesophagus and upper stomach. The anti-reflux procedure must be loose, performed around an F60 bougie if the wrap is complete, and the crural defect must be repaired.

Operations for oesophageal shortening

Oesophageal shortening is the biggest problem. It is usually encountered in patients with long-standing reflux, in children with a history of oesophageal atresia or after multiple previous anti-reflux operations. These operations are best performed in tertiary referral centres with the necessary expertise to deal with these complex and taxing problems as even in these centres these remedial operations carry a significant morbidity. The surgical options include: oesophageal lengthening by means of a Collis gastroplasty combined with either a Belsey or a loose Nissen repair, oeso-phageal resection with interposition of a short segment of colon [52] or jejunum [53,54], or transhiatal oesophagectomy with gastric pull-through and cervical anasto-mosis [55] or long-segment colonic interposition [56]. The relative merits of distal *vs* total resections of the thoracic oesophagus is the subject of continued debate. Theoretical considerations apart, in expert hands the results obtained by the two procedures are similar. Thus the decision is best based on the surgeon's experience with one or other of these approaches.

Another approach favoured by some is vagotomy, antrectomy and Roux-en-Y bile diversion [57,58]. Apart from reduced gastric acid secretion, this procedure diverts bile and pancreatic secretions away from the stomach and oesophagus. The reported experience with this operation is limited though generally favourable. Although it has been used in the primary treatment of reflux disease, and one clinical trial with short follow-up showed it to be superior to fundoplication in patients with severe reflux oesophagitis [59], it is generally regarded as a fall-back option which is indicated in complicated forms of oesophagitis particularly following failed previous anti-reflux surgery in which it is impossible or hazardous to embark on further attempts of this nature. It is also useful in patients developing alkaline or neutral reflux oesophagitis after gastric surgery for peptic ulcer disease. The disadvantage of this operation is the high incidence (20%) of postprandial symptoms [60]. Another late complication which occurs in 5–6% is the development of stomal ulcer. A recently described alternative procedure described by DeMeester *et al.* [61] is the 'duodenal switch operation' (Figure 7.8) which entails a suprapapillary duodeno-jejunal anastomosis in conjunction with a Roux loop. Further assessment of the long-term outcome of this operation is needed before its general use can be recom-mended.

Distal oesophageal resection with intrathoracic oesophagogastrostomy, although practised by some, is a bad operation because it leads to continued severe reflux oesophagitis in a significant majority of patients [49].

Collis–Belsey and Collis–Nissen procedures
Gastroplasty was reported by Collis in 1961 as an anti-reflux method suitable for patients with oesophageal shortening and stricture formation [62]. Although it creates a 'gastric neo-oesophagus' with a stable intra-abdominal segment, the long-term results of this procedure alone have been disappointing. This operation was subsequently modified with the addition of a Belsey procedure – the combined Collis–Belsey procedure [63]. Although this improved the overall results, a high

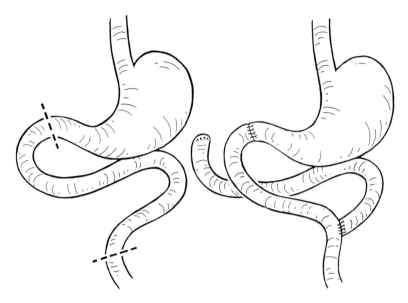

Figure 7.8 The duodenal switch operation recently described by
DeMeester *et al.* [61]

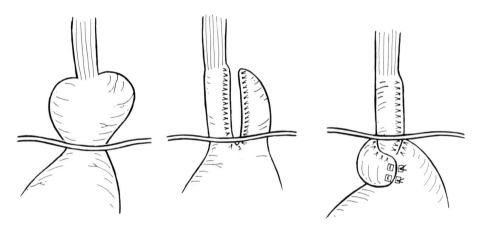

Figure 7.9 Collis–Nissen operation for re-do reflux surgery. The sutures are best tied over Teflon
pledgets because of the oedema of the gastric wall in these revisional cases

incidence of continued or recurrent reflux was reported [64,65]. Total fundoplication
gastroplasty, the combined Collis–Nissen procedure, was therefore introduced to
incorporate the anatomical stability of the Collis procedure and provide a more
effective control of reflux [66]. In general the results of combined Collis–Nissen
procedure for these patients are better than those obtained by the combined Collis–
Belsey procedure [49,67,68]. This is therefore the operation of choice in patients with
one previous failed anti-reflux operation and oesophageal shortening, provided the

dismantling of the original procedure is technically feasible and does not result in devascularization of the fundus. In the author's opinion, the combined Collis–Nissen procedure is best performed through the thoracic approach. The gastroplasty can be performed by hand suturing or stapler guns. It should be of sufficient length to ensure 3–5 cm gastric tube below the diaphragm. The resulting elongated gastric fundus is passed behind the neo-oesophagus and a loose 360° (around an F60 bougie) 2.0 cm wrap performed. As the gastric walls are oedematous and inflamed, the fundoplication sutures should be tied over Teflon pledgets (Figure 7.9). There is one problem concerning oesophageal lengthening by the Collis gastroplasty which has not been sufficiently addressed. This procedure effectively creates an 'artificial Barrett's oesophagus' and fears have been raised regarding the risk of adenocarcinoma and several such cases have been reported although the aetiological relationship between the Collis gastroplasty and the development of the carcinoma remains unproven [69].

Oesophageal resections

These should not be undertaken lightly. The absolute indications are intractable non-dilatable strictures and a persistent fistula after a previous anti-reflux operation. Other considerations which may suggest the need for resection include poor peristaltic activity in the body of the oesophagus and inability to take down a previous repair (particularly a combined gastroplasty fundoplication) or evidence of devascularization when this is completed. The author favours jejunal interposition to colonic segments as the small bowel is a contractile segment whereas the colon is a passive conduit which empties by gravity and predisposes some patients to persistent regurgitation [70]. The technique favoured by the author [54] consists of the isolation of an isoperistaltic segment of jejunum on an eccentrically placed vascular pedicle (Figure 7.10) which is used for replacing the excised distal oesophagus. With the right technique, the jejunum can be brought up to the upper chest if necessary. Redundancy should be avoided as this can cause kinking and obstruction. If the mesentery is too short for the length of jejunum needed, the technique of box resection can be employed to straighten the segment (Figure 7.11). The proximal end of the transposed loop is closed and the anastomosis with the oesophagus is performed in an end-to-side fashion (Figure 7.12). The distal end is invaginated into the proximal stomach thus creating a valve which further limits reflux into the segment (Figure 7.13). Long-term transit studies of oesophageal interposed jejunal segments have shown sustained segmental rather than peristaltic activity but the clinical outcome in terms of absence of reflux symptoms and complete freedom from dysphagia has been excellent. The operation seems ideal for patients who require oesophageal excision for Barrett's columnar cell metaplasia [54].

Transhiatal oesophagectomy with cervical gastric anastomosis or long-segment colonic interposition is popular with some. Transhiatal total oesophagectomy undoubtedly abolishes reflux and utilizes a safe cervical anastomosis which, however, has a tendency to stricture although this can be lessened by constructing the anastomosis around an F46 bougie. The various reports on transhiatal oesophagectomy do not accurately document the incidence of recurrent laryngeal damage following this procedure which, in the author's experience, occurs in 20% with devastating consequences.

The results of re-do anti-reflux surgery are not ideal and carry a significant failure rate of 24% and a high postoperative morbidity [49].

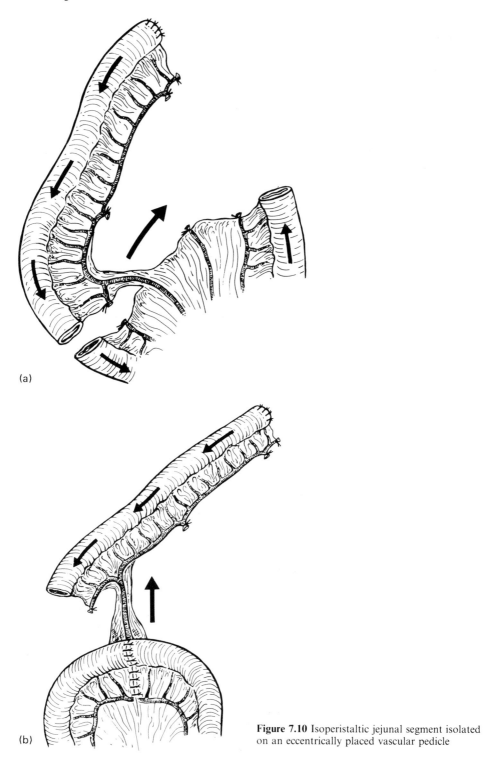

(a)

(b)

Figure 7.10 Isoperistaltic jejunal segment isolated on an eccentrically placed vascular pedicle

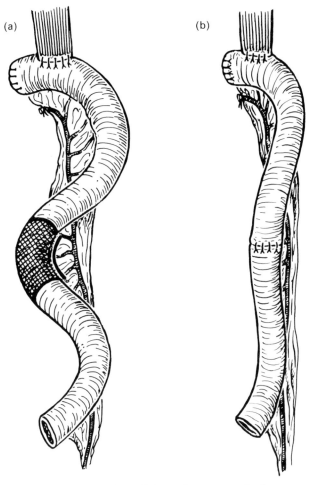

Figure 7.11 Box resection which may be necessary for long-segment replacements to avoid redundancy and kinking of the interposed loop

Reflux disease in infants and children

In general reflux in infants and children has a good outcome and tends to resolve by 2 years. Only a small percentage of patients, approximately 15–20%, require surgical treatment. Management is initially conservative with postural treatment, thickening of feeds and antacid therapy. A clinical trial has shown that oral antacids are as effective as H_2-receptor blockers in the paediatric age group [71]. Other drugs used include prokinetic agents designed to enhance clearance and improve the tone of the lower oesophageal sphincter such as metoclopramide and domperidone. There is an appreciable incidence of neurological disease and other congenital malformations in these children. The most common of these include mental retardation, hypotonia, Down's syndrome and cystic fibrosis.

The clinical presentation differs from that encountered in the adult. The most

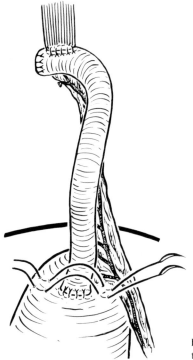

Figure 7.12 End-to-side anastomosis of the proximal end of the isolated jejunal loop to the oesophagus

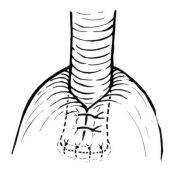

Figure 7.13 The distal anastomosis is invaginated into the stomach thus creating a valve which further limits reflux

common manifestations are vomiting, regurgitation, respiratory problems and failure to thrive. The respiratory sequelae of reflux disease are important and potentially life threatening especially in infancy. They include aspiration pneumonia, asthmatic attacks, bronchopulmonary dysplasia and the apnoea syndrome. Gastrointestinal bleeding and stricture formation are uncommon and encountered in 3%.

The diagnosis is best confirmed by 24-hour pH monitoring [72]. In addition some of these infants have oesophageal and gastric dysmotility and this small subset of patients requires identification preoperatively because this influences the nature of the surgical treatment [73].

Surgery is best delayed because the results in infants are less good than in children and because of the tendency for spontaneous resolution of the reflux. The operation performed for these children is a complete 1.5–3.0 cm wrap which is sutured to the diaphragm. Some advocate approximation of the crura posteriorly [72]. The use of a temporary tube gastrostomy for feeding is advisable [74]. The outcome is good with an overall reported success rate of 90%. Failures are largely confined to infants with neurological disease [75] or delayed gastric emptying when a concomitant pyloroplasty is indicated [73].

Reflux after myotomy for achalasia

One of the well-documented complications of cardiomyotomy for achalasia is the development of oesophageal reflux and some recommend the routine use of an anti-reflux procedure [76–78]. Others consider that reflux is a rare complication after myotomy and argue against the routine use of an additional anti-reflux procedure since it may precipitate obstruction in the presence of an aperistaltic oesophagus [79]. In a recent collective review of 5002 patients reported in the literature [80] the incidence of gastro-oesophageal reflux after myotomy without an anti-reflux procedure performed transthoracically was 7.7%. This was significantly lower than myotomy alone performed through the abdominal route (13.2%) and compared favourably with the incidence of reflux after myotomy combined with an anti-reflux procedure (7.3%). According to this collective review, gastro-oesophageal reflux occurs twice as often after myotomy performed through the abdomen suggesting that damage to the phreno-oesophageal membrane, undue mobilization of the gastro-oesophageal junction and an excessively long myotomy are responsible for the development of this complication. The authors of this review concluded that a carefully executed thoracic cardiomyotomy does not require an anti-reflux procedure. However, when the operation is performed through the abdominal route, an anti-reflux operation may be advisable. The disadvantage of this and other collective reviews, however carefully the reports included are scrutinized, is that the data are retrospective and are thus subject to the effect of uncontrolled variables. Conclusions based on these reports are at best tentative. Prospective studies are needed to deal with this controversy.

The author has changed his practice in recent years from routine to selective use of an anti-reflux procedure in patients undergoing myotomy. Two patients with combined thoracic short myotomy and Belsey Mark IV developed dysphagia and regurgitation with marked transit delay on isotope scintigraphy using a standardized egg bolus test. This experience led to an ongoing study in patients with achalasia who are now investigated with oesophageal transit studies, manometry and 24-hour pH monitoring before and at intervals after short thoracic cardiomyotomy, where the latter does not extend beyond 1.0 cm into the stomach and care is taken to avoid disruption of the cardio-oesophageal junction. To date 15 out of 18 patients did not exhibit reflux before the myotomy and have not developed reflux symptoms or shown any evidence of reflux when tested with 24-hour pH monitoring after their operation. Three patients included in this study exhibited reflux preoperatively and therefore needed partial fundoplication [81]. The preliminary findings of this study suggest that reflux may be present initially in some patients with achalasia [82] and at least in this subgroup may not be a consequence of the myotomy. Preoperative pH monitoring is advisable in patients with achalasia irrespective of surgical approach intended and will identify a group of patients who definitely require an additional anti-reflux procedure. Whether reflux will in time develop after myotomy in patients with an effective anti-reflux mechanism before surgery remains unclear; long-term follow-up of these patients is needed before this dilemma is settled.

Meanwhile, because disruption of the gastro-oesophageal fixation, particularly the insertion of the phreno-oesophageal membrane, is inevitable when cardiomyotomy is performed through the abdominal route, an anti-reflux procedure is a sensible adjunct to this procedure. In view of the impaired peristaltic activity of the oesophageal body, a complete fundal wrap is unwarranted. Instead, a partial wrap (180–200°) as initially recommended by Toupet [17] and more recently by Crookes *et al.* [83] should be performed as this is less likely to disturb oesophageal transit. There is no doubt that gastro-oesophageal reflux is particularly damaging to the oesophagus in patients with achalasia because the absence of effective peristaltic activity leads to a very prolonged contact time between the refluxate and the oesophageal mucosa. It probably accounts for the development of strictures which is well documented in these patients.

Reflux after gastric surgery

Reflux oesophagitis is commonly encountered after gastric surgery and may be acid or neutral (alkaline). The latter occurs notably as a complication of gastrectomy when its incidence depends on the extent of the gastric resection and the type of reconstruction [84,85], although it may complicate vagotomy and other operations, including cholecystectomy [86]. Acid reflux is more often documented after vagotomy.

Reflux symptoms especially heartburn are encountered in 20–40% of patients after vagotomy and drainage and highly selective vagotomy [87–89]. In the past this was interpreted as resulting from damage to the oesophagogastric fixation, vagal denervation of the lower oesophagus and alteration of the cardio-oesophageal angle [90–92]. Recent studies have, however, confirmed what has been suspected for a while. Duodenal ulcer patients have a high incidence of reflux symptoms and oesophagitis proven by endoscopy and 24-hour pH monitoring before their operation [93–95]. Furthermore, there is no evidence that vagotomy influences the reflux symptoms and the incidence of oesophagitis [95]. The question which needs to be addressed concerns the value of routine addition of an anti-reflux procedure in patients requiring highly selective vagotomy for intractable duodenal ulcer [96]. The decrease in the need for surgical treatment of patients with duodenal ulcer following the introduction of effective antacid therapy with H_2-receptor blockers has reduced the scope and feasibility of this study.

Although frequently referred to in the literature as alkaline oesophagitis, this is a misnomer since the pH of the reflux in many of these patients is around neutral and for this reason is missed by 24-hour pH monitoring. The refluxate may contain any of the following: pepsin, activated pancreatic enzymes, bile salts and lysolecithin. However, the main agent and the exact mechanism responsible for the mucosal damage remains unknown despite several clinical and experimental studies [7,97–99]. Indeed recent clinical reports have tended to dismiss bile and bile salts in the aetiology of erosive oesophagitis [100,101]. In one study using the Milk EHIDA test, 20% of normal subjects showed enterogastric bile reflux compared to 80% of patients with truncal vagotomy and drainage and 90% of patients after partial gastrectomy. There was little difference in the extent of enterogastric reflux between symptomatic and symptom-free patients after gastric surgery. However, delayed emptying of the refluxate was encountered only in the symptomatic group [102]. This study suggests that impaired gastric emptying and clearance of the refluxate may be important in the aetiology of bile vomiting and neutral oesophagogastritis. The oesophagitis is usually severe, often haemorrhagic, with chronic blood loss, and leads to severe mural fibrosis and early stricture formation.

In a personal series of 337 patients referred to the author for remedial surgery after gastric operations for peptic ulcer, 49 had biopsy proven oesophagitis (Table 7.2). Twenty-four hour pH monitoring was performed in the last 21 of these. Acid reflux episodes ($< pH$ 4.0) were identified in 4 patients and alkaline peaks (pH > 7.6) were observed in 1 patient. The remainder had neutral reflux.

Table 7.2 Oesophagitis after gastric surgery

Previous or last operation*	Vagotomy and drainage	21
	Vagotomy and antrectomy	5
	HSV	2
	BI resection	6
	BII resection	7
	Subtotal resection	2
	Total resection	6
pH monitoring [21]	Acid reflux	4
	Alkaline reflux	1
	Neutral reflux	16
Oesophagitis	Grade I and II	17
	Grade III and IV	32
Erosive gastritis [41]		41
Abnormal Milk EHIDA [29]		29

* 23 had more than one previous operation.

This experience with this highly selected group of patients can be summarized as follows:

1. Neutral reflux oesophagitis is always accompanied by erosive 'alkaline gastritis' in patients with a residual gastric remnant and in patients with a truncal vagotomy and drainage.
2. Pathological enterogastric reflux exceeding 10% of the administered isotope dose is found on testing with the Milk DISIDA test [102,103].
3. The oesophagitis is often severe, grade III or more.
4. Neutral reflux oesophagitis is most disabling after subtotal to total gastrectomy especially when reconstruction had been performed by a loop jejunostomy with enteroenteric anastomosis. The reported literature supports the view that neutral oesophagitis is more common after gastric resections particularly after total/subtotal gastrectomy [84,85].

The author has had patients who developed symptomatic neutral gastro-oesophageal reflux after cholecystectomy. This was particularly severe in three patients who also had additional surgery for peptic ulcer. Surgeons should be wary of cholecystectomy after a previous gastric resection or vagotomy and consideration should be given to non-surgical treatment such as extracorporeal shock wave lithotripsy or dissolution therapy in these cases. If stones are found at operation for peptic ulcer, it is the author's practice to remove the stones via a cholecystotomy and ensure complete clearance of the biliary tract of stones by cholangiography but to leave the gallbladder *in situ*.

The management of patients with symptomatic reflux after gastric surgery starts with a careful appraisal of their symptoms because, although specific postgastric surgery syndromes are described, in the majority of these patients the clinical picture is mixed and separate diagnostic labels, e.g. dumping, bilious vomiting etc., are misleading and inappropriate. However, each patient usually has a dominant complaint and it is to this that treatment should be targeted after appropriate investigations to determine the altered physiology and pathological anatomy of the gastrointestinal tract.

Patients with reflux symptoms as their dominant complaint should initially undergo upper gastrointestinal endoscopy with multiple biopsies of the stomach and oesophagus. If diagnosis is confirmed in this way, 24-hour pH monitoring is performed to determine whether the reflux is acid or neutral. Patients with acid reflux benefit from combined alginate–H_2-receptor blockade therapy. If this first-line therapy fails, omeprazole may be tried particularly if the patient is elderly or is considered a surgical risk. Operative treatment is indicated only if reflux is not controlled by medical measures.

Medical therapy (bile salt binding agents, prokinetic agents, e.g. metoclopramide, domperidone and cisapride, and mucosal protective agents, e.g. sucralfate and prostaglandin analogues) is ineffective in patients with neutral reflux and these patients should undergo surgical treatment unless this is contraindicated by old age, infirmity or co-morbid disease.

The surgical treatment depends on the nature of the previous operations and the pH of the refluxate. In patients with acid reflux after vagotomy and drainage or PCV, a partial fundoplication or loose 1.0 cm Nissen procedure is the preferred operation if the patient is thin and has a wide subcostal angle, otherwise a Belsey Mark IV should be considered. A fundoplication of any sort is difficult in patients with previous gastric resection as there is not enough slack to allow a loose wrap without tension. The author's choice for this subgroup is Hill's posterior gastropexy performed with intraoperative manometry.

Neutral reflux after vagotomy and gastroenterostomy is best dealt with by takedown of the drainage procedure provided the duodenum is not scarred. Pyloric reconstruction in patients after truncal vagotomy and pyloroplasty, while improving dumping symptoms, does not reduce enterogastric reflux and influence the oesophagitis [104]. In all other instances antrectomy with Roux-en-Y diversion is generally favoured although an isoperistaltic interposition of the segment of jejunum between the stomach remnant and the duodenal stump is a good alternative in the author's experience. The recently described duodenal switch operation [61] may turn out to be useful in some of these patients particularly those with reflux after truncal vagotomy and pyloroplasty.

Conclusions

Although seemingly satisfactory, the treatment of gastro-oesophageal reflux remains problematical. The surgical results are not as good as generally believed and reported and tend to deteriorate with time. Prospective clinical trials are needed to solve existing controversies.

Familiarity with a particular anti-reflux operation is important to ensure consistent and good results. Despite this, patient selection based on certain factors such as the build of the patient, previous surgery etc., is necessary to optimize the results of surgical treatment. Whereas the majority of patients who are not adequately controlled by medical therapy might be well served by an abdominal operation such as a loose short total fundoplication or incomplete wrap, there is no doubt that others require a thoracic approach. Finally, complicated, failed anti-reflux surgery, or reflux after previous gastric surgery pose management and technical problems and these patients should be treated in tertiary referral centres with the necessary expertise.

References

1. Allison, P. R. Peptic ulcer of the oesophagus. *J. Thorac. Surg.* 1946; **15**: 308–317
2. Allison, P. R. Reflux oesophagitis, sliding hiatal hernia and anatomy of repair. *Surg. Gynecol. Obstet.* 1951; **92**: 419–431
3. Mahler, J. W., Hocking, M. P. and Woodward, E. R. Re-operations for esophagitis following failed antireflux procedures. *Ann. Surg.* 1985; **201**: 723–727
4. Eriksen, C. A., Cranford, C., Sadek, S. and Cuschieri, A. Combined cimetidine–alginate antacid therapy versus single agent treatment for reflux oesophagitis: Results of prospective double-blind randomized clinical trial. *Ann. Chir.* 1989; (in press)
5. Klinkenberg-Knol, E. C., Jansen, J. M. B. J., Festen, H. P. M., Meuwissen, S. G. M. and Lamers, C. B. H. W. Double-blind multicentre comparison of omeprazole and ranitidine in the treatment of reflux oesophagitis. *Lancet* 1987; **i**: 349–350
6. Kivilaakso, E., Fromm, D. and Silen, W. Effect of bile salts and related compounds on isolated esophageal mucosa. *Surgery* 1980; **87**: 280–285
7. Lillemoe, K. D., Johnson, L. F. and Harmon, J. W. Alkaline esophagitis: a comparison of the ability of components of gastroduodenal contents to injure the rabbit esophagus. *Gastroenterology* 1983; **85**: 621–628
8. Nissen, R. Gastropexy and fundoplication in surgical treatment of hiatal hernia. *Am. J. Dig. Dis.* 1961; **6**: 954–961
9. Negre, J. B., Markkulh, H. T., Keyrilainen, O. and Matikainen, M. Nissen fundoplication: results of a 10 year follow-up. *Am. J. Surg.* 1983; **146**: 635–638
10. Negre, J. B. Post fundoplication symptoms: Do they restrict the success of fundoplication? *Ann. Surg.* 1983; **198**: 698–700.
11. Low, D. E., Mercer, C. D., James, E. C. and Hill, L. D. Post-Nissen syndromes. *Surg. Gynecol. Obstet.* 1988; **167**: 1–5
12. Cullen, P., Campbell, F. C. and Cuschieri, A. The bloated abdomen after antireflux surgery. *Br. J. Surg.* 1987; **74**: 1161.
13. Rosetti, M. and Hell, K. Fundoplication for the treatment of gastroesophageal reflux in hiatal hernia. *World J. Surg.* 1977; **1**: 439–444
14. DeMeester, T. R., Bonavina, L. and Albertucci, M. Nissen fundoplication for gastroesophageal reflux disease. *Ann. Surg.* 1986; **204**: 9–20
15. Thal, A. P. A unified approach to surgical problems of the gastroesophageal junction. *Ann. Surg.* 1968; **168**: 542–550.
16. Watson, A. A clinical and pathophysiological study of a simple and effective operation for the correction of gastro-oesophageal reflux. *Br. J. Surg.* 1984; **71**: 991.
17. Toupet, A. Technique d'oesophago-gastroplastie avec phrenogastropexie appliquée dans la cure radicale des hernies hiatales et comme complément del'operation d'Heller dans les cardiospasmes. *Mém. Acad. Chir. Paris* 1963; **89**: 384–389
18. Boutelier, P. and Jonsell, G. An alternative fundoplicative maneuver for gastroesophageal reflux. *Am. J. Surg.* 1982; **143**: 260–264
19. Dor, J., Humbert, P., Dor, V. *et al.* L'intérêt de la technique de Nissen modifice dans le prévention du reflux après cardiomiotomie extramuqueuse de Heller. *Mém. Acad. Chir. Paris* 1962; **27**: 877–882
20. Mir, J., Ponce, J., Jaun, M. *et al.* The effect of 180° anterior fundoplication on gastroesophageal reflux. *Am. J. Gastroenterol.* 1986; **81**: 172–175

21. Demos, N. J., Smith, N. and Williams, D. A new gastroplasty for strictured short esophagus. *N Y J. Med.* 1975; **75**: 57–59

22. Bingham, J. A. W. Hiatus hernia repair combined with reconstruction of an antireflux valve in the stomach. *Br. J. Surg.* 1977; **64**: 460–465

23. Henderson, R. D. and Marryatt, G. Total fundoplication gastroplasty. Long-term follow-up of 500 patients. *J. Thorac. Cardiovasc. Surg.* 1983; **85**: 81–87

24. Piehler, J. M., Payne, W. F., Cameron, A. J. and Pairolaoriop, C. T. The uncut Collis–Nissen procedure for esophageal hiatus hernia and its complications. In: Pickleman, J., Ed. *Problems in General Surgery.* New York: Plenum Medical Books. 1984: 1–14

25. Angelchik, J. P. and Cohen, R. A new surgical procedure for the treatment of gastroesophageal reflux and hiatal hernia. *Surg. Gynecol. Obstet.* 1979; **148**: 246–248

26. Wale, R. J., Royston, C. M. S., Bennett, J. R. and Buckton, G. K. Prospective study of the Angelchik anti-reflux prosthesis. *Br. J. Surg.* 1985; **72**: 520–524

27. Pickleman, J. Disruption and migration of an Angelchik esophageal anti-reflux prosthesis. *Surgery* 1983; **93**: 467–468

28. Lilly, M. P., Slapsky, S. F. and Thompson, W. R. Intraluminal erosion and migration of the Angelchik anti-reflux prosthesis. *Arch. Surg.* 1984; **119**: 849–853

29. Gear, M. W. L., Gillison, E. W. and Dowling, B. L. Randomized prospective trial of the Angelchik anti-reflux prosthesis. *Br. J. Surg.* 1984; **71**: 681–683

30. Stuart, R. C., Dawson, K., Keeling, P., Byrne, P. J. and Hennessy, T. P. J. A prospective randomized trial of Angelchik prosthesis versus Nissen fundoplication. *Br. J. Surg.* 1989; **76**: 86–89

31. Hill, L. D. An effective operation for hiatal hernia: an 8-year appraisal. *Ann. Surg.* 1967; **166**: 681–692

32. Hermreck, A. S. and Coates, N. R. Results of the Hill antireflux operation. *Am. J. Surg.* 1980; **140**: 764–767

33. Vansant, J. H. Surgical management of hiatal hernia with esophageal reflux. *Am. Surg.* 1978; **44**: 179–195

34. Baue, A. E. and Belsey, R. H. R. The treatment of sliding hiatus hernia and reflux oesophagitis by the Mark IV technique. *Surgery* 1967; **62**: 396–406

35. Boerma, I. Hiatus hernia repair: repair by right-sided anterior gastroplasty. *Surgery* 1969; **65**: 884–893

36. Narbona, B., Olavarietta, L. and Iloris, J. Hernia hiatal reflux gastro-oesophagico. Rehabilitacion nofegica y resultados con la pexia del ligamento redondo. *Cir. Espanol.* 1979; **33**: 487–495

37. Payne, S. The long term clinical state after resection with total gastrectomy and Roux loop anastomosis. In: Smith, R. A. and Smith, R. E., Eds. *Surgery of the Oesophagus.* Butterworths: London. 1972: 23–28

38. Glick, M. E. Clinical course of esophageal strictures managed by bougienage. *Dig. Dis. Sci.* 1982; **27**: 884–888

39. Lanza, F. and Graham, D. Y. Bougienage is effective therapy for most benign esophageal strictures. *J. Am. Med. Assoc.* 1978; **240**: 844–847

40. Dooner, J. and Cleator, I. G. M. Selective management of benign esophageal strictures. *Am. J. Gastroenterol.* 1982; **77**: 172–177

41. Buchin, P. J. and Spiro, H. M. Therapy of esophageal stricture: a review of 84 patients. *J. Clin. Gastroenterol.* 1981; **3**: 121–128

42. Mercer, C. D. and Hill, L. D. Surgical management of peptic esophageal stricture. Twenty-year experience. *J. Thorac. Cardiovasc. Surg.* 1986; **9**: 371–378

43. Vitale, G. C., Cheadle, W. G., Sadek, S., Michel, M. E. and Cuschieri, A. Computerized 24-hour ambulatory esophageal pH monitoring and esophagogastroduodenoscopy in the reflux patient. *Ann. Surg.* 1984; **200**: 724–728

44. Watson, A. Randomized study comparing medical and surgical reflux control in peptic oesophageal stricture treated by intermittent dilatation. *Gut* 1985; **26**: A553

45. Mahler, J., Hocking, M. P. and Woodward, E. R. Supradiaphragmatic fundoplication: Long-term follow up and analysis of complications. *Am. J. Surg.* 1984; **147**: 181–186

46. Richardson, J. D., Larson, G. M. and Polk, H. C. Intrathoracic fundoplication for shortened esophagus. Treacherous solution to a challenging problem. *Am. J. Surg.* 1982; **143**: 29–35

47. Starnes, V. A., Adkins, R. B., Ballinger, J. F. and Sawyers, J. L. Barrett's esophagus: a surgical entity. *Arch. Surg.* 1984; **119**: 563–567

48. Brand, D. L., Eastwood, I. R., Martin, D., Carter, W. B. and Pope, C. E. II. Esophageal symptoms, manometry and histology before and after antireflux surgery: Long term follow up study. *Gastroenterology* 1979; **76**: 1393–1401

49. Stirling, M. C. and Orringer, M. B. Surgical treatment after failed antireflux operation. *J. Thorac. Cardiovasc. Surg.* 1986; **92**: 667–672

50. Belsey, R. H. R. Gastroesophageal reflux. *Am. J. Surg.* 1980; **139**: 775–781

51. Little, A. G., Ferguson, M. K. and Skinner, D. B. Reoperation for failed anti-reflux operations. *J. Thorac. Cardiovasc. Surg.* 1986; **91**: 511–517

52. Belsey, R. H. R. Reconstruction of the esophagus with left colon. *J. Thorac. Cardiovasc. Surg.* 1965; **49**: 33–35

53. Polk, H. C. Jr. Jejunal interposition for reflux esophagitis and oesophageal stricture unresponsive to valvuloplasty. *World. J. Surg.* 1980; **4**: 731–736

54. Wright, C. and Cuschieri, A. Jejunal interposition for benign oesophageal disease. *Ann. Surg.* 1987; **205**: 54–60

55. Orringer, M. B. Transhiatal esophagectomy for benign disease. *J. Thorac. Cardiovasc. Surg.* 1985; **90**: 649–655

56. Postlethwait, R. W. Colonic interposition as oesophageal substitution. *Surg. Gynecol. Obstet.* 1983; **145**: 377–383

57. Herrington, J. L. and Mody, B. Total duodenal diversion for treatment of reflux oesophagitis uncontrolled by repeated antireflux procedures. *Ann. Surg.* 1976; **183**: 636–644

58. Royston, C. M. S., Dowling, B. L. and Spencer, J. Antrectomy with Roux-en-Y anastomosis in the treatment of peptic oesophagitis with stricture. *Br. J. Surg.* 1975; **62**: 605–607

59. Washer, G. F., Gear, M. W., Dowling, B. L., Gillison, E. W., Royston, C. M. S. and Spencer, J. Randomized prospective trial of Roux-en-Y duodenal diversion versus fundoplication for severe reflux oesophagitis. *Br. J. Surg.* 1984; **71**: 181–184

60. Perniceni, T., Gaget, B. and Fekete, R. Total duodenal diversion in the treatment of complicated peptic oesophagitis. *Br. J. Surg.* 1988; **75**: 1108–1111

61. DeMeester, T. R., Fuchs, K. H., Ball, C. S., Albertucci, M., Smyrk, T. C. and Marcus, J. N. Experimental and clinical results with proximal end-to-end duodenojejunostomy for pathological duodenogastric reflux. *Ann. Surg.* 1987; **206**: 414–426

62. Collis, J. L. Gastroplasty. *Thorax* 1961; **16**: 197–206

63. Pearson, F. G., Langer, B. and Henderson, R. D. Gastroplasty and Belsey hiatus repair: an operation for the management of peptic stricture with acquired short esophagus. *J. Thorac. Cardiovasc. Surg.* 1971; **61**: 50–63

64. Orringer, M. B. and Sloan, H. Complications and failings of the combined Collis–Belsey operation. *J. Thorac. Cardiovasc. Surg.* 1977; **74**: 726–731

65. Henderson, R. D. The gastroplasty tube as a method of reflux control. *Can. J. Surg.* 1978; **21**: 264–267

66. Pearson, F. G., Cooper, J. D. and Nelms, J. M. Gastroplasty and fundoplication in the management of complex reflux problems. *J. Thorac. Cardiovasc. Surg.* 1978; **76**: 665–672

67. DeMeester, T. R., Johnson, L. F. and Kent, A. H. Evaluation of current operations for the prevention of gastroesophageal reflux. *Ann. Surg.* 1974; **180**: 511–525

68. Orringer, M. B. and Sloan, H. S. Combined Collis–Nissen reconstruction of the esophagogastric junction. *Ann. Thorac. Surg.* 1978; **25**: 16–21

69. Pearson, F. G., Cooper, J. D., Patterson, G. A., Ramirez, J. and Todd, T. R. Gastroplasty and fundoplication for complex reflux problems. *Ann. Surg.* 1987; **206**: 473–481

70. Idolauri, J., Reinikainen, P. and Markukkla, H. Functional evaluation of interposed colon in esophagus. Manometric and 24-hour pH observations. *Acta Chir. Scand.* 1987; **153**: 21–24

71. Farrell, M. K. and Balistreri, W. F. The infant seat as treatment of gastroesophageal reflux. *N. Engl. J. Med.* 1984; **310**: 528

72. Randolph, J. Experience with Nissen fundoplication for correction of gastro-esophageal reflux in infants. *Ann. Surg.* 1983; **198**: 579–584

73. Fonkalsrud, E. W., Berquist, W., Vargas, J., Ament, M. E. and Foglia, R. P. Surgical treatment of gastroesophageal reflux syndrome in infants and children. *Am. J. Surg.* 1987; **154**: 11–18

74. St Cyr, J. A., Ferrara, T. B., Thompson, T. R., Johnson, D. E. and Foker, J. E. Nissen fundoplication for gastroesophageal reflux in infants. *J. Thorac. Cardiovasc. Surg.* 1986; **92**: 661–666

75. Dedinsky, G. K., Vane, M. W., Black, C. T., Turner, M. K., West, K. W. and Grosfeld, J. L. Complications and reoperation after Nissen fundoplication in childhood. *Am. J. Surg.* 1987; **153**: 177–183

76. Black, J., Vorbach, A. N. and Leigh-Collis, J. Results of Heller's operation for achalasia of the oesophagus. The importance of hiatal hernia repair. *Br. J. Surg.* 1976; **63**: 949–953

77. Tomlinson, P and Grant, A. F. A reivew of 74 patients with oesophageal achalasia: the results of Heller's cardiomyotomy with and without Nissen fundoplication. *Aust. N.Z. J. Surg.* 1981; **51**: 48–51

78. Gonzales, E. M., Alvarez, A. G. and Garcia, I. L. Results of esophageal achalasia. Multicentre retrospective series of 1856 cases. *Int. Surg.* 1988; **73**: 69–77

79. Ellis, F. H., Gibb, S. P. and Crozier, R. E. Esophagomyotomy for achalasia of the esophagus. *Ann. Surg.* 1980; **192**: 157–161

80. Andreollo, N. A. and Earlam, R. J. Heller's myotomy for achalasia: is an added anti-reflux procedure necessary? *Br. J. Surg.* 1987; **74**: 765–769

81. Cuschieri, A. Reflux after cardiomyotomy. *Br. J. Surg.* 1989; in press

82. Cheadle, W. G., Vitale, G. C., Sadek, S. and Cuschieri, A. Evidence for reflux in patients with achalasia. *Dig. Surg.* 1988; **5**: 1–4

83. Crookes, W. G., Wilkinson, A. J. and Johnston, G. W. Heller's myotomy with partial fundoplication. *Br. J. Surg.* 1989; **76**: 99–100

84. Helsingen, N. Oesophagitis following total gastrectomy – a clinical and experimental study. *Acta Chir. Scand.* 1961; **273**: 1–21

85. Domjan, L. and Simon, L. Alkaline reflux esophagitis in gastro-resected patients: objective detection with a simple isotope method. *Scand. J. Gastroenterol.* 1984; **19**: 245–249

86. Gowen, S. F. Spontaneous enterogastric reflux gastritis and esophagitis. *Ann. Surg.* 1985; **201**: 170–175

87. Goligher, J. C., Hill, G. L., Kennedy, T. F. and Nutter, E. Proximal gastric vagotomy without drainage for duodenal ulcer: results after 5–8 years. *Br. J. Surg.* 1978; **65**: 145–151

88. Dorricot, N. J., McNeish, A. R., Alexandre-Williams, J. *et al.* Prospective randomised multicentre trial of proximal gastric vagotomy or truncal vagotomy and antrectomy for chronic duodenal ulcer: interim results. *Br. J. Surg.* 1978; **65**: 471–478

89. Stoddard, C. J., Vassilakis, J. S. and Duthrie, H. L. Highly selective vagotomy or truncal vagotomy and pyloroplasty for chronic duodenal ulceration: a randomized, prospective clinical study. *Br. J. Surg.* 1978; **65**: 793–796

90. Clarke, S. D., Penry, J. B. and Ward, P. Oesophageal reflux after abdominal vagotomy. *Lancet* 1965; **ii**: 824–826

91. Alexander-Williams, J. and Woodward, D. A. K. The effect of sub-diaphragmatic vagotomy on the function of the gastroesophageal sphincter. *Surg. Clin. N. Am.* 1967; **47**: 1341–1344

92. Temple, J. G. and McFarland, J. Gastro-oesophageal reflux complicating highly selective vagotomy. *Br. Med. J.* 1975; **2**: 168–169

93. Earlam, R. On the origin of duodenal ulcer pain. *Lancet* 1985; **i**: 973–974

94. Earlam, R. J., Amerigo, J., Kakavoulis, T. and Pollock, D. J. Histological appearance of oesophagus, antrum and duodenum and their correlation with symptoms in patients with duodenal ulcer. *Gut* 1985; **26**: 95–100

95. Flook, D. and Stoddard, C. J. Gastro-oesophageal reflux and oesophagitis before and after vagotomy for duodenal ulcer. *Br. J. Surg.* 1985; **72**: 804–807

96. Camula, G. and Jordan, P. H. Is an antireflux procedure necessary in conjunction with parietal cell vagotomy in the absence of preoperative reflux? *Am. J. Surg.* 1987; **153**: 215–220

97. Kaye, M. D. and Showalter, J. P. Pyloric incompetence in patients with symptomatic gastroesophageal reflux. *J. Lab. Clin. Med.* 1974; **83**: 198–206

98. Kivilaakso, E. Fromm, D. and Silen, W. Effect of bile salts and related compounds on isolated esophageal mucosa. *Surgery* 1980; **87**: 280–285

 99. Coursar, C. D., Johnson, L. F. and Harmon, J. W. Aprotinin prevents trypsin-alkaline esophagitis. *Gastroenterology* 1985; **88**: 1356

100. Collins, B. J., Crothers, G., McFarland, R. J. and Love, H. G. Bile acid concentrations in the gastric juice of patients with erosive esophagitis. *Gut* 1985; **26**: 495–499

101. Smith, M., Buckton, G. K. and Bennett, J. R. Bile acid levels in stomach and oesophagus in patients with acid gastro-oesophageal reflux. *Gut* 1984; **26**: A556

102. Mackie, C., Hulks, G. and Cuschieri, A. Enterogastric reflux and gastric clearance of refluxate in normal subjects and in patients with and without bile vomiting following peptic ulcer surgery. *Ann. Surg.* 1986; **204**: 537–542

103. Mackie, C. R., Wisbey, M. L. and Cuschieri, A. Milk ^{99m}Tc-EHIDA test for entero-gastric bile reflux. *Br. J. Surg.* 1982; **69**: 101–104

104. Cheadle, W. G., Baker, P. R. and Cuschieri, A. Pyloric reconstruction for severe dumping after vagotomy and pyloroplasty. *Ann. Surg.* 1985; **202**: 568–572

Chapter 8

Benign strictures and other complications of reflux

T. P. J. Hennessy, A. Cuschieri and J. R. Bennett

Introduction

The inflammatory changes and subsequent fibrosis provoked by gastro-oesophageal reflux are responsible for the majority of benign oesophageal strictures. In a study of the natural history of strictures by Patterson *et al.* [1] around 80% were identified as peptic in origin. Postoperative strictures accounted for less than 10% of the total and corrosive strictures were even less frequent.

The early inflammatory changes in the oesophageal mucosa brought about by reflux have been described by Ismail-Beigi *et al.* [2] and are identified at histological examination which reveals a thickened basal layer with extension of the papillae towards the surface and a loss of surface cells. When inflammation is more advanced, oval or linear ulcers are present in the mucosa interspersed with islands of surviving epithelium. The wall of the oesophagus is oedematous and thickened with narrowing of the lumen. The inflammatory reaction may extend no deeper than the muscularis mucosae or the submucosa may be involved. In severe inflammation the muscle layers are involved. Proliferation of fibroblasts is more prominent in the submucosa where it may progress to connective tissue. With stricture formation collagen is present and the oesophageal wall is grossly thickened and may be shortened. Eventually muscular atrophy may occur due to intravascular thrombosis of mural vessels.

An oesophageal lumen of less than 12 mm will cause dysphagia. Mild strictures of this sort are easily managed with dilatation and medical treatment. A severe stricture with a lumen of less than 3 mm and a vertical length of more than 3 cm is indicative of extensive oesophageal damage and, despite intensive medical treatment or anti-reflux surgery, has a tendency to recur. In the majority of strictures fibrosis is confined to the mucosa and preoperative or intraoperative dilatation is possible. With adequate reflux control by medical treatment or anti-reflux surgery one or two dilatations may suffice to relieve the dysphagia. Even in more severe cases where regular dilatation is necessary, control of the reflux will lead to longer intervals between dilatations. Undilatable strictures with transmural fibrosis are uncommon and resection of benign strictures is much less frequent than formerly. Most reflux-induced strictures occur in the distal few centimetres of the oesophagus. More proximally located strictures are associated with Barrett's oesophagus and are of two types. One is located at the squamocolumnar junction and is the result of reflux oesophagitis. The second type occurs within the columnar lined segment of oeso-phagus at the site of a chronic (Barrett's) ulcer which has healed by scarring [3]. The incidence of strictures in Barrett's oesophagus is generally reported to be between 30% and 40% although some series have noted an incidence of 65–81% [4,5]. While most of these strictures have been identified in the mid-oesophagus, they have also been found in the distal oesophagus.

Despite the more severe reflux associated with columnar lined oesophagus, a comparison between Barrett's and non-Barrett's reflux-induced strictures revealed that the former were more responsive to medical treatment and required fewer dilatations. Patients with benign strictures have increased exposure to acid reflux with a greater number of reflux episodes. The duration of reflux episodes is longer indicating poor oesophageal clearance. The poor clearance is accounted for in part by the high incidence of reflux episodes in the recumbent position. A further contributory factor may be the decrease in oesophageal motility in the elderly who constitute the majority of patients with reflux-induced stricture. A factor of possible significance is the association between reflux and motility disorders.

Reflux episodes are often accompanied by irregular non-peristaltic contractions which may impair acid clearance thus creating a vicious circle in which the injurious effects of reflux are exacerbated by the effects of the reflux on clearance ability. Most reflux strictures are short. Long strictures of several centimetres are occasionally found and tend to be associated with prolonged nasogastric intubation particularly in the recumbent position, although it has been claimed that nasogastric intubation contributes very little to stricture formation unless there is a pre-existing hernia [6] and/or an intrinsic defect in the lower oesophageal sphincter.

Symptoms

The predominant symptom of acid-reflux stricture is dysphagia. The dysphagia may be intermittent at first. Progression is variable. A rapid course is common in children. In adults the dysphagia usually worsens over a period of months or even years. In most patients it is possible to obtain a history of reflux symptoms preceding the onset of obstruction, but often when the dysphagia is established reflux symptoms cease. Weight loss is common. Bleeding and anaemia may occur and are often present in children. Aspiration from the obstructed oesophagus may give rise to recurrent bouts of pulmonary infection.

Investigations

Radiological
Barium swallow will establish the location and extent of the stricture. The distinguishing features of a benign stricture are (1) a narrowed lumen, (2) lack of distensibility and (3) a symmetrical tapering of the moderately dilated proximal oesophagus towards the upper end of the stricture. A sliding hiatus hernia may be visualized immediately distal to the stricture (Figure 8.1). Asymmetrical stenosis and gross irregularity of the mucosal surface within the stricture indicating severe ulceration are suggestive of carcinoma. Benign strictures vary in length and may extend from 2 cm to 7 or 8 cm. The longer strictures are associated with nasogastric intubation. A positive diagnosis of benign stricture cannot be made on radiological examination alone, and endoscopy and biopsy are essential in order to exclude malignancy. A misdiagnosis of benign stricture will be made in between 20% and 25% of patients with oesophageal cancer and 10% of benign lesions may be incorrectly diagnosed as cancer on radiological examination [7].

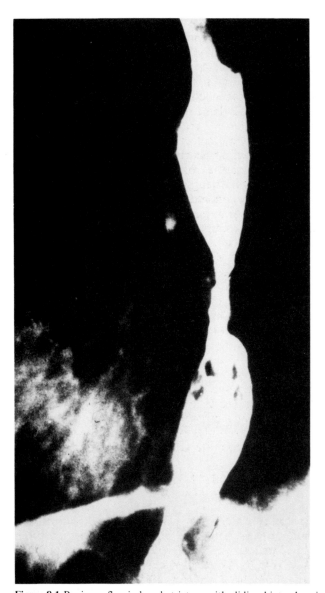

Figure 8.1 Benign reflux-induced stricture with sliding hiatus hernia

Endoscopy
The flexible fibreoptic endoscope has almost completely replaced the rigid instrument in the evaluation of oesophageal stricture. The flexible endoscope has the advantage of avoiding anaesthesia, a negligible risk of perforation and much better visualization. These advantages greatly outweigh the benefits of the rigid oesophagoscope with which luminal debris can be cleared more easily and larger biopsies taken.

Inflammation and ulceration can be readily seen at the site of the stenosis in moderate strictures, but when the stricture is very narrow nothing can be seen beyond the proximal margin of the stricture. In these circumstances it is essential to dilate the stricture sufficiently to pass the endoscope to its lumen so that biopsies may be taken and brush cytology carried out. With flexible endoscopy, biopsy and brush cytology an accurate diagnosis may be anticipated in 95% of cases [8]. It is also of value to carry out a complete endoscopic examination of stomach and duodenum. There is a significant association between duodenal ulcer and reflux disease and the presence of a duodenal ulcer may affect subsequent treatment of the stricture.

Manometry and pH monitoring
These should be carried out to complete the investigations in patients with benign stricture. As already indicated, the pH profile is likely to be abnormal with an increase in the percentage time below pH 4 particularly in the supine position, and poor oesophageal clearance demonstrated by prolonged reflux episodes.

Manometry may demonstrate a weak lower oesophageal sphincter with pressures below 10 mmHg and also reveal abnormal motility patterns with repetitive multi-peaked non-peristaltic contractions.

Conservative treatment

The twin aims of treatment are to relieve the dysphagia and to prevent recurrence of the stricture. A number of options are available but choice of treatment may be dictated by the severity of the stricture or the general condition and age of the patient. The options are:

1. Dilatation of the stricture with subsequent medical and postural treatment and repeat dilatation as indicated.
2. Dilatation and anti-reflux surgery.
3. Resection of the stricture and reconstruction of the oesophagus.
4. Permanent intubation.

Dilatation of strictures

Bougies and dilating systems
Dilatation followed by medical treatment of the reflux is the first line of treatment for any patient. For many years dilatation was performed using gum-elastic and other tapered dilators inserted down a rigid endoscope. With the advent of safer fibreoptic endoscopes, and the availability of bougies which pass over a guide wire inserted through the biopsy channel of such endoscopes, the customary method has changed to one of the many wire-guided bougies. The ideal characteristics of such a dilator are listed in Table 8.1, and those currently available in Table 8.2. The first to be introduced in 1971 were the Eder–Puestow olives [9]. These dilators have a flexible shaft consisting of a tightly coiled spring to which the spindle-shaped metal dilators of graduated diameters can be attached in sequence. The dilators range from 21 Fr (7 mm) to 58 Fr (19.5 mm). A flexible guide wire is passed initially using the fibreoptic endoscope. With the guide wire in position through the stricture, the first dilator is passed over the guide wire and through the stricture. Each successive dilator is two Fr sizes larger and successive dilators are passed until an adequate lumen is obtained. Intravenous benzodiazepine sedation and sometimes local pharyngeal anaesthesia are generally adequate to achieve patient tolerance although

Table 8.1 Characteristics desirable in an ideal dilator

1. Smooth, easy passage through pharynx and stricture and ability to negotiate tortuous strictures:
   (a) Narrow tip
   (b) Tapering contour
   (c) Intermediate 'angle of incidence'
   (d) Smooth passage over guide wire
   (e) Flexible staff or dilator
2. Safe, effective dilatation:
   (a) Wide effective dilating surface
   (b) 'Feel' as dilatation occurs
   (c) Few passages needed but variable size of dilatation permitted
3. Suitable for use in small stomachs
4. No X-rays needed routinely, but dilator is radio-visible and staff is radio-opaque if screening desired
5. Suitable for use in a busy endoscopy list:
   (a) Easy to use and not time consuming
   (b) No need for special room
   (c) Easy to clean
6. Patient acceptability
7. Cost equivalent to other dilators

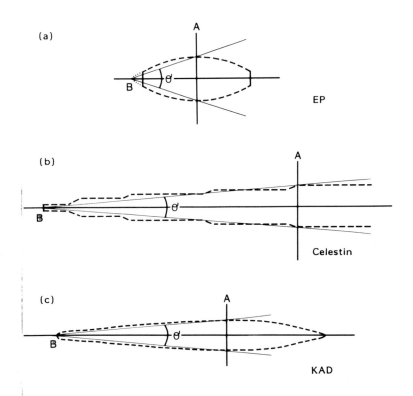

Figure 8.2 The calculated effective angles of incidence (θ) of the Eder–Puestow, Celestin and KAD bougies: θ is formed between the dilator's maximum diameter (A) and its tip (B) or, in the case of the Eder–Puestow bougie, the point at which the contours, if extended, would meet

Table 8.2 Technical characteristics of existing dilators

Dilator	Wire needed?	X-ray needed?	Min. diameter (tip) (mm)	Max. diameter (body) (mm)	(Fr)	Tip to max. diameter[a] (cm)	Angle of incidence[b] (°)	Number of passages[c]
Balloon (Rigiflex)	Yes	Yes	2.8	20	60	8	–	1
Balloon (Rigiflex TTS)	No (inbuilt wire)	No	1.8	20	60	8	–	1
Celestin	Yes	No	3.7	18	54	16	6	2
Eder–Puestow	Yes	No	3.7	19.3	58	2.1	32	Multiple
Hurst	No	No	4.0	19.5	59	14	8	Multiple
KAD	Yes	No	3.0	17.3	52	8.2	12	3 or less
Maloney	No	No	4.4	16	48	11.5	8	Multiple
Pilling	No	No	4.4	19.8	60	14	8	Multiple
Savary	Yes	No	5.0	20	60	17.7	6	Multiple
Tridil	Yes	No	3.7	18	54	2.1	46	3 or less

[a] This length is from the start of the dilator proper (bougie or rod) to the maximum diameter.
[b] The angle of incidence is the angle θ at the start of the dilator, subtended by the maximum diameter of the largest bougie or rod (Figure 8.2).
[c] The number of passages to achieve maximum dilatation depends on the individual circumstances.

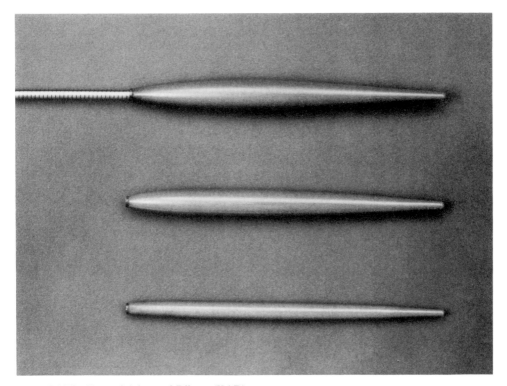

Figure 8.3 The Keymed Advanced Dilator (KAD)

intravenous analgesics may be required. Occasionally general anaesthesia is needed for a nervous patient. Dilatation to 15 mm (45 Fr) will allow normal swallowing. With a dense stricture where resistance to the passage of the dilators is considerable, it is prudent to carry out the dilatation in two or more sessions with an interval of a few days between each dilatation. Such gradual dilatation minimizes the risk of splitting the oesophageal wall. The main disadvantage of these dilators is the discomfort to the patient of repeated passage of the dilators but their efficacy is undoubted [10–12]. An attempt to minimize the number of passages was made by placing three olives on each staff, the Tridil dilator [13] but the blunt olives are sometimes difficult to pass through the pharynx or a tough stricture.

The dilators designed by Celestin [14] offer a significant advantage from this point of view. Only two passages of the dilators are required to reach 18 mm diameter [15]. These dilators consist of long rods of thermal polyvinyl chloride with a central lumen which can be passed over a guide wire. The tubes have a tapered end 20 cm in length. The tip of the tapered end is 4 cm in diameter and gradually increases in size to 12 mm in the first dilator and 18 mm in the second. Thus two passages of the dilators are sufficient to achieve an adequate lumen. However, paradoxically, their innate smoothness diminishes the tactile feel for the stricture so that it is difficult to determine whether resistance is at the stricture or at the pharynx. The length of the

Celestin dilators renders them unsuitable for use in patients with stomachs of small capacity after previous gastric surgery and difficult hiatus hernias.

Savary [16] has produced a set of flexible plastic dilators which are smooth and easier to handle than the Celestin but they require several passages [17].

The safest dilators are the mercury weighted flexible bougies designed by Maloney. When the need for dilatation is frequent these can be passed by the patient himself at home with complete safety and without significant discomfort. Their flexibility is such that they cannot be passed through very narrow strictures and their real value is in maintaining an adequate lumen after dilatation has been achieved using a more rigid system. The Maloney dilators have, however, declined in popularity and use with the advent of the guide wire systems which are undoubtedly more effective and very safe in experienced hands.

The Keymed Advanced Dilator (KAD), shown in Figure 8.3, consists of a spindle-shaped bougie dilator made of medical grade silicone rubber mounted on a flexible steel shaft. There are three sizes of bougie: diameters 6.5–9 mm (20–27 Fr), 6.5–14 mm (20–42 Fr) and 6.5–17.3 mm (20–52 Fr). A larger 6.5–18 mm (20–54 Fr) is currently under evaluation. The bougies are attached to the staff by a simple screw junction. The bougie is barium impregnated for visualization under radiological control and the radio-opaque proximal screw acts as a marker. The tapering ends of these dilators which give them their spindle shape, enhance the natural flexibility of the material. The dilators are used in the usual way over a laser-welded flexible stainless steel guide-wire with the lumen siliconed before use. Because the bougie is flexible, unlike the Eder–Puestow system, there is no need for a distal flexible spring tip. The shape and flexibility of the bougie allow the operator to ease the dilator through the oropharynx without hold-up, but during dilatation the operator still retains the sensation of 'feel' as the maximum diameter passes through the stricture.

Table 8.3 Longevity and cost

Dilator	Length of life in our hands or recommended	Current UK cost per set (VAT included)[a]
Balloon (Rigiflex) 20 mm	Not known 50 cases	£281 (manometer £345 extra)
Balloon (Rigiflex) 20 mm TTS	Not known	£370 (manometer £345 extra)
Celestin	2 years	£141 (2 dilators)
Eder–Puestow	17 years (still in use)	£837 (19 olives)
Hurst	2 years recommended	Priced individually, e.g. £41 each up to 38 Fr £59 for 40 Fr
KAD	Not known	£592 (3 dilators)
Maloney	2 years recommended	Priced individually, e.g. £71 for 44 Fr £103 for 57 or 60 Fr
Pilling	2 years recommended	Priced individually, e.g. £54 for 40 Fr
Savary	3–4 years recommended	£880 (10 dilators)
Tridil	Not known (same construction as Eder–Puestow)	No longer marketed

[a] Guidewire replacements cost: 250 cm steel   £24
                                            400 cm Teflon coated £35

At present, the KAD comes closest to fulfilling the qualities of the ideal dilator (Table 8.3).

Balloon dilators, modelled on polyethylene balloons of the Grunzig angioplasty type, have been used for stricture dilatation [18]. These balloons are inelastic and, when fully inflated, retain their rigid state; increasing the pressure renders the balloon harder but not larger. For oesophageal use, balloons may be passed over a guide-wire, or used under direct vision after insertion down the endoscope, although such 'TTS' balloons are more fragile than those used over guide-wires. Although dilating balloon systems are safe, in a recent controlled trial Cox et al. [19] found that bougies were rather more effective at achieving and maintaining an adequate lumen. For optimum use balloons require radiological control to ensure accurate positioning and full inflation.

Efficacy of dilatation
The size to which a stricture is dilated is usually dictated by the difficulty of dilatation, by the equipment available, by the patient's reaction to the procedure and the operator's whim. Dilatation to a diameter of 15 mm (45 Fr) allows normal swallowing of solids to take place. It has been variously suggested that dilatation should be gradual or rapid, and that it should be to the maximum diameter (17–20 mm) compatible with safety or to modest size only in case wide dilatation should cause ulceration and quicker re-stenosis. Perhaps the most important consideration which is often ignored by the proponents of maximal dilatation is the increased likelihood of oesophageal splitting inherent in this approach. There is a surprising lack of quantitative information about the actual effect of bougie dilatation on stricture size.

The effective diameter of a stricture can be measured in a number of ways, and the authors believe that discussions on the relative merits of various dilatation procedures should be based on such quantitative data. The authors' own preference is to use calibrated spheres but other techniques are available and provide reliable information if used consistently. With the sphere technique, the dilated stricture reaches its maxiumum effective bore about a week after bougienage. This diameter is always smaller than the maximum size bougie used, usually by 4–8 mm

The efficacy and safety of gradual dilatation over several sessions compared with one-session maximal dilatation remain uncertain. Common sense indicates that, if the passage of bougies requires increasing force or if the patient experiences discomfort, then one should desist from further attempts to achieve a greater diameter. By contrast if the dilatation is proceeding easily, then progress to 'maximum' size (18–20 mm) is both safe and effective. The frequency with which dilatation is required is extremely variable and can only be determined by assessing progress and relief of dysphagia in the individual patient. It is reasonable after a first dilatation to repeat the procedure a month later. The degree of narrowing which has occurred by that time is a useful guide to the likely future frequency of dilatation. The tendency with most benign strictures is that the need for dilatation decreases with time, and the intervals can steadily be lengthened [10]. A few resistant strictures can be effectively dealt with only by frequent bougienage – perhaps weekly for several months. Some of these eventually stabilize and come to require less frequent dilatation [20], although Williamson [21] feels that bougienage will rarely cure a fibrous stricture. These patients pose management problems in that, beyond a certain number of dilatations, the cumulative risk of perforation becomes substantial. It is our view that the need for frequent repeated dilatations beyond 3 months is an indication for operative intervention if the patient is considered fit for surgery.

After treatment
Once dilatation has been achieved the aim of subsequent treatment is to minimize
further reflux injury to the oesophageal mucosa. Postural measures and vigorous
medical treatment are given a trial initially. A combination of H_2-receptor antagonists and alginate is the preferred medical regimen.

Complications of dilatation

Endoscopic examination of the gastrointestinal tract carries a measurable risk of
perforation, and this increases if stricture dilatation is performed. Bleeding, although
common at the time of dilatation, is seldom of clinical prominence and when
encountered usually indicates incomplete injuries (mucosal laceration–intramural
haematoma). The incidence of such accidents is low, but it is essential that
endoscopists minimize the risk and be aware of the appropriate management should
perforation occur, since this will vary depending upon the anatomical location,
severity, age of patient etc.

Oesophageal perforation

Incidence
Surveys of endoscopists using fibreoptic instruments in the UK in 1972 [22] and in
the USA in 1974 [23] suggested an overall incidence of complications of about 3 per
1000 examinations. Better instrumentation and training have improved performance
and a 1981 survey of 38 000 examinations by members of the British Society of
Gastroenterology showed an overall perforation rate during fibreoptic oesophago-
gastroduodenoscopy of 0.018% [24]. In this survey the risk for dilatation of strictures
was 0.9%. In the last decade there have been reports of perforation rates with
bougies of 0.63% [15], 2.0% [25] and 3.79% [26]. The risk factors for perforation fall
into three groups: equipment, technique and type of lesion. Familiarity with a
specific dilating system is an important aspect of prevention and, in this respect, the
various quoted rates for different bougies are both irrelevant and suspect. Accidents
are least likely when the procedure is performed by an experienced operator using an
up-to-date fibreoptic endoscope in a well-equipped unit, but senior staff are not
immune from inflicting these complications [27]. Forceful dilatation is hazardous
because it may cause splitting. The dilatation should proceed as long as the dilators
slip through the stricture with relative ease and minimal force (dead weight of the
hand/wrist). The type of lesion for which dilatation is carried out influences the risk
of perforation. The most vulnerable in this respect is chronic lye stricture followed by
achalasia.

Pathology
Most lesions are complete and consist of either perforation of the oesophagus (above
or below the stricture) or splitting of the gullet at the narrowed segment. Incomplete
perforations usually occur in the cervical oesophagus at or just distal to the
cricopharyngeus. These rare lesions are caused by the endoscope. There may or may
not be a re-entry hole lower down. This lesion results in dissection of the oesophageal
mucosa from the muscularis with the development of an intramural haematoma and
a characteristic double-barrel oesophagogram. Incomplete injuries carry a low risk
and are always treated conservatively. Complete cervical and subdiaphragmatic
perforations are less serious than the intrathoracic variety.

Diagnosis of perforation

In most cases the perforation is recognized or suspected at the time of occurrence. No complaint of chest or abdominal discomfort, dyspnoea or pyrexia should be dismissed lightly, and after therapeutic procedures patients should be specifically questioned about such symptoms. They should also be kept under observation without anything by mouth for several hours even if this entails an overnight stay.

Even the remote possibility of perforation is an absolute indication for plain films of the neck (in two planes) and chest X-rays. Air may be seen in the mediastinum or within the soft tissues of the neck. However, these may be normal even if perforation has occurred [28] and continuing suspicion should lead to a water-soluble radio-opaque swallow. With a complete instrumental perforation symptoms usually develop rapidly. Pain exacerbated by swallowing and movement of the neck is often marked in cervical perforation. Pain is also a prominent symptom in perforation of the thoracic oesophagus and is frequently accompanied by dyspnoea. When the perforation is in the lower oesophagus pain is also experienced in the upper abdomen. Subcutaneous emphysema is present early in cervical perforations but may be a late manifestation in damage to the lower oesophagus. Pyrexia and tachycardia occur early. Chemical inflammation of the mediastinum occurs initially due to escape of gastric content into the mediastinum followed by invasion of virulent micro-organisms from the mouth and oesophagus.

Treatment

Instrumental perforation of the oesophagus should be regarded as a surgical emergency and these patients are best managed in a surgical ward. This does not imply that surgical intervention is always necessary or indeed advisable. Consider-able controversy exists regarding the optimum management of these patients and there has been an increasing trend among endoscopists towards conservative man-agement [29–35]. To a large extent these extreme views indicate a lack of appreciation of the varied requirements of these unfortunate patients. The only sensible attitude is that which considers that each patient has to be assessed individually in light of specific circumstances. There is no doubt that conservative management is appropri-ate in certain patients and equally certain is the fact that for others the only hope of survival is immediate surgical intervention, ideally performed within 24 hours of the accident since delay is the single most important factor in influencing survival in these patients [36]. The factors governing the decision on the appropriate management include: type of injury, findings of the contrast examination, age and general condition of the patient and the level of surgical expertise available. With respect to location, the risk of death is highest in intrathoracic perforation. These lesions particularly if early (diagnosed within 24 hours) are best treated surgically by an experienced oesophageal surgeon although small localized leaks are managed con-servatively by some. Lesions of the cervical and lower oesophagus and stomach with localized perforation (as identified by the contrast study) without evidence of established sepsis can be treated conservatively in the first instance provided they are carefully monitored in a surgical ward. Indeed most of these patients do well and few require emergency surgical treatment. This approach is therefore sensible particularly in the aged and the infirm. Likewise all incomplete injuries irrespective of location should be treated conservatively. On the other hand, free perforations with extensive and wide extravasation of the contrast resulting from extensive lacerations and splitting in any segment of the oesophagus require immediate surgical treatment as this provides the only realistic hope of survival.

The principles of conservative management include:

1. Total starvation, nasogastric aspiration using a Salem sump tube (on continuous suction) and intravenous fluid therapy.
2. Systemic broad-spectrum antibiotics, e.g. amoxycillin and an aminoglycoside.
3. Daily haematological, biochemical and radiological monitoring (plain X-rays) and frequent (4–6 hourly) clinical assessment particularly during the first 24 hours.
4. Resort to surgical intervention in the event of deterioration with the development of established sepsis.

The nature of surgical treatment depends on whether the perforation is early when direct suture closure is possible or late when the gross transmural oedema and tissue softening preclude this option. Several procedures are available to seal late perforations such as intercostal muscle flaps, diaphragm flaps, Thal fundal patch etc. In particularly severe injuries the safest approach is closure of the oesophagus above and below the injury by use of bands with tube cervical oesophagostomy and gastrostomy. The latter is used for enteral nutrition until reconstruction which is undertaken at a later stage if the patient survives and after full and complete recovery.

Surgical treatment

Fit patients with an unacceptable frequency of dilatations with medical treatment should undergo an anti-reflux procedure. After successful anti-reflux surgery strictures may undergo spontaneous resolution [37,38]. A success rate of 75% was reported by Watson with anti-reflux surgery and a single dilatation [39].

Anti-reflux surgery

There are no controlled trials evaluating the merits of different anti-reflux procedures in the treatment of oesophageal strictures. In patients without shortening of the oesophagus either the Nissen fundoplication or the Hill posterior gastroplexy may be used. The Belsey Mark IV operation may be appropriate where there is some degree of oesophageal shortening. It is usually possible to reduce the sliding hernia and carry out the Belsey repair after mobilization of the lower oesophagus through a left thoracotomy.

If adequate oesophageal lengthening cannot be achieved by mobilization the cut Collis cardioplasty is probably the procedure of choice with the addition of a Nissen fundoplication or the Belsey procedure.

Nissen fundoplication

The superiority of the Nissen fundoplication in controlling reflux has been demonstrated by DeMeester *et al.* [40]. For this reason and because of its technical simplicity, low morbidity and minimal mortality, the loose short Nissen fundoplication is one of the procedures of choice for dilatable strictures. Herrington *et al.* [41] and Naef and Savary [37] reported satisfactory results from Nissen fundoplication. No dilatation was necessary after fundoplication in the latter series.

Hill posterior gastropexy
Hill *et al.* [42] reported satisfactory results in 85% of patients with stricture after posterior gastropexy. Digital dilatation was carried out via a gastrotomy in patients with strictures at the gastro-oesophageal junction. Patients with higher strictures had a columnar lined lower oesophagus. Acquired shortening of the oesophagus was not seen, and adequate length of intra-abdominal oesophagus was obtained in every case.

Angelchik prosthesis
Satisfactory results can be achieved in some patients using the Angelchik prosthesis [43]. However, the tendency for progressive dysphagia to occur due to fibrous capsule formation around the prosthesis makes it an unsuitable operation for stricture.

Gastroplasty
The Collis cardioplasty [44] was designed to provide a tubular segment of stomach which would function like the intra-abdominal oesophagus albeit without a sphincter. The acute angle between it and the newly fashioned fundus served as an anti-reflux valve. Collis reported a 40% incidence of reflux after this operation. The addition of a Belsey procedure by Pearson reduced the incidence of postoperative reflux to 6.5% [45,46]. Henderson [47] added a complete Nissen fundoplication to the cardioplasty with excellent results. Of 44 strictures followed up for 6 years only one had residual dysphagia. The Collis cardioplasty may be constructed without dividing and separating the tubular portion (uncut Collis, Bingham cardioplasty). Although this modification gives excellent results in the control of reflux [48] it is less satisfactory when used for patients with stricture [49].

Thal procedure
This procedure involves dividing the stricture and using the gastric fundus as a patch over the defect. A skin graft may be added to protect the gastric serosa. Thal's original procedure [50] gave rise to severe reflux but satisfactory reflux control was obtained by Woodward by the addition of a full fundoplication. However, the Thal procedure with or without full fundoplication makes it necessary to bring the fundus of the stomach into the chest. Mansoor *et al.* [51] have documented the severe complications which may develop in these circumstances. They include intrathoracic gastric rupture with gastrobronchial fistula, lesser curve ulceration and herniation of the fundoplication. Two fatalities occurred in his series from intrathoracic rupture of the gastric wrap.

Resection

Resection of the strictured segment of the oesophagus and replacement by mobilized stomach with oesophagogastric anastomosis is likely to lead to further reflux and stricture formation. Belsey [52] reported an incidence of 27% re-stenosis within 6 months of resection and oesophagogastric anastomosis. Better results may be obtained if the oesophagogastric anastomosis is accompanied by a 360° wrap to prevent reflux.

Jejunal interposition
Replacement with an isoperistaltic jejunal segment was reported by Merendino [53,54]. The 4 cm segment below the diaphragm acted as a reflux barrier. The mortality was 4%. All surviving patients were relieved of their dysphagia although

some complained of delay in swallowing which obliged them to eat more slowly. Weight gain was significant in 70% of patients. Dumping and diarrhoea occurred in a number of patients but the symptoms were transient in most. These symptoms were attributed to the vagotomy and pyloroplasty included in the procedure. Polk carried out jejunal interpositions on 28 patients with either undilatable stenosis or intractable reflux. He compared the outcome with that of eight patients with equally severe symptoms in whom he elected to perform a further anti-reflux procedure. One death occurred in the jejunal transposition series. All patients with jejunal replacement were relieved of their symptoms but four of the eight patients who underwent repeat fundoplication continued to have dysphagia or reflux.

Wright and Cuschieri [55] reported excellent long-term results in 30 patients with one death from anastomotic leakage and sepsis. Although no postoperative patients complained of dysphagia for either liquids or solids, radionuclide transit studies showed segmental rather than peristaltic contractions and delayed transit times.

Colon interposition
Belsey [52] found jejunal transposition unsatisfactory for two reasons – the precarious blood supply in children and the development of an alkaline oesophagitis proximal to the oesophagojejunal anastomosis in some cases. He reported his experience with 105 colon transpositions, 82 of which were for benign fibrous strictures of the oesophagus. The preferred segment was the left half of the transverse colon and splenic flexure pedicled on the left colic artery which facilitates placement in an isoperistaltic position. Postoperative mortality in resections for fibrous strictures was 3.6%. The functional results were excellent with no evidence of recurrence of reflux or stenosis during the follow-up period. Henderson [47] recommended maintaining a 10 cm segment of colon in the abdominal cavity. Redundant colon may cause bolus obstruction and reflux may persist in some patients. Postlethwait [56] noted that although transit through the transposed colonic segment was due to gravity rather than peristalsis reflux was rare in an isoperistaltic segment. The most dangerous complication was colonic necrosis and leakage at the proximal anastomosis.

Transhiatal oesophagectomy
Some centres advocate transhiatal oesophagectomy with cervical anastomosis of the transposed stomach. As this procedure avoids thoracotomy, it is well tolerated by these patients (see Chapter 7).

In summary most benign strictures associated with reflux are dilatable and should not be considered undilatable until intraoperative stretching, either digitally or using a Hegar dilator, has been tried. In the majority of strictures the associated hernia is reducible with proper mobilization. Most strictures can, therefore, be treated initially by an anti-reflux procedure and dilatation. Cardioplasty and anti-reflux procedure may be used when the hernia cannot be reduced. Distal resection and replacement with a segment of jejunum or colon or transhiatal oesophagectomy with cervical anastomosis of the transposed stomach should be reserved for patients with undilatable strictures. The importance of excluding malignancy in undilatable strictures has been repeatedly emphasized.

Procedures which involve antrectomy, vagotomy and Roux loop division may be occasionally indicated particularly in patients with multiple previous unsuccessful operations but should not be advocated as first-time operations.

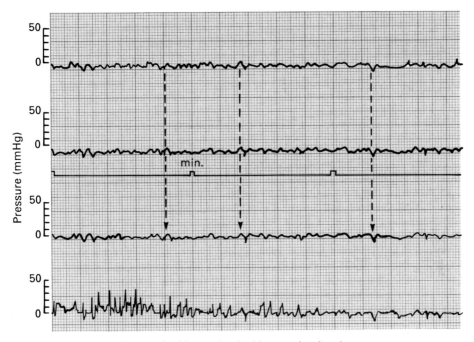

Figure 8.4 Almost complete aperistalsis associated with systemic sclerosis

Strictures associated with systemic sclerosis

When systemic sclerosis involves the oesophagus, peristalsis is lost due to atrophy and fibrinoid degeneration of oesophageal smooth muscle. Lower oesophageal sphincter function is abolished allowing free reflux of gastric contents. The combination of severe reflux and poor oesophageal clearance gives rise to inflammation and ulceration of the oesophageal mucosa and stricture formation (Figure 8.4). Although intermittent bougienage may relieve the dysphagia, reflux symptoms tend to persist despite intensive medical treatment. Care must be exercised in selecting patients for more aggressive treatment. If prognosis is poor due to cardiomyopathy or incipient renal failure a conservative approach is indicated but when the outlook is more optimistic, anti-reflux surgery can confer great benefit by relieving the reflux symptoms. In Orringer's view [57] the more frequently employed anti-reflux procedures such as the Nissen fundoplication, the Hill posterior gastropexy or the Belsey Mark IV procedure are unsuitable for use in systemic sclerosis as the fibrinoid degeneration in the lower oesophagus makes it unsuitable for the insertion of stitches. He advocates the Collis cardioplasty in combination with the Belsey procedure or a full 360° wrap. Comparing these two procedures he found that 17% of Collis–Belsey repairs continued to have moderate to severe reflux. In the Collis–Nissen group only 5% continued to have significant reflux symptoms. Resolution of strictures was complete in six of the nine in the Collis–Belsey group and partial in three; in the Collis–Nissen group resolution was complete in four and partial in three. Technical points stressed by Orringer are the construction of the cardioplasty with a

46 Fr dilator in place and the construction of a loose wrap of no more than 3 cm in vertical length. In a group of 37 patients mortality was nil and no problems with wound healing were encountered.

Postmyotomy strictures

The incidence of reflux oesophagitis and stricture following Heller's myotomy for achalasia varies from series to series but is around 5–6% overall, and to some extent is related to the technique employed. Ellis [58] emphasizes that if the myotomy extends distally no further than the oesophagogastric junction the risk of postoperative reflux is reduced to a minimum. In a group of 103 patients treated by this technique and followed for an average of 6.75 years only 4 developed significant reflux oesophagitis. Tomlinson and Grant [59] noted oesophagitis in 12 and strictures in 8 out of a total of 39 patients undergoing myotomy. When fundoplication was added to the myotomy the incidence of complications was significantly reduced. Belsey [60] treated 62 patients with myotomy and the Mark IV plication. Although he routinely extended the myotomy onto the stomach wall none of the patients developed symptoms of reflux or stricture during a follow-up period of 8 years. Mansour *et al.* [61] reported complete relief of symptoms in nine myotomized patients with reflux and three with stricture when an anti-reflux procedure was subsequently carried out.

From a review of the literature between 1970 and 1985 involving 5002 cases, Andreollo and Earlam [62] concluded that oesophageal myotomy carried out through the abdomen was twice as likely to give rise to reflux as a transthoracic myotomy. However, when an anti-reflux operation was added to the transabdominal myotomy the incidence of reflux was the same as in the transthoracic approach. The incidence of peptic structure in these 75 reports was 3%

Alkaline reflux

The term 'alkaline reflux oesophagitis' is something of a misnomer suggesting that the alkalinity of the refluxate is responsible for the inflammatory changes. There is no evidence that this is so and it would seem probable that pancreatic proteolytic enzymes and bile salts are the injurious agents. Gillen *et al.* [63] demonstrated that significant concentrations of bile acids may be present in gastric content without being detectable on oesophageal pH monitoring. Although most reports of alkaline reflux oesophagitis refer to postoperative patients who have undergone procedures such as Billroth II gastrectomy, total gastrectomy with oesophagojejunostomy or vagotomy and pyloroplasty [64] the condition may also occur in non-operated patients [65]. While the majority of patients demonstrate varying grades of oesophagitis ulceration and stricture formation also occur. Antrectomy and Roux loop diversion of duodenal contents is the procedure of choice. The duodenojejunal segment should be anastomosed to the jejunum 40–60 cm distal to the gastrojejunal anastomosis.

Schatzki ring

The Schatzki ring [66] is an annular stricture located in the distal 1 or 2 cm of the

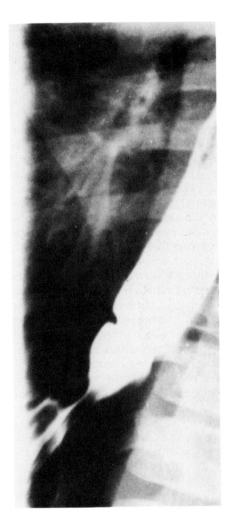

Figure 8.5 Schatzki ring which gives rise to intermittent bolus obstruction

oesophagus (Figure 8.5). The stricture is confined to the mucosa and submucosa, and is lined with squamous epithelium on its upper surface and columnar epithelium on its lower surface. It projects into the lumen of the oesophagus at right angles to the long axis and radiologically presents the appearance of a web or membrane with a central opening. Histologically the ring is infiltrated with lymphocytes and plasma cells. Dysphagia occurs as acute episodes of bolus obstruction with pain due to muscular spasm and profuse salivation. Episodes of dysphagia may become more frequent if the lumen becomes progressively more narrow. Schatzki noticed this tendency in around 20% of his patients [66].

Postlethwait and Masser [67] have concluded that these rings are a manifestation of localized oesophagitis but there is no consensus on this point. There is usually a hiatus hernia present and gastro-oesophageal reflux is a common finding. If obstructive episodes are rare and resolve spontaneously either by regurgitation or passage of the bolus, no intervention is necessary. However, frequent or progressive dysphagia is best treated by dilatation. Dilatation may have to be repeated at intervals. Sometimes the ring is too fibrotic to respond to dilatation and in these circumstances excision of all or part of the ring via a gastrotomy may be carried out with the addition of an anti-reflux procedure. In Eastridge's [68] series 65 of 88 patients responded to dilatation. Repeat dilatation was necessary in nine and two required operation for reflux. Of the 18 patients who were initially treated by operation all had disruption or excision of the ring and an anti-reflux procedure. Only one patient had recurrence of the ring with mild symptoms and another developed recurrent reflux and a stricture.

Motility disorders associated with reflux

Patients with gastro-oesophageal reflux may also experience motility disorders such as diffuse oesophageal spasm or symptomatic oesophageal peristalsis. Sometimes the spontaneous attacks of pain are accompanied by the characteristic motility patterns of diffuse spasm or nutcracker oesophagus and sometimes by a fall in the intraoeso-phageal pH. In these patients an accurate diagnosis may be impossible. Provocation tests may add to the confusion. In patients whose spontaneous pain may be associated with a motility disorder the acid perfusion test may be positive and the edrophonium test may produce a motility disorder in patients whose spontaneous pain is accompanied by a fall in intraoesophageal pH. These patients have been classified as having an irritable oesophagus [69]. Clearly, if reflux is the basic problem a myotomy to relieve the motility disorder would be a disaster. On the other hand an anti-reflux procedure alone may not be sufficient to relieve symptoms in a patient whose oesophageal motility pattern is unstable.

Complications of reflux in children

Gastro-oesophageal reflux is a common disorder in infancy and childhood. Typical symptoms of regurgitation and vomiting after meals may begin in the neonatal period or arise later. A hiatus hernia may or may not be demonstrable. In the majority of these children improvement will occur with time and conservative measures such as attention to posture and thickening of feeds. Antacids, metoclopra-mide and H_2-receptor antagonists may help the child's progress towards spon-taneous resolution but should be used with caution. Persistent vomiting and failure to gain weight, persistent oesophagitis with bleeding and anaemia and recurrent respiratory infections are indications of failed medical treatment and anti-reflux surgery may have to be considered. The association of apnoea, cyanosis and 'near miss'sudden infant death episodes and the presence of gastro-oesophageal reflux is controversial. The incidence of stricture in children with gastro-oesophageal reflux is around 5%. Most strictures will respond to anti-reflux surgery and subsequent bougienage. Dense fibrous strictures with shortening of the oesophagus will require more direct intervention. An acceptable procedure is vertical division of the stricture and a Thal fundic patch accompanied by a Nissen fundoplication. In some severe strictures resection of the affected segment of the oesophagus and replacement with isoperistaltic colon may be the only option.

Reflux oesophagitis and carcinoma

An association between hiatus hernia, gastro-oesophageal reflux and carcinoma of the cardia has long been suspected but little evidence to support this view has been forthcoming. Tanner reported that in a small series of 16 patients with carcinoma of the cardia 4 had an associated hiatus hernia. The association between Barrett's oesophagus and adenocarcinoma of the oesophagus is well known and the relationship between achalasia and squamous cell oesophageal cancer has been recognized for many years. Similarly the chronic irritation induced by corrosive strictures of the gullet is known to increase the risk of oesophageal cancer. The possibility that oesophagitis might be associated with an increased incidence of oesophageal cancer was examined by Kuylenstierna and Munch-Wikland [70]. In a retrospective study of 163 oesophageal cancers they found that 10% had a history of oesophagitis. Of the 51 patients with lower oesophageal cancer 13 (25%) had oesophagitis while none of the patients ($n = 47$) with cervical or upper oesophageal cancer had a history of oesophagitis. Although the incidence of tobacco and alcohol abuse in the whole group was higher than in the normal population it was less in patients with lower oesophageal cancer than in the group with upper oesophageal neoplasms. The majority of patients in this report had squamous carcinoma but it is not clear how many of the six patients with adenocarcinoma had a preceding history of reflux oesophagitis.

References

1. Patterson, D. J., Graham, D. Y., Smith, J. L. *et al.* Natural history of benign esophageal stricture treated by dilatation. *Gastroenterology* 1983; **85**: 346–350
2. Ismail-Beigi, F., Horton, P. F. and Pope, C. E. Histological consequences of gastro-esophageal reflux in man. *Gastroenterology* 1970; **58**: 163–174
3. Atkinson, M. and Robertson, C. S. Benign oesophageal stricture in Barrett's columnar epithelialised oesophagus and its responsiveness to conservative management. *Gut* 1988; **29**: 1721–1724
4. Burgess, J. N., Payne, W. S., Anderson, H. A., Weiland, I. H. and Carlson, H. C. Barret esophagus: the columnar epithelial lined esophagus. *Mayo Clinic Proc.* 1971; **46**: 728–734
5. Robbins, A. H., Hermos, J. A., Schimmel, E. M., Friedlander, D. M. and Messian, R. A. The columnar lined oesophagus. *Radiology* 1977; **123**: 1–7
6. Hussain, R. Esophageal stricture following use of indwelling Ryle's tube. *Br. J. Surg.* 1964; **51**: 525–528
7. Eastman, M. C., Gear, M. W. L. and Nicol, A. An assessment of the accuracy of modern endoscopic diagnosis of oesophageal stricture. *Br. J. Surg.* 1978; **65**: 182–185
8. Glick, M. E. Clinical course of esophageal stricture managed by Bougienage. *Dig. Dis. Sci.* 1982; **27**: 884–888
9. Lily, J. O. and McCaffery, T. D. Oesophageal stricture dilatation. A new method adapted to the fibreoptic oesophagoscope. *Am. J. Dig. Dis.* 1971; **16**: 1137
10. Price, J. D., Stanciu, C. and Bennett, J. R. A safer method of dilating oesophageal strictures. *Lancet* 1974; **i**: 1141–1142
11. Rago, E., Boesby, S. and Spencer, J. Results of Eder–Puestow dilatation in the management of esophageal peptic strictures. *Am. J. Gastroenterol.* 1983; **78**: 6–8
12. Hine, K. R., Hawkey, C. J., Atkinson, M. and Holmes, G. K. T. Comparison of the Eder–Puestow techniques for dilating benign oesophageal strictures. *Gut* 1984; **25**: 1100–1102
13. Goldberg, R. I., Manten, H. O. and Barkin, J. S. Oesophageal bougienage with triple metal olive dilators. *Gastrointest. Endosc.* 1986; **32**: 226–268
14. Celestin, L. R. and Campbell, W. B. A new and safe system for oesophageal dilatation. *Lancet* 1981; **i**: 74–75
15. Fellows, I. W., Raina, S. and Holmes, G. K. T. Celestin dilatation of benign oesophageal strictures: a review of 100 patients. *J. Gastroenterol.* 1986; **81**: 1052–1054
16. Savary, M. Cours d'endoscopie de la clinique. *O.R.L. de Lausanne*, September 15–18, 1980
17. Dumon, J-F., Meric, B., Sivak, M. V. and Fleischer D. A new method of oesophageal dilatation using Savary–Gilliard bougies. *Gastrointest. Endosc.* 1985; **31**: 379–382

18. Gotberg, S., Afzelius, L., Hambraeus, G. *et al.* Balloon catheter dilatation of strictures in the upper digestive tract. *Radiology* 1982; **22**: 479–483

19. Cox, J. G. C., Winter, R. J., Maslin, S. C. *et al.* Balloon or Bougie for dilatation of benign oesophageal stricture? An interim report of a randomised controlled trial. *Gut* 1988; **29**: 1741–1747

20. Wesdorp, I. C. E., Bartelsman, J. F. W. M., den Hartog Jeger, P. C. A., Huibregtse, K. and Tytgat, G. N. Results of conservative treatment of benign oesophageal strictures. *Gastroenterology* 1982; **82**: 487–493

21. Williamson, R. C. N. The management of benign oesophageal stricture. *Br. J. Surg.* 1975; **62**: 448–454

22. Schiller, K. F. R., Cotton, P. B. and Salmon, P. R. The hazards of digestive fibre-endoscopy: a survey of British experience. *Gut* 1972; **13**: 1027

23. Mandelstam, P., Sugawa, C., Silvis, S. E., Nebel, O. T. and Rogers, B. H. G. Complications associated with esophagogastroduodenoscopy and with esophageal dilatation. *Gastrointest. Endosc.* 1976; **23**: 16–19

24. Dawson, J. and Cockel, R. Oesophageal perforation at fibreoptic gastroscopy. *Br. Med. J.* 1981; **283**: 583

25. Reiertsen, O., Skjoto, J., Jacobsen, C. D. and Rosseland, A. R. Complications of fibreoptic gastrointestinal endoscopy – five years experience in a central hospital. *Endoscopy* 1983; **19**: 1–6

26. Nashef, S. A. M. and Pogliero, K. M. Instrumental perforation of the esophegus in benign disease. *Ann. Thorac. Surg.* 1987; **44**: 360–362

27. Skinner, D. B., Little, A. G. and DeMeester, T. R. Management of esophageal perforation. *Am. J. Surg.* 1980; **139**: 760–765

28. Han, S. Y., McElvein, R. B., Aldret, J. S. and Tisker, J. M. Perforation of the oesophagus: correlation of site and cause with plain film findings. *Am. J. Roentgenol.* 1986; **145**: 537–540

29. Goldstein, L. A. and Thompson, W. R. Esophageal perforations: a 15 year experience. *Am. J. Surg.* 1982; **143**: 495–503

30. Van der Zee, D. C., Sloof, M. J. H. and Kingma, L. M. Management of oesophageal perforations: a tailored approach. *Netherlands J. Surg.* 1986; **38**: 31–35

31. Mengoli, L. R. and Klassen K. P. Conservative management of esophageal perforation. *Arch. Surg.* 1965; **91**: 238–240

32. Fiasse, R., Goncette, L., Pringot, J. *et al.* Traitement des perforations oesophagiennes instrumentales. *Acta Gastroenterol. Belg.* 1981; **44**: 430–447

33. Wesdorp, I. C. E., Bartelsman, J. F. W. M., Huibregtse, K., den Hartog Jeger, F. C. A. and Tytgat, G. N. Treatment of instrumental oesophageal perforation. *Gut* 1984; **25**: 348–404

34. Mee, A. S. Traumatic oesophageal perforation (letter). *Hosp. Update* 1986; **12**: 601

35. Rogers, B. H. G. In: Hunt, R. D. and Waye, J. D., Eds. *Colonoscopy.* London: Chapman and Hall. 1981; 231–264

36. Silvis, S. E., Nebel, O., Rogers, G., Sugawa, C. and Mandelstam, P. Endoscopic complications: results of the 1974 American Society for Gastro-intestinal Endoscopy Survey. *J. Am. Med. Assoc.* **235**: 928–930

37. Naef, A. P. and Savary, M. Conservative operations for peptic esophagitis with stenosis in columnar lined lower esophagus. *Ann. Thorac. Surg.* 1972; **13**: 543–551

38. Seaman, W. B. and Wiley, R. H. Observations on the nature of the stricture in Barrett's esophagus (Allison and Johnstone's anomaly). *Radiology* 1966; **87**: 30–32

39. Watson, A. Randomised study comparing medical and surgical reflux control in peptic oesophageal stricture treated by intermittent dilatation. *Gut* 1985; **26**: A553

40. DeMeester, T. R., Johnson, L. F. and Kent, A. H. Evaluation of current operations for the prevention of gastro-oesophageal reflux. *Ann. Surg.* 1974; **180**: 511–525

41. Herrington, J. L. Jr, Wright, R. S. and Edwards, W. H. Conservative surgical treatment of reflux esophagitis and esophageal stricture. *Ann. Surg.* 1975; **181**: 552–556

42. Hill, L. D., Gelfand, M. and Bauermeister, D. Simplified management of reflux esophagitis with stricture. *Ann. Surg.* 1970; **172**: 638–646

43. Stuart, R. C., Dawson, K., Keeling, P., Byrne, P. J. and Hennessy, T. P. J. A prospective randomised trial of Angelchik prosthesis versus Nissen fundoplication. *Br. J. Surg.* 1989; **76**: 86–89

44. Collis, J. L. Gastroplasty. *Thorax* 1961; **16**: 197

45. Pearson, F. G. Surgical management of acquired short oesophagus with dilatable peptic stricture. *World J. Surg.* 1977; **1**, 463–472

46. Pearson, F. G., Cooper, J. D. and Nelems, J. M. Gastroplasty and fundoplication in the management of complex reflux problems. *J. Thorac. Cardiovasc. Surg.* 1978; **76**: 665–672

47. Henderson, R. D. Management of the patient with benign esophageal stricture. *Surg. Clin. N. Am.* 1983; **63**: 885–903

48. Bingham, J. A. W. Hiatus hernia combined with the construction of an anti-reflux valve in the stomach. *Br. J. Surg.* 1977; **64**: 460–465

49. Keenan, D. J. M., Hamilton, J. R. L. Gibbons, J. and Stevenson, H. M. Surgery for benign esophageal stricture. *J. Thorac. Cardiovasc. Surg.* 1984; **88**: 182–188

50. Jones, E. L., Booth, D. J., Cameron, J. L. *et al.* Functional evaluation of esophageal reconstruction. *Ann. Thorac. Surg.* 1971; **12**: 331–334

51. Mansour, K. A., Barton, H. G., Miller, J. I. and Hatcher, C. R. Complications of intrathoracic Nissen fundoplication. *Ann. Thorac. Surg.* 1981; **32**: 173–178

52. Belsey, R. Reconstruction of the esophagus with left colon. *J. Thorac. Cardiovasc. Surg.* 1965; **49**: 33–55

53. Merendino, K. A. and Dillard, D. H. The concept of sphincter substitution by an interposed jejunal segment for anatomic and physiologic abnormalities at the esophagogastric junction with special reference to reflux esophagitis cardio spasm and esophageal varices. *Ann. Surg.* 1955; **142**: 486–509

54. Merendino, K. A. and Thomas, G. I. The jejunal interposition operation for substitution of the esophagogastric sphincter. *Surgery* 1958; **44**: 1112–1115

55. Wright, C. and Cuschieri, A. Jejunal interposition for benign esophageal disease. *Ann. Surg.* 1987; **205**: 54–60

56. Postlethwait, R. W. Colonic interposition for esophageal substitution. *Surg. Gynecol. Obstet.* 1983; **156**: 377–383

57. Orringer, M. Surgical management of scleroderma reflux esophagitis. *Surg. Clin. N. Am.* 1983; **63**: 859–867

58. Ellis, F. H. Short oesophago myotomy – thoracic approach. In Jamieson, G. G., Ed. *Surgery of the Oesophagus.* Edinburgh: Churchill Livingstone. 1988: 783–788

59. Tomlinson, P. and Grant, A. F. A review of 74 patients with oesophageal achalasia: the results of Heller's cardio myotomy with and without Nissen fundoplication. *Aust. N.Z. J. Surg.*, 1981; **51**: 48–51

60. Belsey, R. H. Functional disease of the oesophagus. *J. Thorac. Cardiovasc. Surg.* 1966; **52**: 164–188

61. Mansour, K. A., Synbas, P. N., Jones, E. L. and Hatcher, C. R. A combined surgical approach in the management of achalasia of the esophagus. *Ann. Surg.* 1976; **42**: 192–195

62. Andreollo, N. A. and Earlam, R. J. Heller's myotomy for achalasia: is an added anti-reflux procedure necessary? *Br. J. Surg.* 1987; **74**: 765–769

63. Gillen, P., Keeling, P., Byrne, P. J., Healy, M., O'Moore, R. R. and Hennessy, T. P. J. Implication of duodenogastric reflux in the pathogenesis of Barrett's oesophagus. *Br. J. Surg.* 1988; **75**: 540–543

64. Wickbon, G., Bushkin, E. L. and Woodward, E. R. Achaline reflux esophagitis. *Surg. Gynecol. Obstet.* 1974; **139**: 267–271

65. Scudamore, H. H., Echstam, E. E., Fencil, W. G. *et al.* Bile reflux gastritis. Diagnosis medical and surgical therapy. *Am. J. Gastroenterol.* 1973; **60**: 9

66. Schatzki, R. The lower esophageal ring. *Am. J. Roentgenol.* 1963; **90**: 805–808

67. Postlethwait, R. W. and Masser, A. W. Pathology lower oesophageal web. *Surg. Gynecol. Obstet.* 1967; **120**: 571–574

68. Eastridge, C. E., Pate, J. W. and Mann, J. A. Lower esophageal ring: experience and treatment of 88 patients. *Ann. Thorac. Surg.* 1984; **37**: 103–107

69. VanTrappen G., Janssens, J. and Ghillebert, G. The irritable oesophagus – a frequent cause of angina-like pain. *Lancet* 1987; **i** 1232–1234

70. Kuylenstierna, R. and Munch-Wickland, E. Esophagitis and cancer of the esophagus. *Cancer* 1985; **56**: 837–839

Index